fourth edition

A Concise Handbook of

RESPIRATORY
DISEASES

fourth edition

A Concise Handbook of

RESPIRATORY DISEASES

Sattar Farzan, MD, FACP, FCCP
Clinical Professor Emeritus of Medicine, State University of New York at Buffalo
Consultant, Erie County Medical Center
Consultant, Buffalo VA Medical Center
Buffalo, New York

with the assistance of
Doris A. Farzan, MS, RN

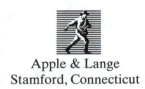

Apple & Lange
Stamford, Connecticut

97 98 99 00 01 / 10 9 8 7 6 5 4 3 2 1

Prentice Hall International (UK) Limited, *London*
Prentice Hall of Australia Pty. Limited, *Sydney*
Prentice Hall Canada, Inc., *Toronto*
Prentice Hall Hispanoamericana, S.A., *Mexico*
Prentice Hall of India Private Limited, *New Delhi*
Prentice Hall of Japan, Inc., *Tokyo*
Simon & Schuster Asia Pte. Ltd., *Singapore*
Editora Prentice Hall do Brasil Ltda., *Rio de Janeiro*
Prentice Hall, *Upper Saddle River, New Jersey*

Library of Congress Cataloging-in-Publication Data
Farzan, Sattar, 1932–
     A concise handbook of respiratory diseases / Sattar Farzan : with the assistance of Doris A. Farzan. — 4th ed.
          p.   cm.
     Includes bibliographical references and index.
     ISBN 0-8385-1493-6 (alk. paper)
     1. Respiratory organs—Diseases—Handbooks, manuals, etc.
I. Farzan, Doris A.   II. Title.
     [DNLM: 1. Respiratory Tract Diseases.   WF 140 F247c 1997]
RC731.F37   1997
616.2—dc21
DNLM/DLC
for Library of Congress   96-40177
                                                                        CIP

Acquisitions Editor: Kimberly Davies
Production Service: Spectrum Publisher Services
Designer: Libby Schmitz

ISBN 0-8385-1493-6

PRINTED IN THE UNITED STATES OF AMERICA

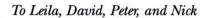

To Leila, David, Peter, and Nick

Contents

Preface

This thoroughly revised fourth edition of *A Concise Handbook of Respiratory Diseases* was prepared with the intent to produce a text that reflects recent advances in knowledge and understanding of the practical aspects of respiratory medicine. Extensive research and review of the current clinically relevant medical literature have been the stepping-stones of this revision. As with the previous three editions, by setting a high standard for this up-to-date work, the author has adhered to the guiding principles of accuracy, informativeness, conciseness, and readability. The educational needs of the readers, especially students and trainees in respiratory care, were carefully considered throughout the revision process. Suggestions by readers and reviewers were most helpful in this endeavor. By emphasizing the essentials and avoiding the esoteric subjects, the book has remained relatively small despite its rather comprehensive coverage of clinically and practically important topics on respiratory diseases. Each chapter has been fastidiously reviewed and the appropriate changes made. Some of the chapters were rewritten entirely. Several new illustrations and tables also were added for further clarification of related subjects.

Despite extensive revision and many major text changes, the basic format established with the third edition has been maintained. The content is again arranged in 12 sections. The number of chapters has, however, increased from 26 to 29. A new chapter was written on postoperative pulmonary complications (Chapter 19). Because of the size of the chapter on respiratory failure (Chapter 26), two separate chapters were arranged to include ARDS (Chapter 27) and mechanical ventilation (Chapter 28). Appendix I, Essential Pharmacology of Respiratory Disease, and Appendix J, Normal Values of Commonly Used Blood Tests, were added. With the inclusion of many new items resulting from the revision, the Glossary has remained a convenient source of ready information.

I want to express my appreciation to the many readers and reviewers for their useful suggestions. I also would like to thank the editorial staff at Appleton & Lange for their thoughtful guidance and cooperation.

Sattar Farzan, MD, FACP, FCCP

Respiration, in a broad sense, is the combination of various physical and chemical processes by which oxygen is supplied to the living cell for its metabolic needs, and carbon dioxide, a product of oxidation, is removed from it. In simple organisms, such as protozoa, the exchange of these gases is by the basic physical process of diffusion that takes place directly between them and their environment. However, in larger and more complex organisms, including humans, it is accomplished by more elaborate coordinated functions of (1) the *circulatory system,* which provides a means of carrying these gases in a special medium, *blood,* and (2) the *respiratory system,* which obtains the necessary oxygen from, and eliminates carbon dioxide to, the atmosphere. Although all of these functions are essential for cellular respiration and should always be taken into account when dealing with respiratory diseases, in this book the primary concern is the *respiratory system.*

The main function of the respiratory system, the delivery of oxygen to and removal of carbon dioxide from the blood, is accomplished and regulated by an intricate set of structures. These structures include (1) the lungs, which provide the gas-exchanging surface; (2) the conducting airways, which convey the air into and out of the lungs; (3) the thoracic wall, which supports and protects the lungs and, at the same time, acts as a bellows through the ability to change its volume; (4) the respiratory muscles, which create the energy necessary for the movement of air into and out of the lungs; and (5) the respiratory centers with their sensitive receptors and communicating nerves, which control and regulate ventilation.

The transfer of oxygen and carbon dioxide between the blood in the pulmonary capillaries and the alveoli takes place by diffusion through an extremely thin but vast membrane. The difference in the partial pressures of these gases across the alveolar-capillary membrane determines the direction of movement: oxygen moves from the alveoli to the capillaries, and carbon dioxide moves from the capillaries to the alveoli.

Ventilation, the flow of air into and out of the lungs with each breath, keeps the alveolar gases at a fairly constant concentration, thus preventing the exhaustion of oxygen and the accumulation of carbon dioxide. Air, like any fluid, flows from a region of higher pressure to one of lower pressure. During inspiration, contraction of the inspiratory muscles increases the thoracic volume and hence reduces the intrathoracic pressure. The reduction of the intrathoracic pressure enlarges the alveoli, expands the alveolar gas, and therefore, lowers its pressure to less than atmospheric. Air flows from the outside (higher pressure) to the alveoli (lower pressure) until pressures equalize. With increasing cross-sectional areas of air passages from the central to peripheral regions, the flow of air slows down progressively toward the gas-exchanging units. At the end of inspiration, potential energy created by contraction of the inspiratory muscles is stored in the elastic tissues of the lungs and chest wall. During expiration, relaxation of these muscles allows the lungs and thorax to recoil, resulting in reduction of their volumes. Pressure in the alveoli becomes higher than atmospheric, causing the air to flow from the alveoli (higher pressure) to the outside (lower pressure) until the pressures become equal. For further increase in alveolar pressure, such as during cough, the expiratory muscles are also activated.

The flow of air into and out of the lungs encounters only a small amount of resistance. The inspired air is warmed, humidified, and filtered in the upper air passages before reaching the lower airways and alveoli.

Blood reaches the alveolar units through a series of branching pulmonary arteries and arterioles, leading to a vast network of capillaries where slower blood flow allows enough time for gas exchange between the blood and alveolar air.

The regulation of ventilation is operated by a complex system of sensitive interconnecting structures that sense the need for adjusting ventilation under various physiologic conditions. The activities of respiratory muscles are controlled through their nerve supply by the respiratory centers, which receive and integrate impulses from various receptors and other neurologic centers.

Elaborate and highly effective defense systems of the airways and lungs protect them against different pathogenic organisms and various noxious respirable agents to which they are constantly exposed.

As respiratory dysfunction may result from structural and functional abnormalities in *any* of these components of the respiratory system, the possibility of involvement of any of them should be considered. This monograph adheres to this important principle.

I

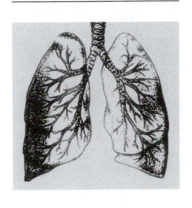

CLINICAL MANIFESTATIONS, DIAGNOSTIC STUDIES, FUNCTIONAL ASSESSMENT, AND MONITORING

The Patient with Respiratory Disease

Patients with respiratory disease, as with any other medical condition, consult health-care professionals mainly because they, their family members, or friends have noted or suspected a certain deviation from normal health. They may be suffering from uncomfortable symptoms or fear a serious and potentially incapacitating illness. Naturally, they expect a clear and satisfactory explanation of their condition and look for relief and reassurance.

A patient is not just a collection of certain symptoms, signs, damaged organs, and disturbed function. He or she is human, and has feelings, emotions, hopes, and fears. Health professionals dealing with a patient should use not only their scientific knowledge and technical skill, but also their human understanding, sympathy, and tact. Developing a good rapport with the patient by gaining and maintaining his or her confidence and demonstrating concern and compassion are essential for successful patient care.

Proper care of the patient with respiratory disease necessitates identifying the specific problems and diagnosing the underlying organic or functional disorder. This can be achieved only after adequate information is obtained from various sources and by various means. Taking a history, doing a physical examination, obtaining radiographic studies, assessing the various functions, and performing other diagnostic procedures are methods used to provide this information.

■ TAKING A HISTORY

The history should contain all the pertinent facts about the patient's illness. The characteristics of the main complaint and other associated symptoms should be ascertained. The date and the time of the onset of these symptoms, their severity and duration, the circumstances leading to or aggravating them, and the factors alleviating them should be determined. Other essential parts of taking a thorough history include the state of the patient's health prior to the present illness; previous diseases, surgeries, and injuries; occupational, environmental, and travel history; allergies; health of family; smoking and other habits; and intake of medication.

Despite remarkable progress in methods of objective evaluation and the availability of sophisticated laboratory tests for patients with respiratory diseases, the importance of history taking has not diminished. This is particularly true in regard to the occupational and environmental history, which is crucial in evaluating the patient with respiratory disorder and, in many instances, is the key to a correct diagnosis.

The common and important symptoms of respiratory diseases are limited in number. These symptoms are cough, expectoration, dyspnea, hemoptysis, chest pain, and wheezing.

Cough

Cough, one of the important body reflexes, is primarily intended to maintain airway patency by eliminating materials accumulated or deposited on the mucosa of the respiratory tract, such as tracheobronchial secretions, blood, aspirated substances, and other foreign bodies. However, not infrequently, cough is produced by irritation of the airways with nothing to be expectorated. Hyperreactivity of the irritant receptors on the respiratory tract mucosa, resulting from inflammation or other pathologic processes, may enhance the cough reflex to the extent that even a mild irritation can

trigger it. The most sensitive areas of the respiratory tract for the cough reflex are the larynx, carina, trachea, and major bronchi. In addition to the airways, irritation of the pleura, tympanic membrane, and occasionally other viscera may produce cough.

The cough reflex is mediated through sensory nerve endings of cranial nerve X (vagus nerve) and motor nerves of the larynx and respiratory muscles. The reflex center is in the medulla. Cough also may be initiated and partially inhibited voluntarily. The mechanism of cough is as follows (Fig. 1–1): after a rapid inspiration of a fairly large amount of air, the glottis is tightly closed by the vocal cords for a short period of time while the expiratory muscles, particularly the abdominals, contract vigorously. The intrathoracic pressure is markedly increased, and the trapped air in the lungs is compressed. The sudden opening of the glottis results in an explosive outflow of air with high velocity, carrying the secretions or other materials with it. Transient narrowing of the large intrathoracic airways on opening of the glottis, which results mainly from inward bulging of their membranous portion, contributes to clearing of these airways. The high shearing force of airflow strips the secretions from the airway wall. Successive coughs following a single deep inspiration results in decreasing lung volumes, which allows clearing of more peripheral airways. The characteristic noise of cough is due mostly to vibration of vocal cords and sometimes to vibration of secretions. Although normal function of larynx is essential for forceful cough, glottic closure is not absolutely necessary for an effective cough. Cough in many patients who have tracheostomy may serve the purpose of clearing the airways. The ability to take a deep breath and gen-

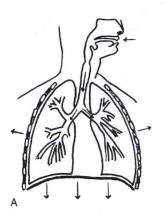
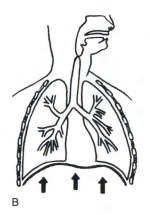
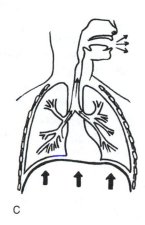

A   B   C

Figure 1–1. Mechanism of cough. (a) Rapid inspiration of fairly large amount of air. (b) The glottis is tightly closed while the expiratory muscles, particularly the abdominals, contract; the intrathoracic pressure is markedly increased and the trapped air in the lungs is compressed. (c) The sudden opening of the glottis results in an expulsive outflow of air with high velocity, carrying the secretions.

erate a high expiratory pressure is also an important determinant of a forceful and effective cough. Patients with weak respiratory muscles (inspiratory or expiratory) are therefore at a significant disadvantage.

Although a very common symptom, cough has limited diagnostic value; however, it may be the only indication of a serious bronchopulmonary disease. The most common and clinically significant cause of acute cough is viral tracheobronchitis. Other acute inflammatory disorders of the respiratory tract of infectious or noninfectious etiology are most often associated with cough. Alteration of the surface epithelium, by exposing the nerve endings, makes the airways very sensitive to the cough-provoking effect of commonly occurring mild irritants such as dusts, cold air, rapid or deep breathing, talking, and even laughing. In addition, increased tracheobronchial secretions stimulate coughing. Acute cough may also result from inhalation of irritant gases or aspiration of liquid or solid matters. Heart failure not uncommonly may cause cough.

Chronic cough, defined as a cough lasting for more than 3 weeks, usually indicates structural changes of the respiratory tract or persistence of other cough-producing factors. Cough is so prevalent among smokers that they are often oblivious to its presence. Only changes in the characteristics of cough or expectoration may concern them. Such changes are frequently due to an infection, but it may be an indication of the occurrence of a malignant neoplasm, a fairly common disease of smokers. When there is no clinically or radiographically identifiable reason for chronic cough, determination of its cause becomes quite a challenge. Airway hyperreactivity, the hallmark of asthma, is a common cause of chronic or recurrent cough in otherwise healthy persons; therefore, it may be the sole manifestation of asthma.

Gastroesophageal reflux disease (GERD) should also be considered when dealing with unexplained chronic cough. Cough reflex in this disorder originates from the distal esophagus. Chronic postnasal drip and recurrent aspiration of upper airway secretions are other causes of chronic cough. Pertussis infection, a cause of whooping cough in children, may also be a cause of persistent cough in adults. Cough may be a prominent clinical manifestation of chronic left-side heart failure. Foreign-body aspiration should always be kept in mind in differential diagnosis of chronic cough. After an initial episode of an acute cough spell or choking sensation at the time of aspiration, cough may resume and persist long after the incident. The angiotensin-converting enzyme inhibitors such as captopril and enalapril, drugs used for treatment of hypertension and heart failure, may result in a dry annoying cough, which stops after discontinuation of the drugs. A **psychogenic** or even intentional cough should be seriously considered when organic causes are properly excluded.

The intensity of cough has no relationship to the severity or seriousness of underlying bronchopulmonary disease. It is not unusual for a patient with serious, even fatal, pulmonary disease to have minimal or no cough. On the other hand, a mild viral infection involving the trachea or the bronchi may cause the most troublesome cough. In certain conditions, the cough may have characteristic features. For example, the characteristics of cough in pertussis (whooping cough) and croup are quite distinctive. Chronic cough productive of very large amounts of sputum is often indicative of bronchiectasis. Voluntary hawking (clearing the throat) is a common sign of postnasal drip.

Although cough is very important in protecting the lungs, clearing the airways, and assuring their patency, it may be an annoying symptom when dry and nonproductive. Moreover, it may occasionally prove to be harmful. Spread of infection, airway injury, hemoptysis, pneumothorax, rib fractures, syncope, and aggravation of heart failure have

been attributed to both severe and persistent cough. At times the mechanical irritation of cough itself brings about more coughing.

Respiratory therapists and nurses have the opportunity as well as the responsibility to observe and report the type of cough and expectoration of the patient. From the therapeutic point of view, an effective cough is important in adequate tracheobronchial hygiene. In many patients it is important to encourage cough and expectoration by appropriate instruction, particularly when they are unable to do so spontaneously. This may or may not be combined with measures such as intermittent positive pressure breathing (IPPB), humidity therapy, or postural drainage.

Expectoration

Expectoration is defined as the act of coughing up and spitting out material raised from the respiratory tract. This material is called *sputum*. Normally, sputum consists of secretions formed continuously by the mucous glands and the goblet cells of the tracheobronchial tree. Forming a thin mucous blanket, these secretions move slowly toward the pharynx with the help of cilia. Cilia are microscopic hairlike processes that extend from the free surfaces of the mucosal lining cells and vibrate rhythmically, propelling the overlaying mucous coating. With proper balance between its formation and elimination, a thin protective layer of mucus is maintained for trapping and removing impurities of inspired air, while excessive accumulation of secretions is prevented.

In pathologic conditions, increased tracheobronchial secretions may be due to the stimulation of normal secretory cells or to an increase in the number of these cells. In acute situations, increased sputum production is mainly the result of transient stimulation of mucous glands and goblet cells, while their chronic irritation, in addition, causes their hyperplasia. Chronic bronchitis is a good example; prolonged irritation of bronchial glands and cells by cigarette smoke results in an increase in their number and activities.

In addition to mucus, expectorated material may contain other fluids transuded or exuded from the various sites of the respiratory tract, including the alveoli. It may contain white blood cells accumulated for the purpose of defense against infection, necrotic material from tissue death, blood, aspirated vomitus, and, rarely, other indigenous or foreign matters.

The quantity of expectoration varies from scant to several hundred milliliters or more per day. The patient should be asked about the appropriate amount of sputum produced in a 24-hour period and about the other characteristics of expectoration, such as its color and consistency as well as the time of its production. Expectoration in most patients is more abundant on arising in the morning. It should be remembered that some people, particularly children and sometimes women, have difficulty in expectorating and have a tendency to swallow their sputum. Objective evaluation of sputum is discussed in Chapter 2.

Dyspnea

Dyspnea is an uncomfortable awareness of breathing. The patient suffering from dyspnea may describe it as chesttightness, shortness of breath, choking, or inability to get enough air. Dyspnea is generally believed to be due to increased work of ventilation out of proportion to the level of activity. However, the clinical observation that dyspnea develops with respiratory muscle fatigue and weakness suggests that an increase in the efferent neuronal output, rather than actual muscular work of breathing, is the mechanism by which this distressful symptom develops.

The disagreeable awareness of breathing may range in intensity from a mild discomfort to extreme distress. Visual analogue scales have been used to quantify the degree of dyspnea. However, dyspnea, similar to pain, is a *subjective* symptom, and thus likely to be influenced by the patient's reaction, sensitivity, and emotional state. The degree of dyspnea, therefore, may be quite different in two individuals with similar conditions.

Although dyspnea is a subjective symptom, the patient may be described as dyspneic when there is enough objective evidence to indicate labored and distressful breathing. Patients having a severe asthma attack or with acute pulmonary edema readily appear dyspneic, as they breathe with difficulty and seem in obvious distress. However, a simple increase in rate or depth of breathing, disturbances of rhythm, or changes in other characteristics of respiration do not necessarily indicate dyspnea. In these situations, the terms that exactly characterize the breathing patterns should be used. Various patterns of respiration are discussed on page 17.

Dyspnea as a result of increased work of breathing is seen under numerous clinical conditions. Some of the basic causes are increased airway resistance, such as in upper airway obstruction, asthma, and other chronic obstructive pulmonary diseases; reduced pulmonary compliance as a result of pulmonary fibrosis, congestion, edema, and a variety of other parenchymal lung diseases; mechanical interference with the expansion of the lungs due to massive pleural effusion or pneumothorax; and abnormality of chest wall and respiratory muscles resulting in inefficient and wasteful respiratory efforts.

Dyspnea due to heart disease usually is directly related to changes in the lungs as a result of pulmonary congestion and/or edema characteristic of cardiac failure. Inadequate blood supply to the exercising muscles, including the respiratory muscles, is another factor in producing shortness of breath in heart failure. In patients with severe physical debility, the weakness of respiratory muscles is the main cause of their breathlessness. The same is true in severe anemia, in which there is also increased work of breathing.

Certain patients may complain of shortness of breath with no evidence of organic disease to explain it. These patients often suffer from an anxiety state or panic disorder and have a tendency to hyperventilate (see page 22). They usually state that they are unable to get enough air and frequently sigh. The psychogenic nature of dyspnea becomes more evident when such patients indicate that they are more aware of this symptom at rest than during physical activity. This is the opposite of the organic causes of dyspnea, in which the severity of shortness of breath is directly related to the amount of exertion.

In evaluating for dyspnea, it is important to determine whether it is chronic or acute. When acute, it indicates a recent acute, often serious, event has occurred. The circumstances in which a patient's dyspnea develops should also be determined.

Breathlessness may occur with certain body positions. **Orthopnea** refers to dyspnea on lying down, which is a characteristic symptom in heart failure. However, some patients with advanced pulmonary disease may also be more short of breath when lying flat. Bilateral diaphragmatic paralysis is another cause of orthopnea. **Platypnea** is the opposite of orthopnea, in which dyspnea on upright position improves by lying down. It is usually due to certain vascular abnormality of the lung. **Trepopnea** indicates that the patient breathes more comfortably when lying on one side or the other. **Paroxysmal nocturnal dyspnea** is the sudden onset of shortness of breath in the middle of the night in a cardiac patient after he or she has been in bed for a few hours. It probably results from acute and usually transient pulmonary congestion or edema.

The majority of patients with cardiopulmonary disease have *exertional* dyspnea. The amount of exertion resulting in dyspnea helps in determining its severity. Severity of exertional dyspnea can be determined by the distance the patient can walk in 6–12 minutes (walk test). It also can be quantified by the kind of exertion that causes it. A patient who becomes short of breath on walking a short distance on a level surface has a more severe condition than if he were dyspneic on climbing stairs. The change of dyspnea with progression of disease or response to treatment is also judged by the change in the amount of exertion required to induce shortness of breath. It should, however, be remembered that with a slow deterioration of lung function, patients may adjust their physical activities in order not to experience dyspnea. In chronic pulmonary disease, such as emphysema, patients become short of breath with less and less effort with the progression of the disease, so that, in the advanced stage, they become dyspneic even at rest. A recent increase in dyspnea in the patient with chronic respiratory disease is indicative of an acute event. This may be due to increased airway resistance such as with bronchospasm, secretions, and infection or reduced pulmonary compliance such as with pulmonary congestion or edema. Other causes of sudden dyspnea, which may also occur in otherwise healthy individuals, include spontaneous pneumothorax, pulmonary embolism, and upper airway obstruction.

Hemoptysis

Although *hemoptysis* means spitting blood (*hemo-*, blood; *-ptysis*, spitting), it generally refers to the expectoration of blood that originates from the respiratory tract below the pharynx. It may consist of pure blood or it may be mixed with sputum, causing blood-tinged or blood-streaked expectoration. The amount of bleeding indicates the severity of hemoptysis. Massive hemoptysis is the expectoration of 600 milliliters (mL) or more of blood within 24 hours.

Few symptoms force a patient to seek medical advice as readily as hemoptysis. This alarming symptom not only may be life-threatening by its own merit, but it also frequently indicates a serious underlying disease, which may be a real challenge to diagnose. The causes of hemoptysis are multitudinous, and almost any pulmonary lesion may result in hemoptysis. A significant number of patients may actually have no demonstrable evidence of cardiopulmonary disease to explain this symptom. The three major basic underlying pathologic conditions are infec-

tion, neoplasm, and cardiovascular disorders.

Common infectious causes of hemoptysis are bronchitis, pneumonia, tuberculosis, bronchiectasis, and lung abscess. Fungus infection and parasitic lung diseases may also result in hemoptysis. The latter conditions are some of the most frequent causes of pulmonary hemorrhage in endemic areas of the world.

Among the neoplastic diseases of the lung, bronchogenic carcinoma is the most common cause of hemoptysis. Approximately 50% of patients with lung cancer will have bloody expectoration in the course of their disease. Benign endobronchial tumors may also bleed readily.

Certain cardiovascular diseases manifest with hemoptysis. Pulmonary embolism is frequently associated with bleeding from the respiratory tract. Vascular malformations of the lung should be suspected in patients with hemoptysis without obvious cause. Heart failure may be accompanied by hemoptysis. Among the valvular heart diseases, mitral stenosis is well known for its propensity for hemoptysis.

The immediate danger of hemoptysis is related to airway obstruction. This risk is much greater than that of blood loss. If the rate of bleeding is more than its removal by expectoration or suctioning, the lungs will be flooded. The spread of infection, particularly from a tuberculous lesion, is another potential complication of hemoptysis.

In a patient who gives a history of spitting blood, it should be determined whether the blood is actually coming from the respiratory tract. It is not uncommon for the frightened patient to be confused regarding the source of bleeding. Therefore, it should be ascertained that blood is actually coming from the airways and is not vomited from the gastrointestinal tract. Furthermore, bleeding from the nose, mouth, and throat should be looked for and properly excluded.

Once it is determined that the source of bleeding is the respiratory tract below the pharynx, the rate of bleeding and the amount of blood loss should be estimated from the patient's history, close observation, vital signs, and blood count. The nurse or respiratory therapist will have the opportunity to observe the patient and report the occurrence and the characteristics of bloody expectoration.

In the management of the patient with hemoptysis, the immediate task should be directed toward maintaining a patent airway. The patient's bedside should be equipped with a suction machine, tracheal intubation set, and equipment for respiratory assistance. Bed rest, reassurance, mild sedation, and close observation are measures that should be followed. If the bleeding side is known, the patient is positioned with that side dependent. Hemoptysis will usually stop spontaneously, but occasionally operative procedures will be necessary.

Although a careful history, physical examination, and chest x-ray or chest computed tomography (CT) are most helpful in identifying the cause of hemoptysis, bronchoscopy frequently will be required. In some instances, for a more definitive diagnosis, specialized radiologic examinations such as radioisotopic studies or angiography will be necessary.

Chest Pain

Chest pain is one of the symptoms that causes alarm to the patient and concern to the health-care team. It may be due to a variety of conditions, ranging from a transient and insignificant event to a most serious and life-threatening medical catastrophe. As with pain anywhere else, the patient's pain response is unpredictable. The same disease with similar severity may cause minimal discomfort to one patient and excruciating pain to another.

The thorax is made of and contains many structures that may be the site of the pain's origin. The thoracic wall is the most common source of chest pain; skin, muscles, nerves, and bones may be its cause in association with various clinical conditions. The lung parenchyma itself is insensitive to painful stimuli, and only the parietal layer of pleura is very pain sensitive. Its direct or indirect involvement by various pathologic processes is a frequent cause of chest pain. Pain in pneumonias and other inflammatory diseases of the lung is usually due to pleural reaction. In lung cancer, the chest pain is frequently indicative of pleural and/or chest-wall invasion. However, certain patients with lung cancer will have a heavy sensation in the chest without such an invasion.

Pulmonary arterial hypertension sometimes causes chest pain, which may be due to increased tension of arterial walls or secondary to myocardial ischemia from right ventricular strain. The sudden and transient chest pain of pulmonary embolism probably occurs through a similar mechanism. However, more persistent "pleuritic" pain following pulmonary embolism is secondary to pleural reaction. In acute inflammation of the trachea and major bronchi (tracheobronchitis), a scratchy feeling behind the sternum is common.

Pleuritic pain refers to chest pain that is produced or aggravated by deep breathing and other chest-wall movement. It is not exclusive to pleural disease, but may also be a manifestation of painful conditions of the chest wall. The lack of chest pain does not exclude the presence of lung disease; many serious pulmonary lesions produce no pain.

Other intrathoracic organs and structures may be the source of chest pain. Pain originating from the heart and its major blood vessels is a common occurrence, particularly the pain of myocardial ischemia, which is known as angina pectoris. Myocardial infarction; pericarditis; rupture, dissection, or distension of the aorta; disease of the mediastinum; and esophageal disorders are other important causes of chest pain.

Because of the multiplicity of causes of chest pain, it is often a diagnostic challenge. A careful history, thorough physical examination, proper radiographic studies, electrocardiography, and other appropriate tests usually help to identify the underlying cause of chest pain.

Other Respiratory Symptoms

Wheezing, as a symptom, is heard by the patient as a whistling sound in association with asthma. It may also be present in conditions such as acute bronchitis and other causes of bronchial narrowing. Many patients are aware of the presence of wheezing, but others may not notice it. Auscultation of the chest will be necessary to detect or confirm the wheezing. This is discussed in the "Physical Examination" section that follows. **Stridor** is a noisy breathing characterized by a harsh inspiratory sound secondary to narrowing of an extrathoracic portion of the upper airway. Abnormal **snoring** is usually a complaint of a roommate or bed companion rather than the snorer. This symptom is important in evaluation for sleep-related respiratory disorders (Chapter 24).

Hoarseness, varying from roughen-

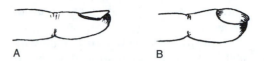

Figure 1–2. Normal finger (A); clubbed finger (B).

ing of the voice to its total loss, is indicative of laryngeal disease, such as inflammation, tumor, vocal cord paralysis, and overuse or misuse of vocal cords, or it may be secondary to tracheal intubation.

■ PHYSICAL EXAMINATION

The physical examination of patients with pulmonary disease should not be limited to the respiratory tract, but should include other organ systems. This will not only enable one to detect concomitant abnormalities, but will also help to identify conditions that may be the cause or result of respiratory disorders. For example, recognition of signs of heart disease may explain a patient's breathlessness, or demonstration of peripheral thrombophlebitis will suggest pulmonary embolism in a patient with a compatible clinical picture. Clubbing of fingers and toes (Fig. 1–2) may be a manifestation of lung disease, or cyanosis of fingers and lips may suggest respiratory pathology. The determination of body temperature and other vital signs is indispensable in evaluating patients with respiratory disease.

Remarkable progress in various diagnostic techniques, particularly radiology, and their ready availability have resulted in slackened emphasis on the importance of physical diagnosis. We believe that this is unfortunate. Taking a good history and performing a proper physical examination provide valuable information not only necessary for accurate diagnosis, but also essential for rational choice and more precise interpretation of diagnostic procedures.

The four fundamental components of the physical examination that are applicable to the examination of patients with respiratory disease are *inspection, palpation, percussion,* and *auscultation.*

Inspection

In performing a physical examination we use our sense organs, the most important being our eyes. Examination by looking is called inspection, which is the most informative phase of a physical examination. This applies to the examination of most areas of the body, as well as to the respiratory system. Students of the health sciences should develop the ability and the habit of becoming astute observers, and they should familiarize themselves with simple and easily acquired techniques of inspection. By simple inspection, a great amount of valuable information can be obtained on a patient's general health. His or her general appearance, developmental and nutritional state, color, complexion, degree of illness and distress, posture, gait, and behavior can be readily assessed.

Inspection in relation to the respiratory system should include observation of the patient's chest and its movement. Shape of the chest and its symmetry, deformities, breathing pattern, rhythm, rate, sighing, use of accessory respiratory muscles, chest excursion, symmetry of expansion, paradoxical movements, retraction between the ribs and above the clavicles, and presence of scars of prior surgery and previous tracheotomy should be carefully noted.

Of particular importance is the observation of paradoxical movement of the chest and the abdomen, which is a fairly common but often overlooked finding in ventilatory failure in patients with a weak or fatigued diaphragm. Instead of simultaneous expansion of the abdomen and the chest during inspiration, the abdominal wall is sucked inward while the thorax is expanding (Fig. 1–3).

Observation of the patient while he or she takes a deep breath will give some idea about the ventilatory ability of the lungs. Bedside performance of a forced expiratory maneuver may give a rough estimate of the degree of airway obstruction. Respiration should be observed for rate and rhythm without the patient's awareness; otherwise the pattern and rate of breathing might change. This can be done by pretending that the examiner is

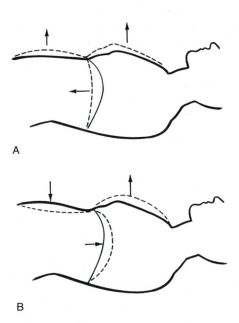

A

B

Figure 1–3. Relationship between abdominal and rib cage motions with respiration. Dashed lines and arrows denote directions of movements of the chest wall, diaphragm, and abdomen on inspiration. Normally, the movements of the chest wall and abdomen are in the same direction (A). With a paralyzed or weak diaphragm, there is a paradoxical motion; while the rib cage is expanding, the abdomen is being sucked in (B).

counting the pulse or making some other observation while actually concentrating on the patient's respiration. Respiratory patterns are discussed on page 17.

Palpation

In palpation, the tactile sense is used to determine the physical characteristics of organs and tissues. Their shape, size, consistency, tenderness, temperature, smoothness or roughness, movement, and movability are thus examined.

Palpation of the chest is mainly used for evaluation of the degree and symmetry of respiratory movements and for determination of *vocal fremitus*. For the purpose of elicitation of thoracic expansion and comparison of two sides, the hands are placed symmetrically over the patient's chest at various locations, and the movement of the underlying chest wall is felt while the patient takes deep breaths (Fig. 1–4). Vocal fremitus is the tactile perception of vibration set by the larynx on phonation and transmitted to the chest wall. It is determined by placing the

palms lightly on the patient's chest while he or she is repeating certain words or numbers in a loud, deep voice. The significance of this examination lies in the comparison of two corresponding sides of the chest.

Reduced ventilation of a lobe or a whole lung due to various pathologic conditions will result in reduced thoracic expansion over that area. The presence of air or fluid between the lung and chest wall, or any obstacle to transmission of voice vibration, including airway obstruction, will cause diminution or absence of vocal fremitus. However, the consolidation of lung tissue without obstruction to its bronchus, as in pneumonia, will facilitate the transmission of vibration and, thus, will increase vocal fremitus.

Palpation will also allow the examiner to locate the cervical position of the trachea and larynx, elicit chest wall tenderness, evaluate any masses or swellings, and detect subcutaneous accumulations of air (subcutaneous emphysema).

Percussion

Examination by percussion has been compared to a radar or sonar detection system. Tapping on the chest produces vibration of the chest wall and the underlying lung, which is reflected and picked up by the examiner's auditory and tactile senses. The note and the loudness of sound will depend on the force of percussion and the characteristics of the underlying tissues. Percussion over solid or liquid-containing organs, such as the upper part of the liver or the heart, results in a low-amplitude, high-frequency short sound without any resonance; this is a *dull* percussion note. Flat percussion note indicates absolute dullness when there is no air under the percussed area, such as ar-

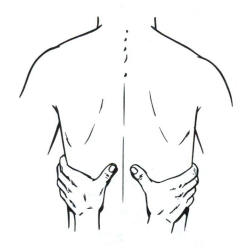

Figure 1–4. Palpation of the chest for an evaluation of its expansion.

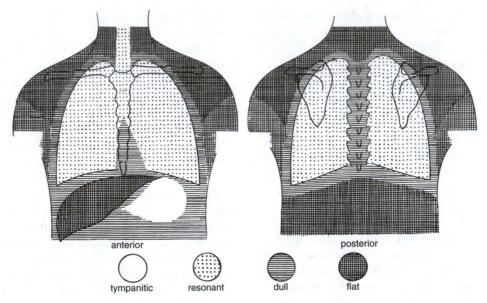

anterior   posterior

tympanitic   resonant   dull   flat

Figure 1–5. Diagrammatic demonstration of percussion notes of the chest and upper abdomen, which shows resonance of lung fields contrasting with dullness and flatness over solid structures. Tympanitic note over the air-containing stomach is also shown.

eas over the shoulders or lower part of the liver. Percussion over an air-containing viscus, such as the lung, produces a *resonant* note, which has a higher amplitude, lower pitch, and longer duration. Tympanitic note sounds like a drum, and is normally detected over the gas-filled stomach below the left lung base anteriorly (Fig. 1–5).

The most commonly used method of percussion is as follows: the palmar surface of the middle finger of one hand is firmly applied against the chest wall, while the tip of the middle finger of the other hand strikes upon it with short, quick, and uniform vertical blows delivered from the wrist (Fig. 1–6). This is repeated by changing the location of percussion to various regions of the chest, always comparing corresponding areas of two sides. The vibrations produced by percussion are not only heard but also felt by the fingers applied over the chest.

Percussion notes vary among normal individuals, and in the same individual,

over different areas of the chest. This is because of variations in the thickness of the tissues surrounding the lungs in different people and different lung regions and also because of the presence and the position of other intrathoracic structures, as well as unevenness of the thickness of the underlying air-containing lung tissues. However, with few exceptions, the percussion note is equal over the symmetrical areas of the two hemithoraces, which is why percussion notes should be

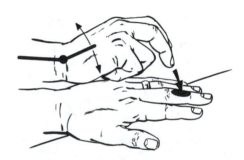

Figure 1–6. Technique of percussion.

compared over the two corresponding sides. Because of the presence of the liver, the right lung base is dull to percussion. The height of this dullness helps in the estimation of liver size. The position of the heart in the chest, which is close to the anterior wall and somewhat to the left, makes this area relatively dull to percussion.

Increased lung inflation, as during deep inspiration or in patients with emphysema and asthmatic attacks, will cause increased resonance (hyperresonance). Sometimes the presence of a large amount of air in the pleural cavity (pneumothorax) will result in a tympanitic note. The replacement of air in the lung by solid tissue or liquid material will reduce the resonance. Over a completely airless lung, or when there is a significant amount of fluid in the pleural cavity, percussion notes will be dull or even flat.

Percussion is also useful for delineation of the level of the diaphragm, which roughly corresponds to the line on the chest wall where the normal resonance changes to dullness. Diaphragmatic excursion during a maximum respiratory cycle can be determined by measuring the difference between the levels of the diaphragm at the end of a deep inspiration and after a complete expiration.

Auscultation

Sense of hearing is an important tool for the examination of the respiratory system. The vibration produced by percussion is primarily perceived as sound. Laryngeal disease is usually suspected by a change in voice quality. *Stridor*, a harsh, high-pitched, and loud inspiratory sound, is an important diagnostic sign of upper airway obstruction. Sounds of coughing in certain respiratory diseases, such as whooping cough, are characteristic. In asthmatics during an attack, wheezing may be heard at a distance. Although all these sounds are appreciated by hearing, *auscultation* is commonly referred to as the act of listening for sounds within the body either by the direct application of an ear over the area or, more conveniently, by a *stethoscope*.

The movement of air in and out of the lung normally produces sound vibration as a result of turbulence of flow with sudden changes in the lumen of the airways and their direction. Breath sounds have two basic components, which are discussed as follows (Fig. 1–7).

1. **Bronchial** sounds, which are produced in the proximal airways— that is, the larynx, trachea, and large bronchi—have a higher pitch and are harsh and loud. They are heard equally well during both inspiration and expiration, with a distinct short pause in between. Pure bronchial breath sound is closely approximated by the sound heard when the stethoscope is applied directly over the trachea.

2. **Vesicular** sounds are soft and have a lower pitch and a hissing quality. These sounds are heard mostly during inspiration, dying away rapidly in the early part of expiration. Vesicular sounds, without interfering bronchial sounds, are best heard in the lower lung fields. The long-held general view that vesicular sounds are produced by the passage of air through the bronchioles and alveolar ducts has recently been questioned. There is increasing evidence that they are large airway sounds that are filtered on their way through the lungs, resulting in reduction and elimination of their certain components.

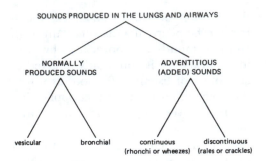

Figure 1–7. Major sounds originating from the lungs in normal and diseased states.

In the upper lung regions, the breath sounds are a combination of or intermediate between the bronchial and vesicular sounds. They are known as **bronchovesicular** sounds. Under normal conditions, pure bronchial breath sounds should not be heard in any lung areas, and bronchovesicular sounds are considered abnormal in the lower lung fields.

The transmission of breath sounds will depend on the physical characteristics of the tissues through which they traverse. They are usually louder in children and lean individuals, but they are diminished and appear distant in obese people. Presence of air or fluid in the pleural cavity will interfere with the transmission of breath sounds. Reduced ventilation of the lung units will also cause diminution of breath sounds. In certain pathologic conditions in which transmission of bronchial sounds is facilitated, bronchial breath sounds will be heard. Consolidation of the lung with pneumonia is a typical example of this phenomenon.

In addition to the breath sounds mentioned previously, other sounds may be produced in the lungs under certain abnormal conditions. As they do not occur normally, they are **adventitious,** or added sounds (see Fig. 1–7). The adventitious sounds produced by air flow are divided into continuous sounds, or **rhonchi,** and discontinuous sounds, or **rales.** Rhonchi, also known as wheezes, are produced by the passage of air through bronchi that are narrowed by swelling, secretions, bronchospasm, foreign body, or a growth. They have a more or less musical quality with a distinguished pitch and are heard mostly during expiration. Rhonchi due to secretions usually will change or disappear with coughing.

Rales, also known as crackles, are brief and explosive rather than musical, and are heard mostly during inspiration. Although the mechanism of their production is not entirely clear, they are often related to the presence of fluid inside the bronchi and the collapsed distal airways and alveoli. Depending on their site of origin, rales have various qualities. They are divided into fine, medium, and coarse. Fine rales are probably the result of opening of the distal small airways with the flow of air during inspiration. Medium and coarse rales are produced by the passage of air in fluid-containing bronchi. It seems that the coarser the rales, the larger are the airways in which air and fluid come in contact.

In describing these sounds, other qualities such as their intensity, location, and timing in the respiratory cycle should be noted. As the intrathoracic airways are narrower during expiration, the rhonchi are best heard during this phase of respiration; however, they are not limited to it. During an asthma attack they may be heard during both phases of respiration, but more during expiration. *Rhonchus* is a Latin word for wheezing and, therefore, they are synonymous. In general usage, however, higher-pitched rhonchi are referred to as wheezes. A phenomenon in which there is an alteration of transmitted voice sounds is known as **egophony** (bleeting sound of a goat). It is characterized by change of a long *E* sound to a long *A* sound while listening with a stethoscope. It occurs when there is a combination of pulmonary consolidation with or without pleural effusion.

Another important adventitious sound is the *pleural rub.* This is a grating sound produced by movement and friction of roughened pleural surfaces. It is a diagnostic sign of pleuritis.

■ RESPIRATORY PATTERNS

Valuable information can be obtained by the careful observation of breathing patterns. In normal individuals at rest, respiration is more or less regular, at a rate between 12 and 20 breaths per minute (in adults), and the respiratory movements are evident over both the chest and abdomen. Although as a general rule males have predominantly *diaphragmatic* or abdominal breathing and females tend to use *costal* breathing, there are wide individual variations even among a healthy population. Normally, inspiration lasts about half as long as expiration.

Changes in respiratory patterns may be related to the rate, depth, rhythm, ratio of expiration to inspiration, and alternation between abdominal and rib cage breathing.

Rapid breathing, known as **tachypnea** or **polypnea,** is usually indicative of reduced pulmonary or thoracic compliance, and is seen in such conditions as pneumonia, pulmonary congestion and edema, and a variety of other restrictive chest diseases. It may or may not result in increased alveolar ventilation, depending on the depth of breathing and the volume of dead space. This can be judged more accurately by the arterial carbon dioxide tension. **Bradypnea** is abnormal

slowness of the respiratory rate. It is seen in patients with respiratory center depression, such as in narcotic drug overdoses. In extreme situations there may be **apnea,** which is the absence of respiration for at least 10 seconds. Apneic episodes are frequently observed during sleep and are hallmarks of sleep apnea syndrome (see Chapter 25).

Increased respiratory depth, frequently accompanied by rapid rate, is characteristic of **Kussmaul's breathing,** which is seen in patients with severe metabolic acidosis. Increased depth of breathing is indicative of increased alveolar ventilation unless dead-space ventilation is significantly high. The amount of alveolar ventilation can only be accurately determined by alveolar or arterial carbon dioxide and its rate of elimination. *Hyperventilation* generally refers to excessive *alveolar* ventilation. The causes of hyperventilation are discussed on page 22.

Shallow respiration is usually due to restrictive pulmonary or thoracic conditions. It is almost always compensated by an increased rate of breathing. Conditions resulting in "stiff" lungs, impairing thoracic expansion and, therefore, causing shallow respiration, are numerous. Severe pulmonary fibrosis and other parenchymal diseases, marked thoracic deformities, massive pleural effusion, increased intra-abdominal pressure, significant chest-wall or pleural pain, and respiratory muscle weakness or fatigue are among conditions that may be associated with shallow, rapid breathing.

In severe obstructive bronchopulmonary disease, the ratio of expiration to inspiration may be significantly increased. This is commonly seen in patients during asthma attacks or with advanced emphysema.

Disturbances of respiratory rhythm

are usually due to central nervous system diseases affecting the regulation of respiration. Although other less common respiratory arrhythmias may occur, the most significant and prevalent abnormal respiratory rhythm is the periodic breathing of Cheyne-Stokes.

Cheyne-Stokes respiration is characterized by alternate waxing and waning of the depth and the rate of breathing. Typically, periods of apnea of various durations are interposed between the cycles. The apneic period is terminated by respirations of gradually increasing depth and frequency until a peak is reached, which is followed by gradually diminishing respiratory effort until the next apneic phase. Cheyne-Stokes respiration may occasionally be observed during sleep in normal persons, particularly among newborns and elderly persons. It commonly

occurs in high altitudes or following forced hyperventilation.

The clinical importance of Cheyne-Stokes ventilation, however, is related to its association with certain central nervous system disorders and cardiac failure. Both abnormal response of the respiratory centers and prolonged circulation time have been implicated in its production. Frequently, it seems that the combination of these two mechanisms is operative. It is the disturbance of *coordination* of factors, which normally control the rhythmic respiration, that results in periodic breathing. It appears that hyperexcitability of the respiratory centers alternates with their depression. Toward the end of apnea a rise in arterial Pco_2 and, more importantly, a fall in arterial Po_2 stimulate the central and peripheral chemoreceptors to a point of overshooting hyper-

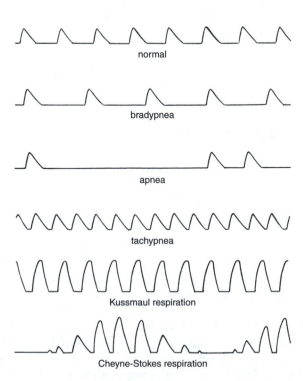

Figure 1–8. Schematic demonstration of commonly occurring respiratory patterns.

ventilation. The latter results in the restoration of oxygenation and the reduction of arterial P_{CO_2}, which in turn suppresses ventilatory drive to the point of its complete cessation (apnea), and the cycle repeats itself. This instability in ventilatory control systems may be the result of prolonged circulation time, which causes a delay in sensing the chemical changes in the blood returning from the lungs. Frequently, however, there is impairment of the sensitivity of the ventilatory control centers. Figure 1–8 shows some of the respiratory patterns. Paradoxical respiration is discussed on page 12.

■ SYSTEMIC MANIFESTATIONS OF RESPIRATORY DISORDERS

Significant alteration of respiratory function may result in systemic manifestations, primarily through the impairment of oxygenation and/or carbon dioxide elimination. Because the regulation of arterial oxygenation and carbon dioxide removal is the main function of the lungs, its derangement is the most important indication of abnormal respiratory function. Due to its significant functional reserve, however, the respiratory system is capable of regulating and maintaining the arterial blood gases in spite of the presence of pathologic conditions. Therefore, the lack of an abnormality in the blood gases does not exclude respiratory disease.

Hypoxemia and Hypoxia

Hypoxemia means low blood oxygen, and commonly refers to decreased arterial blood oxygen tension (P_{O_2}) or saturation below normal levels. **Hypoxia** is a more general term, and signifies low oxygen in tissues or cells resulting from inadequate oxygen delivery to meet their oxidative requirements. **Anoxia,** which means absence of oxygen, is the extreme degree of hypoxia.

The adequate oxygenation of tissue depends on its blood supply containing a sufficient *amount* of oxygen. The amount of oxygen carried in the blood is a function of its oxygen tension, or saturation, and hemoglobin available for its transport. Low hemoglobin levels in anemia and reduced available hemoglobin for binding oxygen in carbon monoxide poisoning are conditions in which the arterial blood oxygen content is decreased while its partial pressure remains normal. Therefore, tissue hypoxia may result not only from arterial hypoxemia, but also from the reduction of tissue blood supply and from the diminished oxygen-carrying capacity of the blood. Moreover, delivery of oxygen to tissues is also influenced by the affinity of hemoglobin to oxygen. This particular and important characteristic of hemoglobin determines its ability to bind and release oxygen under various circumstances, and is the basis for construction of the oxygen-hemoglobin dissociation curve. The subject of oxygen transport is discussed further on page 46.

The basic respiratory *causes of hypoxemia* are reduced inspired oxygen tension, alveolar hypoventilation, impairment of diffusion, ventilation-perfusion mismatching, and venous-to-arterial shunting. They are discussed in Chapter 26 (Respiratory Failure). The most reliable indicator of hypoxemia is the arterial blood P_{O_2} determination. Most symptoms and signs of hypoxemia will not be present unless it is severe.

Cyanosis. Cyanosis is commonly considered to be an important sign of hypoxemia. This time-honored clinical sign, however, is fraught with pitfalls and misinterpretations. Cyanosis by definition is the bluish discoloration of skin and mucous membranes due to the presence of an adequate amount of deoxygenated hemoglobin or certain other hemoglobin compounds in the *capillary blood*. Discoloration due to deposition of certain pigments can be readily differentiated from true cyanosis by pressing over the discolored area—cyanotic skin blanches, pigmented skin does not.

It has been estimated that the presence of at least 5 grams (g) of deoxygenated hemoglobin, 1.5 g of methemoglobin (a hemoglobin compound with ferric instead of ferrous iron), or 0.5 g of sulfhemoglobin (derived from the combination of ferric iron of methemoglobin with hydrogen sulfide) in 100 mL of *capillary* blood is required for the occurrence of cyanosis. The latter two hemoglobin compounds may be occasional causes of cyanosis, whereas cyanosis due to unoxygenated blood in the capillaries is a common occurrence.

Several factors result in increased amounts of deoxygenated hemoglobin in capillary blood. Arterial hypoxemia causes cyanosis when the oxygen content is low enough to result in a significant amount of deoxygenated hemoglobin. The capillary blood flow and the extraction of oxygen by tissues will, however, determine how much more hemoglobin will be deoxygenated while in the capillaries. This is one of the reasons that some patients appear more cyanotic than others with the same degree of arterial

hypoxemia. Arterial hypoxemia need not even be present for the development of cyanosis. Marked reduction in capillary blood flow will allow for enough oxygen extraction by the tissues for cyanosis to appear. Bluish discoloration of the nose and fingertips in very cold weather is a common observation.

In clinical conditions in which peripheral blood flow is diminished as a result of systemic shock or local factors, cyanosis may be observed. This type of cyanosis, in which the arterial blood oxygen content is normal, is called *peripheral* cyanosis, in contradistinction to *central* cyanosis in which arterial blood oxygen is low. Although this differentiation can be unequivocally made only by measurement of arterial blood Po_2, it may also be made in some instances on clinical grounds. Cold extremities with diminished pulse in cyanotic areas but normal color in warm regions suggest peripheral cyanosis; warm extremities and more uniform distribution of cyanosis suggest a central type. However, it should be emphasized that in many clinical situations cyanosis is the result of both arterial hypoxemia and circulatory disorders.

Severely anemic patients may have a markedly low arterial Po_2 without apparent cyanosis, as these patients will not have enough deoxygenated (absolute sense) hemoglobin. On the other hand, patients with polycythemia (increased hemoglobin level above normal) may seem cyanotic even without hypoxemia.

Systemic manifestations of hypoxemia are related to inadequate oxygen delivery to various organs or tissues. Hypoxemia, however, may not be associated with tissue hypoxia, particularly when it is of long duration. There are individuals, such as inhabitants in high-altitude locations who, despite significant arterial hypoxemia, are entirely asymptomatic. Several compensatory and adaptive mechanisms, such as an increase in red blood cells and an alteration in hemoglobin-oxygen affinity as well as a change in blood flow, will assure adequate tissue oxygenation.

As the brain is the organ most sensitive to lack of oxygen, symptoms of cerebral malfunction are the most common manifestations of hypoxemia. Acute cerebral hypoxia usually results in impaired judgment, clumsiness, and a feeling of drunkenness. If severe, mental confusion, coma, and death will occur. Chronic long-standing hypoxia manifests with fatigue, apathy, reduced attention, drowsiness, and muscle twitching.

Hypoxia has a significant effect on the cardiovascular system. It increases the cardiac output and heart rate. Cardiac arrhythmias are common in severe hypoxemia. In extreme hypoxemia, the heart rate slows down before stopping. It dilates peripheral and cerebral blood vessels and is a potent constrictor of the pulmonary arteries. Chronic pulmonary hypertension and cor pulmonale are important complications of long-standing hypoxemia. As discussed in Chapter 21, it is the alveolar hypoxia that causes pulmonary vasoconstriction rather than low blood O_2. As a result of stimulation of red blood cell production, chronic hypoxemia may cause secondary polycythemia.

Hypoxemia is an important respiratory stimulant through the peripheral chemoreceptors. In patients with concomitant hypercapnia, administration of an inappropriate amount of oxygen may result in further carbon dioxide retention by removing the hypoxemic ventilatory drive. Recent studies, however, indicate that oxygen-induced hypercapnia may be due to further impairment of gas ex-

change when the ratio of dead space to total ventilation increases.

Severe hypoxemia resulting in inadequate tissue oxygenation may cause anaerobic metabolism (metabolism in the absence of oxygen). The waste product of such metabolism includes lactic acid, accumulation of which results in metabolic acidosis.

Hypercapnia

The metabolic production of carbon dioxide and its elimination by the lungs determine its partial pressure (Pco_2) in arterial blood. Normally the lungs are capable of regulating their ventilation through a very sensitive control system, according to the amount of carbon dioxide production. As a result, arterial carbon dioxide tension is maintained within a narrow normal range. Hypercapnia or hypercarbia is an increase in arterial blood Pco_2 above 45 torr, the upper limit of normal.

Effective alveolar ventilation is that portion of ventilation that participates in gas exchange; it is inversely related to arterial blood Pco_2. Doubling alveolar ventilation will result in halving the arterial blood Pco_2, and vice versa (see Appendix E). Effectiveness of alveolar ventilation, therefore, is judged by arterial blood carbon dioxide tension. Hypercapnia thus indicates inadequate alveolar ventilation in relation to metabolic production of carbon dioxide.

There are numerous causes of carbon dioxide retention. These are discussed in Chapter 26.

Variable degrees of hypoxemia are always present in patients with hypercapnia, unless a high concentration of oxygen is administered. In clinical situations, therefore, the manifestations of hypercapnia are often combined with manifestations of hypoxemia. A clinical picture of pure hypercapnia may be experimentally demonstrated in individuals breathing CO_2 mixtures. Increased pulse rate and blood pressure, dizziness, headaches, mental clouding, visual difficulty, muscle twitching and tremor, and mental depression are frequently observed. Severe hypercapnia may result in loss of consciousness, which is commonly known as *CO_2 narcosis.* Carbon dioxide dilates cerebral blood vessels, resulting in increased blood flow to the brain. It has a constricting effect on pulmonary vessels.

An acute accumulation of carbon dioxide results in an increased hydrogen ion concentration (acidosis), which is at least partly responsible for most of the harmful effects of CO_2 retention. Slow and gradual increases in the P_{CO_2}, as seen in patients with chronic ventilatory failure, will allow for metabolic compensation by the elevation of serum bicarbonate and, therefore, will prevent or at least slow down the changes in pH. This is further discussed in Chapter 2.

In patients with acute respiratory failure, when there is a combination of hypercapnia and hypoxemia, a clinical picture characterized by headaches, somnolence, mental confusion, weakness, fatigue, irritability, and involuntary muscle movements is commonly observed. In more severe cases, loss of consciousness, paralysis, coma, and death may supervene.

Hypocapnia

Hypocapnia is the reverse of hypercapnia and signifies low arterial blood carbon dioxide tensions. It indicates an increased ventilation out of proportion to the metabolic production of carbon dioxide. This excessive alveolar ventilation is commonly known as *hyperventilation.* Although hyperventilation may be suspected clinically, it can only be confirmed by demonstration of a low arterial blood P_{CO_2}.

Acute reduction of arterial blood P_{CO_2} results in respiratory alkalosis, which is at least partly responsible for clinical manifestations of the *hyperventilation syndrome.* They include lightheadedness, fatigue, irritability, inability to concentrate, sense of unreality, tingling, muscle twitching, and impaired consciousness. The most common cause of hyperventilation is anxiety reaction, including panic attack, but it may also be due to central nervous system disease, severe anemia, shock, high fever, septicemia, alcohol intoxication, severe liver disease, aspirin poisoning, and several other conditions.

In many patients with respiratory disease, particularly in patients with hypoxemic respiratory failure, hyperventilation may be part of the clinical picture. It may be due to hypoxemic stimulation of the chemoreceptors, but it is often due to increased responsiveness of certain reflexes originating in the lungs. Hyperventilation as a result of mechanical ventilation is a common occurrence, which may be inadvertent or intentional.

BIBLIOGRAPHY

Anthonisen NR. Hypoxemia and O_2 therapy. *Am Rev Respir Dis.* 1982; 126:729–733.

Branch WT, McNeil BJ. Analysis of the differential diagnosis and assessment of pleuritic chest pain in young adults. *Am J Med.* 1983; 75:671–679.

Cahill BC, Ingbar DH. Massive hemoptysis: assessment and management. *Clin Chest Med.* 1994; 15(1):147–168.

Cohen CA, Zagelbaum G, Gross D, et al.

Clinical manifestations of inspiratory muscle fatigue. *Am J Med.* 1982; 73:308–316.

Farzan S. Cough and sputum production. In: Walker HK, Hall WD, Hurst JW, eds. *Clinical Methods.* 3rd ed. Boston, Mass: Butterworth; 1990; 207–210.

Forgacs P. The functional basis of pulmonary sounds. *Chest.* 1978; 73:399–405.

Gardner WN. The pathophysiology of hyperventilation disorders. *Chest.* 1996; 109:516–534.

Goldman, JM. Hemoptysis. *Emerg Med Clin North Am.* 1989; 7:325–338.

Irwin RS, Curley FJ, French CL. Chronic cough: the spectrum and frequency of causes, key components of the diagnostic evaluation, and outcome of specific therapy. *Am Rev Respir Dis.* 1990; 141:640–647.

Irwin RS, French CL, Curley FJ, et al. Chronic cough due to gastroesophageal reflux:clinical, diagnostic, and pathogenetic aspects. *Chest.* 1993; 104:1511–1517.

Loudon RG. The lung exam. *Clin Chest Med.* 1987; 8:265–272.

Loudon RG, Murphy RLH Jr. Lung sounds. *Am Rev Respir Dis.* 1984; 130:663–673.

Manning HL, Schwartzstein RM. Pathophysiology of dyspnea. *N Engl J Med.* 1995; 333:1547–1553.

McParland C, Krishnan B, Wang Y, Gallagher CG. Inspiratory muscle weakness and dyspnea in chronic heart failure. *Am Rev Respir Dis.* 1992; 146:467–472.

Pratter MR, Bartter T, Akers S, DuBois J. An algorithmic approach to chronic cough. *Ann Intern Med.* 1993; 119:977–983.

Schneider RR, Seckler SG. Evaluation of acute chest pain. *Med Clin North Am.* 1981; 65(1):53–66.

Sebastian JL, McKinney WP, Kaufman J, Young MJ. Angiotensin-converting enzyme inhibitors and cough. *Chest.* 1991; 99:36–39.

Smoller JW, Pollack MH, Otto MW, et al. Panic anxiety, dyspnea, and respiratory disease. *Am J Respir Crit Care Med.* 1996; 154:6–17.

Tobin MJ, Chadha TS, Jenouri G, et al. Breathing patterns. *Chest.* 1983; 84:202–205, 286–294.

Wasserman K, Casaburi R. Dyspnea: physiologic and pathophysiologic mechanisms. *Annu Rev Med.* 1988; 39:503–515.

Weinberger SE, Schwartzstein RM, Weiss JW. Hypercapnia. *N Engl J Med.* 1989; 321: 1223–1231.

Wolkove N, Dajczman E, Colacone A, Keisman H. The relationship between pulmonary function and dyspnea in obstructive lung disease. *Chest.* 1989; 96:1247–1251.

Diagnostic Methods, Functional Assessment, and Monitoring

The diagnosis of respiratory diseases and the evaluation of their functional effect sometimes may be made by appropriate history taking and physical examination. However, in most instances, applicable laboratory, radiographic, and/or bedside procedures are necessary for a definitive diagnosis, accurate functional assessment, and close monitoring. This chapter deals with these ancillary studies. It should be emphasized that information obtained by history taking and physical examination is essential for proper selection and effective utilization of such studies. The results of these studies should always be interpreted in light of clinical information and by considering their accuracy, sensitivity, and specificity.

■ SPUTUM EXAMINATION

Expectoration is a significant manifestation of many respiratory disorders, and information obtained from sputum ex-amination may be necessary for their diagnosis and management. Sputum examination is particularly helpful in the evaluation of respiratory-tract infections for bacteriologic identification and selection of the proper antibiotic. It is important in assessment of therapy in patients with tuberculosis, chronic bronchitis, asthma, lung abscess, and many other pulmonary diseases. The diagnosis of lung carcinoma and several other conditions is frequently made by or suspected from sputum examination.

Obtaining a proper sputum sample is most important for a successful sputum examination. It is most commonly done by collecting the *expectorated* sputum in a sterile bottle. Unfortunately, this simple task is often fraught with misinformation and mishandling. The respiratory therapist or nurse should be well informed about the proper technique for sputum collection. The sputum sample must represent secretions from the lower respiratory tract; nasal secretions and saliva are not acceptable. The patient should be observed and helped during sputum collection. First, the mouth should be cleared of food particles and rinsed with water. The patient is then asked to take a few deep breaths, and, at the end of the last inspiration, he is instructed to perform a series of gentle, short coughs. Often, following several deep breaths, the secretions will be mobilized more proximally, and the ensuing cough will be more effective in expelling them. The patient should be cautioned not to swallow the sputum, but rather to expectorate it into the specimen bottle. This procedure is repeated until an adequate sample is obtained. It is often easier to collect sputum in the morning as the patient wakens.

Sometimes it is not possible to obtain a sputum sample by cough and expectoration because of dry cough or the thick and tenacious nature of the secretion. The use of aerosolized solutions, such as saline, propylene glycol, acetylcysteine, and others, may help to induce sputum production and expectoration. Systemic hydration is important in dehydrated patients for sputum production. Sputum induction in patients with acquired immunodeficiency syndrome (AIDS), when *Pneumocystis carinii* pneumonia is suspected, is a simple and effective way of making a specific diagnosis (see Chapter 6).

Tracheobronchial suctioning, through the nose or the mouth, is an important way of obtaining a sample of secretions, particularly in obtunded or debilitated patients. Occasionally, secretions are obtained by transtracheal aspiration. With local anesthesia and sterile technique, a small catheter is passed via a large-bore needle inserted into the lumen of the trachea, entering percutaneously through the cricothyroid membrane. The secretions aspirated with this technique, which bypasses the mouth and the pharnyx, are most suitable for anaerobic bacterial culture. With the use of fiberoptic bronchoscopy, usually an adequate amount of secretion can be obtained. It also allows for the study of samples selectively collected from desired lobar or segmental bronchi. Aspiration of the stomach by a nasogastric tube, before arising in the morning, may yield tracheobronchial secretions swallowed during the preceding night. This method is used to obtain a sample for identification of tubercle bacilli in patients suspected of having pulmonary tuberculosis, but unable to expectorate, or as a supplement to sputum examination. Gastric aspiration is particularly useful in children who have difficulty producing sputum.

After collection of an adequate sputum sample, its gross appearance may provide useful information. The color of sputum varies from white, yellow, and green to brown or red, and its consistency varies from watery to thick to semisolid. Mucus with its translucent appearance should be differentiated from mucopurulent or purulent secretions. Yellow or green sputum indicates the presence of large numbers of white blood cells, which are the major component of pus. Red or brown sputum is usually due to the presence of red blood cells.

The specimen should be taken to the appropriate laboratory for its desired examination. This should be done promptly when bacteriologic studies are intended. Sputum is usually examined for its cell content, particularly the amount and type of white blood cells. The presence of alveolar macrophages in sputum is an important indication that its origin is the lung. Squamous epithelial cells indicate the presence of secretions from areas above the larynx, and thus are unsuitable for bacteriologic examination. Significant numbers of polymorphonuclear neutrophils suggest bacterial infection, whereas eosinophils often are indicative of an allergic process such as asthma. Bacteriologic studies include smear and special staining, as well as culturing on special media, depending on the organisms that are suspected. Sputum is also examined for malignant cells in patients suspected of having neoplastic lesions of the respiratory tract.

■ RADIOGRAPHIC EXAMINATION OF THE CHEST

Radiographic examination plays a most important role in studying patients with respiratory disorders and in diagnosing unsuspected lung diseases. Without a chest x-ray, examination of such patients is considered incomplete. A number of pulmonary conditions would be either undiagnosed or misdiagnosed without radiographic study. Many cases of pulmonary malignancy, early tuberculosis, and a variety of other lesions may be completely unrecognized until discovered by a chest x-ray. Radiographic examination is commonly used for screening asymptomatic individuals to detect tuberculosis and, sometimes, other lung diseases.

In patients with respiratory disease, x-ray examination enables better identification of a lesion, more correct assessment of its extent, and its more precise localization. It also helps in following the patient's progress and response to therapeutic measures. In addition, x-ray film is an important medical document, particularly useful as a comparison for future studies. Based on standard chest x-ray examination, special views or body-section radiography, such as plain or computed tomography, may be necessary.

Principles of Radiographic Study of the Chest

Because of differences in the density of its various structures, the chest is very suitable for radiographic examination. There is enough contrast between most of these structures to allow for their delineation on the x-ray film. The air-containing lungs, having the least density, do not significantly interfere with the passage of roentgen rays, causing dark prints on the film. The bones, because of their high density, impede the traverse of x-rays, and therefore prevent its impression on the film, which remains white. The heart, blood vessels, mediastinum, and diaphragm, which have a density greater than air but less than bone, cause differing shades of white and gray on the x-ray film. In addition to their density, the thickness of various structures is an important factor in affecting the x-ray penetration.

The ribs and other bones can be easily identified from the surrounding soft tissue and the lungs. The silhouette of the heart and its major blood vessels, which are flanked by the lungs, is clearly outlined. The diaphragm, with its underlying abdominal organs, contrasts with the air-containing lungs above it. The trachea, because of its air content, is visualized in the middle of the upper mediastinum. The pulmonary blood vessels are traceable from the hili, branching and tapering toward the lung periphery.

Because of the superimposition of certain structures and for better localization of the lesions, usually at least two radiographic views are obtained: (1) the pos-

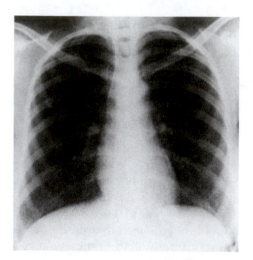 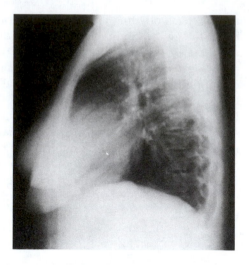

Figures 2–1 and 2–2. Normal posteroanterior and lateral chest roentgenograms.

teroanterior (PA), or occasionally antero-posterior (AP), view; and (2) the lateral (right or left) view. Sometimes other projections such as obliques may be necessary.

The standard projection, which is the cornerstone of radiographic examination of the chest, is obtained by placing the patient in front of the radiographic cassette so that the front of the chest touches it. The x-ray tube is located behind the patient at a distance of about 2 meters. The beam of radiation from the x-ray tube passes through the patient's back in a direction perpendicular to the film. This is intended to minimize distortion and magnification effects. The x-ray is usually taken at the end of inspiration while the patient is temporarily holding his or her breath. The exposure time, voltage, and current are individualized according to the patient's age, thickness of the chest wall, and particular purpose of the study. In certain situations, radiographic studies are done in a AP view, upright or supine, or lateral decubitus position (done across the table while the patient is lying on his or her side).

Reading a Chest X-Ray. In reading a radiographic picture of the chest, the following observations are made (Figs. 2–1 and 2–2):

1. Soft tissues surrounding the bony thorax, including breast shadows.
2. Bony structures; counting and identifying the individual ribs, looking for fractures, deformity, and other lesions; spinal curvature.
3. Diaphragm, its position, comparing the two sides (usually the right hemidiaphragm is slightly higher than the left), its contour, sharpness of its angles with the chest wall (costophrenic or CP angles). A small amount of pleural effusion would obliterate these angles.
4. The mediastinum, including the heart, its position, width, and contour; heart size, configuration, and the ratio of its width to the inner thoracic diameter (cardiothoracic ratio is normally less than $\frac{1}{2}$). Trachea and mainstem bronchi are easily identified, and their posi-

tion in relation to other thoracic structures is defined. In a PA projection of the chest, the outline of the mediastinum on the right side is made by (from above downward) the innominate vein, superior vena cava, right atrium, and, sometimes, the inferior vena cava. On the left, it is made by (from above downward) the subclavian vessels, aorta, pulmonary artery trunk, and the left ventricle (Fig. 2–3).

5. The lungs, their volume, background density, shadows of various lesions; pulmonary blood vessels, their size and direction; and hili, their position, size, and sharpness. The background lung density is normally due to the presence of blood in the pulmonary capillaries, while the larger vessels create the visible lung markings. Normally, the bronchi, beyond a short distance from the tracheal bifurcation, are not visible. The hilum in a chest film refers to the area of the lung where the pulmonary blood vessels converge; it also contains some lymph nodes, which are not normally discernible, but they may become quite large and readily identifiable in certain pathologic conditions. The right hilar position is normally slightly lower than the left.

6. Pleura, its thickness, presence of fluid or air in the pleural cavity; interlobar fissures. Normally, the pleura does not cast any identifiable shadow, but the fissure may be seen as linear densities. The major fissures are usually seen on a lateral chest x-ray film; the minor or horizontal fissure may be seen on both PA and lateral views. Presence of a small amount of fluid causes blunting of the normally sharp angle between the diaphragm and the chest wall (CP angle). A lateral decubitus film may be necessary to confirm the presence of fluid.

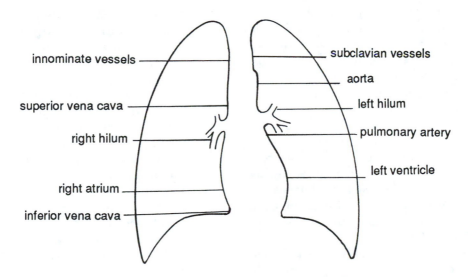

innominate vessels

superior vena cava

right hilum

right atrium

inferior vena cava

subclavian vessels

aorta

left hilum

pulmonary artery

left ventricle

Figure 2–3. Components of the mediastinal borders in a normal chest.

The characteristics of any abnormality observed on a chest x-ray film should be described (e.g., its location, density, size, configuration, and effect on the lung and other adjacent structures). Adequate knowledge of bronchopulmonary segments is necessary for proper localization of lesions seen on a chest radiograph. There are numerous descriptive radiologic terms. Some of the important ones used in interpretation of a chest x-ray are as follows:

- **Radiolucency** is the property of being radiolucent, that is, allowing for the passage of x-rays. This is a relative term used in defining darker areas on a chest x-ray, such as radiolucency of an emphysematous lung or of the inside of a cavity.
- **Radiodensity** is the opposite of radiolucency. It is used to describe dense shadows that look whiter on x-ray film.
- **Consolidation** is a pathologic term that indicates a solid-appearing lung due to pneumonia. It is also used in radiology to describe a radiodensity characteristic of pneumonia.
- **Infiltration** is a loose radiologic term that usually indicates any ill-defined radiodensity, often due to an inflammatory process.
- **Interstitial density** describes density due to thickening of the interstitial tissue of the lung, which often appears as diffuse ground glass, reticular (netlike), or nodular shadow. Coarse reticular density is usually called **honeycombing. Miliary** density refers to the diffuse punctate shadows such as seen in miliary tuberculosis.
- **Alveolar** or **airspace density** is due to the presence of denser substances replacing the air in the alve-

oli. Alveolar edema gives rise to this type of radiographic change. Pulmonary consolidation is a confluent airspace density.

- **Homogeneous density** is characteristic of uniformly dense lesions, such as a solid tumor, fluid-containing cyst, or collection of fluid in the pleural space.
- **Pulmonary mass** is a large, 6 cm or more in diameter, demarcated radiodensity. It often indicates a neoplastic lesion. **Mediastinal mass** is a similar shadow in the mediastinum.
- **Pulmonary nodule** is a smaller, less than 6 cm, circumscribed density, which may be single, and then is called a solitary pulmonary nodule or "coin" lesion.
- **Pleural density** is a radiodensity due to pleural inflammation, fluid, tumor, or scarring.
- **Cavity** refers to a radiolucent lesion surrounded by denser tissue. It is due to a localized necrotic lung lesion that has sloughed off. It is the hallmark of a lung abscess. A fluid level may be seen inside a cavity.
- **Air cyst** or **bulla** is a thin-walled radiolucent area surrounded by more or less normal lung. **Bleb** refers to a superficial lung bulla abutting the pleura.
- **Calcification** indicates the presence of calcium salt deposited in certain lesions. It has a density similar to bone.
- **Volume loss** signifies reduction of volume of a whole lung or part of it as seen on a chest x-ray film. Depending on its location, it is usually manifested by displacement of the mediastinum, trachea, diaphragm, hilum, and interlobar fissures toward the involved area and approximation of the ribs.

- An **air bronchogram** outlines the air-containing bronchial tree beyond its normally visible portion. It results from an infiltration or consolidation that surrounds the bronchi, making their contrasting air columns visible.
- **Silhouette sign** is a term used when a part of the border of the heart or mediastinum is obscured by a radio-dense lesion that abuts that border. The sign helps to determine the lo-cation of such a lesion in a single view radiograph.

Computed Tomography

Computed tomography (CT) is an imaging technique in which radiologic and computer technologies are combined to enable the reconstruction of pictures showing transverse cross sections of the body as thin slices (Fig. 2–4). As in standard radiographic study, CT is based on

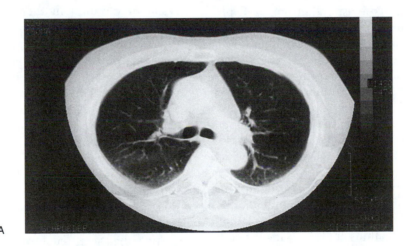

Figure 2–4. A photograph (A), and its diagrammatic drawing (B), of a normal chest CT scan at the level of the carina.

contrasting various structures in the slice that have different specific gravities. This contrast may be enhanced by the intravenous injection of a radiopaque material, which increases the density of tissues proportional to their vascularity. It also outlines blood vessels in the mediastinum and hili, thus allowing differentiation from tumors or enlarged lymph nodes.

Thoracic CT scan is supplementary to the standard radiographic studies. It is most useful for additional delineation of mediastinal and hilar structures, intrapulmonary nodules, and pleural disease; for staging intrathoracic malignancies; and for precise localization of intrathoracic lesion for needle aspiration biopsy. It provides valuable information in patients with mediastinal mass or its other abnormalities. Chest CT with contrast is an excellent way for studying an enlarged hilum and distinguishing masses or lymphadenopathy from blood vessels. It may demonstrate lesions inside major bronchi or trachea. Pulmonary nodules or masses are well suited for CT scanning, which provides more detailed information on their structure and allows for determination of their densities. Pleural diseases such as effusions, thickening, plaques, and calcifications are readily identified by CT scan. Metastatic involvement of the chest wall, including ribs, can be diagnosed by CT when it is missed by conventional radiography. Further refinement of CT technology and development of thin-section, high-resolution CT (HRCT) have improved the capabilities of CT imaging and have allowed better definition of parenchymal lesions in interstitial lung diseases. Bronchiectasis, when suspected on clinical grounds and/or by plain chest film, is another condition that CT scan, especially HRCT, is most useful for its definitive diagnosis or its exclusion.

Magnetic Resonance Imaging

Very briefly, and rather simplistically, MRI technology is based on the characteristics of nuclei of atoms of certain elements in the body tissues (mostly protons of hydrogen atoms) that can be magnetized when placed in a strong magnetic field. These magnetized nuclei are then energized by a radiofrequency pulse. The stored radio signal emitted by the protons is then used by highly specialized equipment to make sectional images of the body. Contrast between the images of different types of tissues made by MRI is the result of variation in their composition and concentration of protons, not from differences in the densities, which are the cause of contrast in CT scanning. MRI is capable of producing images not only of transaxial sections but also sagittal and coronal slices. It has proven its superiority over CT scanning for imaging the brain, spinal cord, and musculoskeletal system. Its role for studying intrathoracic structures is limited. As rapidly flowing blood will have no signal with MRI, and because there are large blood vessels in the mediastinum and hilum, MRI is superior to CT for imaging these structures for detection of abnormal soft tissue masses or lymph nodes. Absence of ionizing radiation and lack of need for injection of contrast material with MRI are other advantages of this imaging technique.

Ultrasonography

Because ultrasound, at the frequency used, does not pass through air or bone, the air in the lungs and ribs in the thoracic wall are the limiting factors for usefulness of ultrasonography in pulmonary diseases. It can, however, demonstrate lesions in contact with the chest wall and between the ribs. This imaging technique is therefore used for detection of fluid in the pleural space when conventional radiographic studies cannot differentiate between a loculated fluid from pleural thickening or other soft tissue mass lesions. Ultrasonography also is used as a guide for thoracentesis when the fluid is small or loculated.

Pulmonary Angiography

Pulmonary angiography is the radiographic study of pulmonary vessels, which are opacified by injection of a contrast material into a peripheral vein, the vena cava, the right chambers of the heart, or the pulmonary artery. The main purpose of this study in pulmonary medicine is to investigate for obstructive lesions. It is particularly useful in pulmonary embolism whenever the diagnosis is in doubt and confirmation is essential for a major therapeutic decision. Occasionally, pulmonary angiography is done for investigation of hemoptysis of unknown cause, for evaluation of vascular malformation, and for study of patients with lung cancer for its resectability.

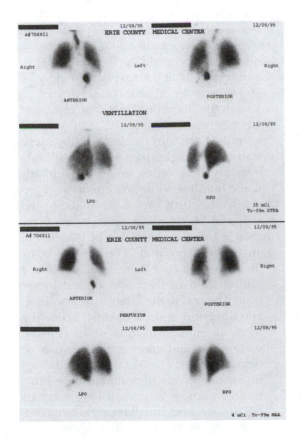

Figure 2–5. Normal ventilation and perfusion lung scans. Note that there is almost complete matching of ventilation and perfusion demonstrated in all four views. LPO, left posterior oblique; RPO, right posterior oblique.

Radionuclide Lung Scanning

The radioisotope scanning in respiratory disease is an important diagnostic tool, particularly in thromboembolic disorders. Perfusion lung scanning, which is the most commonly used radioisotope study, examines the distribution of blood flow to different lung regions. It is usually done by intravenous injection of a substance tagged with radioactive material. Human albumin, which is processed to form into particles or microspheres large enough to be blocked in the pulmonary capillaries, is the most commonly used vehicle. It is labeled with radioactive technetium ($99^{m}Tc$) or other radionuclides. After injection, radioactivity of the lung fields is studied by a counter or, more conveniently, by a special camera over the anterior, posterior, and both lateral surfaces of the chest.

A defect in a lung scan is indicative of perfusion impairment, which may be primary and due to obstruction of a branch of the pulmonary artery, such as in pulmonary embolism, or secondary and due to reduction or cessation of perfusion as a result of a diseased lung. It is always necessary, therefore, to have a concomitant chest x-ray film for proper interpretation of a lung scan.

A *ventilation* lung scan with a radioactive gas, such as xenon and crypton, or aerosolized radioactive material, such as technetium-labeled DTPA, is used for determining the distribution of ventilation in various lung regions and also for ascertaining whether or not reduced perfusion is the result of diminished ventilation of a corresponding lung region. Therefore, by combining ventilation with perfusion scan ($\dot{V}/\dot{Q}$ scans), the specificity and diagnostic value of perfusion scan are increased. Figure 2–5 shows a normal ventilation and perfusion lung scanning.

■ BRONCHOSCOPY

One of the important methods of examination of the respiratory tract is endoscopy, which is direct inspection inside the suspected areas. Viewing the upper airways with instruments such as a rhinoscope to look inside the nasal passages; laryngoscopic mirror to inspect the nasopharynx, hypopharynx, epiglottis, and vocal cords; and direct laryngoscope for visualization of the larynx and passage of an endotracheal tube, is a form of endoscopy. However, the most important endoscopic examination of the respiratory tract is by a bronchoscope, which, in addition to its main purpose of looking inside the bronchi, will allow for examination of the upper air passages.

The development of the *fiberoptic bronchoscope* has revolutionized the field of endoscopic examination by its ease of insertion, acceptability by the patients, and versatility in visualizing all segmental and subsegmental bronchi.

In the fiberoptic bronchoscope, as in any fiberscope, tightly packed fiberoptic bundles (specially processed fiberglass) transmit the light from an external high-intensity light source, and other similarly made bundles, with the help of an objective lens, return the visual image to the eyepiece of the instrument. Its tip is remotely controlled and can be directed to any desired position. The flexible optic fibers, straight or bent, will allow the transmission of light and optical image from one end to the other in any position and direction. A small channel inside the scope permits instillation of anesthetics, suctioning, and passing of a brush or biopsy forceps. The diameter of a fiberoptic bronchoscope, despite all these functioning parts, is very small (5–6 mm). Its advantages over the older rigid bronchoscope are, therefore, quite evident.

The *rigid bronchoscope* is made of a straight metallic tube with a light at its end. It is still used in some instances, such as for removal of certain foreign bodies, suctioning large amounts of thick and inspissated secretions, and studying the source of severe or massive hemoptysis. Otherwise, the flexible fiberscope has replaced the rigid bronchoscope.

Fiberoptic bronchoscopy is usually done under local anesthesia with mild or no sedation. The bronchoscope may be passed through the mouth, nose, or a tracheal tube. The upper air passages, vocal cords, trachea, carina, and bronchi down to the subsegmental bronchi are methodically studied. Observation is made on the characteristics of mucosa, secretions, orientation of airways, external compression, and internal obstructing and nonobstructing lesions. Material for bacteriologic, pathologic, and cytologic studies is often obtained during bronchoscopy.

Indications for bronchoscopy are as follows:

1. Clinically or radiographically suspected bronchial obstruction. Bronchoscopy not only identifies the cause of obstruction but it may also be therapeutic when it is due to retained secretions.
2. Evaluation of suspicious lesions, particularly when carcinoma or other endobronchial lesions are suspected. Bronchoscopic biopsy and other techniques for obtaining pathologic samples are performed when such lesions are found.
3. Investigation of patient for unexplained hemoptysis.
4. As part of staging for lung cancer and for preoperative evaluation for lung resection.
5. Suspected foreign-body aspiration and its removal.
6. Bronchial suctioning when secretions cannot be cleared by simpler means.
7. To obtain bacteriologic and pathologic specimens in a variety of localized or diffuse lung diseases, in which a specific diagnosis is not possible by less invasive methods.
8. For studying the airways following inhalation of smoke and other noxious gases and fumes.
9. To facilitate tracheal intubation in difficult cases.
10. To perform bronchoalveolar lavage (BAL).

Specimens are usually procured bronchoscopically by suctioning, bronchial washing, endobronchial or transbronchial biopsy, needle aspiration, and BAL. By sampling intraalveolar contents, BAL is most useful for the diagnosis of *P carinii* pneumonia in AIDS patients (see Chapter 6). BAL is also performed for diagnosis of ventilator-associated pneumonia.

■ PULMONARY FUNCTION STUDIES

Pulmonary function tests (PFTs) provide objective means for determination of the presence or absence of functional impairment of the respiratory system and allow assessment of its severity, progression, and response to therapeutic measures. These tests are essential in the diagnosis and management of asthma.

As the main functions of the lungs are oxygenation of blood and removal of carbon dioxide from it, determination of arterial blood gases seems to be the most important functional evaluation of the

TABLE 2–1. COMMON INDICATIONS FOR PULMONARY FUNCTION TESTING

Evaluation of patients with chronic dyspnea
Determination of response to therapeutic measures
Assessment of severity of respiratory impairment
Diagnostic evaluation for certain abnormal laboratory findings such as hypoxemia, acid-base disturbance, and polycythemia
Evaluation of patient with occupational exposure to agents known to affect the lungs
Determination of respiratory impairment in neuromuscular disorders
Assessment of disability and suitability to certain occupations
Evaluation of adverse reaction to drugs known to affect the lungs

respiratory system. In view of the significant reserve capacity of lung function, however, alteration of blood gases need not be present with reduction of functioning lung units. For instance, surgical removal of a significant portion of the lung may have no effect on the arterial blood oxygen and carbon dioxide if the remaining lung continues to maintain adequate alveolar ventilation and blood perfusion for gas exchange. In such a case, lung volumes and pulmonary diffusing capacity will be reduced. Therefore, although abnormal blood gases are generally indicative of impaired respiratory function, normal values do not necessarily signify normal lungs.

Numerous tests may identify functional impairment of the respiratory system at a more or less early stage of respiratory disease. Commonly performed pulmonary function studies are measurements of lung volumes, forced expiratory flow rates, diffusing capacity, and arterial blood gases. Additional tests, such as measurement of inspiratory and expiratory pressures, determination of closing volume, assessment of regional ventilation and perfusion, bronchial provocation, exercise test, and sleep studies are sometimes performed. Routine PFTs may be performed with simple spirometric devices or by advanced sophisticated instrumentation available in modern pul-

monary function laboratories. As lung volumes and flow rates are usually the most useful and informative parameters to be measured, simple spirometry will suffice in most situations. The common indication for PF testing is depicted in Table 2–1.

In this section, certain principles and clinical uses of pulmonary function tests are discussed. Predicted normal values, nomograms, and formulas are presented in Appendix B.

Lung Volumes

Total lung capacity is the volume of air in the lungs at the end of a maximum inspiration. It is made up of four volumes (Fig. 2–6):

1. **Residual volume (RV)** is the volume of air that remains in the lungs after a maximum expiration.
2. **Expiratory reserve volume (ERV)** is the maximum volume of air that can be exhaled after expiration of tidal volume.
3. **Tidal volume (TV)** is the volume of air inspired and expired with each normal breath.
4. **Inspiratory reserve volume (IRV)** is the maximum volume of air that one can breathe in after inspiration of tidal volume.

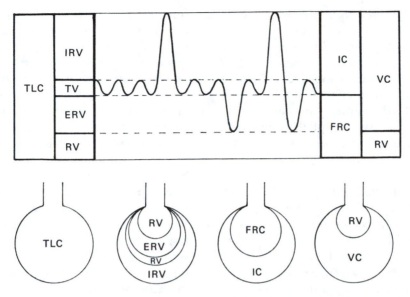

Figure 2–6. Lung volumes and capacities. ERV, expiratory reserve volume; FRC, functional residual capacity; IC, inspiratory capacity; IRV, inspiratory reserve volume; RV, residual volume; TLC, total lung capacity; TV, tidal volume; VC, vital capacity.

Combining two or more of these volumes makes the following four capacities (see Fig. 2–6):

1. **Functional residual capacity (FRC)** is the total of RV and ERV; therefore, it is the volume of air remaining in the lungs at the end of expiration of TV. This is the *resting end-expiratory position.*

2. **Inspiratory capacity (IC)** is the sum of TV and IRV; therefore, it is the maximum volume of air that can be inspired from the *resting end-expiratory position.*

3. **Vital capacity (VC)** is the total of ERV, TV, IRV, or the sum of ERV and IC. It is the maximum volume of air that can be exhaled by forceful effort following a maximum inspiration.

4. **Total lung capacity (TLC)** is the sum of RV, ERV, TV, and IRV, or total of IC and FRC, or sum of VC and RV.

Among the eight lung volumes and capacities, four are most useful in PF study. They are VC, RV, FRC, and TLC. Lung volumes and capacities that do not include the RV can be easily measured from a spirometric tracing (see Fig. 2–6) obtained by a simple spirometer or by one of the currently available electronic, computerized systems. The Wright respirometer is used as a bedside method for measurement of VC and TV. This small gadget is particularly useful when frequent measurements of VC and TV are necessary in the management of patients with respiratory failure.

Special equipment will be required for measuring RV and, therefore, FRC and TLC. Although *closed circuit helium equilibration* or *nitrogen washout methods* may be used for measurement of these volumes, body plethysmography is the preferred technique. Integrated in a computerized system, plethysmographic method is easier to perform and more accurate for measurement of intrathoracic gas volume.

The physical principle of body plethysmography is based on Boyle's law of the relationship between changes of pressure and the volume of a gas. The subject sits inside the airtight box, equipped with a sensitive manometer, breathing air about him or her with a mouthpiece connected to another manometer or pressure transducer. At a desired position of the respiratory cycle (usually FRC), the mouthpiece is occluded by a remote-controlled shutter while the patient continues to breathe against an obstruction (Fig. 2–7). This will result in a reduction of intrathoracic pressure measured by another manometer (or pressure transducer) between the patient's mouth and the shutter, while the pressure inside the body box, read from its manometer, increases as a result of thoracic expansion. From these pressure changes the original thoracic gas volume is calculated, using Boyle's equation. With a computerized system, the information from pressure transducers are processed to compute the thoracic gas volume, which appears in a printout.

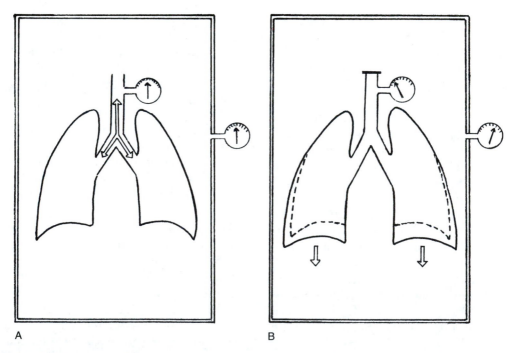

Figure 2–7. Schematic demonstration of measurement of intrathoracic gas volume by body plethysmography. (A) Quiet breathing with airway open, (B) inspiration against closed airway.

Forced Expiratory Flow Rates

The volume of a forceful expiration in relation to time, measured from a maximal inspiratory position, allows for the evaluation of airflow in the respiratory tract. It is the most commonly performed pulmonary function study essential for the assessment of airway resistance. This test is usually done by a recording spirometer.

The subject initially takes a maximally deep breath, holds it for a short while, and then expires as rapidly and forcibly as possible into the spirometer, which records volume versus time (Fig. 2–8). The tracing thus obtained is called a *forced spirogram* and the total volume expired is known as *forced expiratory vital capacity* (FVC). As the FVC is the basis for measurement of expiratory flow rates, it should be performed with utmost care to ensure that the patient is making maximum effort. The analysis of the forced spirogram is one of the most useful pulmonary function studies. Measurements of specifically selected portions of the curve will allow the determination of flow rates at different times of forced expiration. FEV_1, one of the most important

measurements, is the forced expiratory volume in the first second. The volumes expired in the first 0.5, 0.75, 2.0, or 3.0 seconds can also be calculated. The values obtained are expressed in an absolute term and a percentage of vital capacity (FEV_1/FVC). FEV_1/FVC ratio is primarily used for detection of obstructive airway disease and quantification of its severity.

Maximum mid-expiratory flow (MMF), commonly known as $FEF_{25\%-75\%}$, is the average flow rate for the middle two-quarters of the FVC. The volume-time curve is graphically demonstrated and individual components are automatically calculated and displayed by most modern computerized spirometers. With integration of instantaneous flow measurements throughout the forced expiration, a flow-volume curve is also constructed simultaneously (see later in this chapter).

Peak expiratory flow rate, which is the highest flow at any time during a forced expiration, is usually measured by a peak flow meter. It can also be determined from a maximum expiratory flow-volume curve. Self-measurement of peak flow by patients with asthma, using one of the small inexpensive meters on the market, is con-

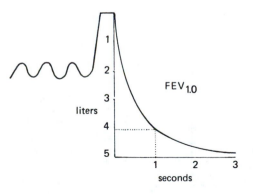
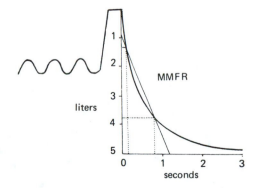

Figure 2–8. Forced expiratory spirogram in a normal individual (volume/time curve). As demonstrated in Figure 2–10, volume-time curves in most current spirometric tracings appear reversed and the curves begin from the crossing point of X and Y axes.

sidered to be essential for proper outpatient management. They have also facilitated objective assessment of the severity of asthma in emergency rooms and its response to therapeutic measures.

Maximal Expiratory Flow-Volume Curve. By studying a forced spirogram, it is evident that the flow rates are higher shortly after the beginning of expiratory effort, when lung volume is large, and decrease progressively toward the end as lung volume diminishes. Plotting expiratory flow rates, measured instantaneously, against lung volume (a forced vital capacity maneuver) will result in a curve known as the *maximal expiratory flow-volume curve* (Fig. 2–9). The summit of the curve indicates the peak expiratory flow, which takes place earlier at a volume close to TLC, followed by progressive reduction of flow until it ceases at the RV. As in the forced spirogram, the maximal expira-

tory flow-volume curve measures the forced vital capacity and gives information on airway function. It offers, however, an added feature for better understanding of airway dynamics.

The airflow in the early portion (about the first one-third) of the curve, which includes the peak flow, is markedly influenced by the intrathoracic pressure and, therefore, is effort dependent. In the remaining portion (last two-thirds of the curve), the maximum flows are reached rapidly with an effort of less than one-third of the maximum expiratory muscle force and, therefore, cannot be increased by further effort. This can be explained by narrowing of the airways with increasing intrathoracic pressure, which offsets the beneficial effect of higher driving pressure, and thus limits the airflow. The mechanical characteristics of the airway influence the position and the configuration of this portion

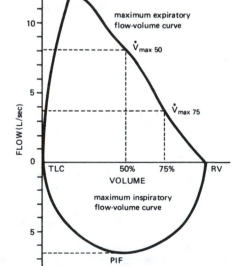

Figure 2–9. Maximum flow-volume loop made of maximum expiratory and inspiratory flow-volume curves.

of the maximal expiratory flow-volume curve and allow determination of airway abnormalities. For a numerical recording, flow rates at 50% and 75% of the expired vital capacity, respectively known as $\dot{V}_{max50}$ and $\dot{V}_{max75}$, are more commonly measured.

Flow-Volume Loop. Maximal inspiratory flow is also usually measured by taking a forceful inspiration from the position of residual volume after a forced expiration. Its recording, plotted against lung volume, produces the inspiratory flow-volume curve. This curve is entirely effort dependent. When combined with the expiratory flow-volume curve, it makes a loop known as the flow-volume loop (see Fig. 2–9). The inspiratory limb is fairly symmetrical with the peak flow occurring at midpoint. Peak inspiratory flow is normally less than peak expiratory flow. The maximal-effort flow-volume loop is especially helpful for diagnosis as well as characterization of obstruction of central or upper airways, as discussed in Chapter 7.

Both volume-time curves and flow-volume loop are simultaneously depicted by many modern automated and computerized pulmonary function machines. These tracings together with numerical determinations of various flow rates as well as lung volumes provide enough information to meet the needs of most clinical situations in which pulmonary function studies are indicated. Based on the results of these tests, two basic patterns of pulmonary function abnormalities can be identified:

1. **Obstructive pattern.** This pattern is characterized by low expiratory flow rates. Although FVC may also be reduced, reduction of FEV_1 is

out of proportion to that of FVC; as a result, FEV_1/FVC ratio is always lower than predicted normal. Expiratory flow-volume curve shows characteristic changes—after a fairly rapid (but lower than normal) peak, expiratory flow rates decline rapidly and continue to remain low throughout the expiration. The descending portion of the curve becomes concave upward, slowly approaching the volume axis. The volume-time curve is a slowly rising curve that does not reach a plateau, as seen in a normal tracing (Fig. 2–10). In obstructive ventilatory impairment, TLC may be higher than normal, but RV is almost always significantly increased. As a result, TV/TLC ratio is also increased.

Reversibility of obstruction from diffuse airway disease can be determined by changes of flow rates after (about 15 min) inhalation of a bronchodilator, such as albuterol.

2. **Restrictive pattern.** This pattern is characterized by reduced lung volumes, especially VC and TLC. With normal airway resistance, it takes shorter time for completion of a forced expiration. Therefore, despite reduced absolute value of FEV_1, FEV_1/FVC ratio is at least normal, but often increased. Expiratory flow-volume curve appears narrow and tall. Volume-time curve is of short duration with a rapid rise, reaching a plateau quickly (see Fig. 2–10). Reduction in lung volumes often includes low residual volume.

In many clinical situations, a combination of obstructive and restrictive ventilatory

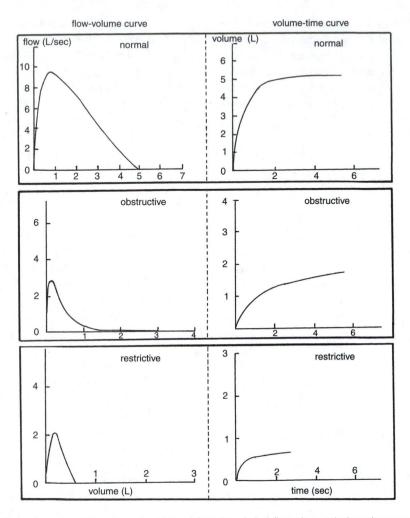

Figure 2–10. Obstructive and restrictive patterns of ventilatory defects shown by both flow-volume and volume-time curves. Normal tracings are also shown for comparison.

defects, in which the pattern of PFTs is a mixed one, may be seen. That is, there is both reduced FEV_1/FVC ratio and reduced lung volumes (which should include TLC).

Normal predictive values for FVC, FEV_1, and other expiratory flow rates are shown in Appendix B.

Diffusing Capacity

Diffusion is the random molecular motion by which matter is transported from a region of higher concentration to one of lower concentration. In the lungs, the net movement of gases by diffusion between the alveolar air and the capillary blood takes place as a result of their pressure gradient: oxygen moves from the alveoli into the pulmonary capillaries, and carbon dioxide moves in the opposite direction.

Diffusing capacity is defined as the movement of a gas (in milliliters, or mL) that crosses the alveolar-capillary membrane every minute for each millimeter (mm) of mercury (mm Hg) pressure difference of that gas in the alveoli and capillaries. Its unit, therefore, is mL/min/mm Hg. Although it is the diffusing capacity of oxygen that is clinically important, because of the closeness of diffusion behavior of carbon monoxide (CO) to oxygen, the former is more widely used for measurement of diffusing capacity.

Both single-breath and steady-state methods, commonly used for determination of CO diffusing capacity (DL_{CO}), are based on the same principle. For its calculation, two measurements are necessary: the amount of CO passing from the alveoli to the blood each minute, and the difference between its partial pressure (P_{CO}) in the alveoli and pulmonary capillaries. The amount of CO transferred is measured by determination of the difference of CO concentrations in inspired and expired air. As the amount of CO used for the test is small and it is taken up by the hemoglobin as soon as it enters the blood, P_{CO} in the capillary blood will be negligible. Therefore, the mean alveolar P_{CO} is the only other measurement needed in the equation:

$$DL_{CO} = mL\ CO\ transferred/min/\\ mm\ Hg\ mean\ alveolar\ P_{CO}$$

The mean alveolar P_{CO} is determined by sampling the alveolar gas.

Diffusing capacity is affected by several physiologic and pathologic factors.

The concentration of hemoglobin in blood, the volume of blood in pulmonary capillaries, the rate of blood flow, the surface area where the capillary blood and alveolar air are in close proximity, and the characteristics of the alveolar-capillary membrane, particularly its thickness, are all important in this regard. Therefore, alteration of diffusing capacity does not indicate a specific anatomic or physiologic abnormality. It may be reduced in a variety of pathologic conditions of the lung. In a patient with known pulmonary disease, however, measurement of diffusing capacity is one of the more useful methods for assessment of its severity, follow-up of disease progress, and determination of response to therapy. It may also be helpful as a sensitive test in demonstration of an abnormality when the result of other studies is equivocal, as in sarcoidosis or in the early course of *P carinii* pneumonia in AIDS. For reference values for diffusing capacity, see Appendix B.

Ventilation

The volume of air inspired, or expired, every minute at a resting state is called *resting minute ventilation,* which is the product of tidal volume and rate of breathing (provided that tidal volumes are equal and the rate is regular). For the bedside need, the Wright respirometer is quite adequate and easy to use. The problem with measurement of minute ventilation is due to the fact that, once the patient is aware of his breathing, it is no longer a purely unconscious process; therefore, both the rate and the depth of breathing may change.

Minute ventilation is composed of *dead-space ventilation* and *alveolar ventilation.* The space occupied by the air that does not exchange with capillary blood is called *dead space,* and the remainder of the air volume that is in the alveoli, and which therefore participates in gas exchange, is called *alveolar space.* Ventilation of these two spaces is called, respectively, dead-space ventilation and alveolar ventilation.

Anatomic and Physiologic Dead Spaces. The anatomic dead space is the internal volume of the conducting airways from the nose and mouth down to the respiratory bronchioles. It is usually estimated from the body height or weight. The ratio of anatomic dead space to tidal volume is not affected by height or weight, but rather by age as shown in Appendix B. The physiologic dead space is more closely related to the efficiency of ventilation, as it includes not only the volume in the conducting airways, but also the volume of gas ventilating the alveoli that do not contribute to gas exchange with blood. It is measured by Bohr's equation described in Appendix F. Dead-space ventilation is determined by multiplying physiologic dead space by the respiratory rate.

Alveolar Ventilation. Effective alveolar ventilation is part of the minute ventilation that participates in gas exchange; therefore, it is the difference between minute ventilation and dead-space ventilation. Alveolar ventilation can also be calculated from an equation derived from carbon dioxide elimination and arterial P_{CO_2} (see Appendix E).

Distribution of Ventilation: Closing Volume. Normally, alveolar ventilation in various lung regions is not uniform but shows a gradual vertical decrement from the base of the lungs to their apexes when the subject is in a standing or sitting position. In pathologic states there is a marked derangement of ventilation distribution. Maldistribution of ventilation is often suspected by physical examination or radiographic studies. For its more precise determination, however, certain laboratory tests are necessary. The ventilation lung scan (page 33) is one such method. Regional differences of distribution of ventilation can also be determined by single-breath nitrogen test, which is the basis for measurement of closing volume.

Pleural pressure at the lung bases is positive at the end of maximal expiration (residual volume), thus exceeding the airway pressure and leading to closure of distal airways. In normal young individuals, the small airways at the lung bases do not start to close until the volume of the lungs is reduced to less than FRC. The volume of the lungs at which the small airways begin to close is known as *closing volume.* This volume normally is between FRC and residual volume.

The small airway closure occurs at higher volumes with aging and various pathologic conditions. The closing volume is, therefore, increased in these situations, reaching and even surpassing the FRC. Determination of closing volume is a particularly sensitive test for identification of obstructive lung disease at its early stage, when the usual flow studies are not conclusive.

The principle of measurement of closing volume is based on variation of the concentration of a tracer gas continuously determined throughout a slow vital-capacity expiration. Nitrogen existing in the lungs after a vital-capacity inspiration of pure oxygen may be conveniently used for this purpose. This method is referred to as a *single-breath nitrogen test*. Throughout the slow expiration to the residual volume position, the concentration of nitrogen and volume of expired air are measured and recorded. The curve thus obtained will demonstrate changes in nitrogen concentrations at various lung volumes, showing four different phases (Fig. 2–11). Phase I represents gas from dead space only, which is filled with oxygen without nitrogen. Phase II shows a rapid rise in nitrogen concentration and represents a mixture of dead space and alveolar gas. Phase III is the alveolar plateau with slight fluctuations and a small positive slope. Phase IV demonstrates a sudden increase in the nitrogen concentration due to closure of airways in the dependent lung regions and contribution of alveoli relatively rich in nitrogen (upper lung zones). The beginning of phase IV, therefore, represents the closing volume.

An increase in closing volume, especially when it is larger than the FRC, indicates premature closure of intrapulmonary airways as a result of the narrowing of small airways or reduced elastic recoil. Closing volume is considered to be a sensitive indicator of small airway disease, which is believed to represent the early stage of pathologic changes in smokers. The slope of phase III provides information on distribution of ventilation; the more uneven the distribution, the steeper the slope.

Maximum Inspiratory and Expiratory Forces

Assessment of the strength of inspiratory and expiratory muscles in respiratory disorders is of paramount importance, particularly in conditions known to affect these muscles. In recent years, the realization that inspiratory muscle weakness and fatigue play a significant role in perpetuating respiratory failure from various causes has resulted in a renewed interest in this area. In evaluating the need for mechanical ventilatory support, in following patients on ventilators, and in serving as a guideline for proper weaning time

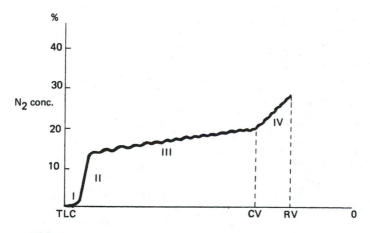

Figure 2–11. Measurement of closing volume (CV) by single-breath nitrogen test.

and method, the measurement of respiratory muscle strength has become a common practice.

The simplest method for determining respiratory muscle strength is the use of a special manometer capable of measuring both negative and positive pressures (Fig. 2–12). The inspiratory and expiratory forces are measured during static effort when no air is flowing. For determining the maximum inspiratory pressure (PI_{max}), the subject, after breathing out fully, holds the wide mouthpiece of the manometer tightly against the lips and makes a greatest possible inspiratory effort. The maximum expiratory pressure (PE_{max}) is obtained by exhaling forcibly, after a full inspiration. The values, usually in cm H_2O, are read directly. For more accurate results, the best of three consecutive PI_{max} and/or PE_{max} efforts is chosen and recorded.

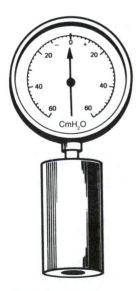

Figure 2–12. Manometer for measuring maximum inspiratory and expiratory pressures.

■ ARTERIAL BLOOD STUDIES

As was briefly mentioned earlier, the main function of the respiratory system is to maintain arterial blood oxygen and carbon dioxide within a physiologic range. It is also essential for regulation of acid-base balance. Measurement of the arterial blood oxygen, carbon dioxide, and pH, therefore, seems to be a most logical approach to evaluation of respiratory function. However, because of the large pulmonary reserve and effective adjustment of ventilation and perfusion within the lungs, normal blood gases do not exclude the presence of pulmonary disease. Their abnormality, however, unless due to extrapulmonary conditions such as right-to-left cardiac shunt or metabolic derangement, is a definite indication of impaired respiratory function. Arterial blood studies performed routinely consist of the measurement of partial pressure of oxygen (Po_2), partial pressure of carbon dioxide (Pco_2), and pH. The bicarbonate level and the oxygen content are usually calculated. From the Pao_2, $Paco_2$, and inspired O_2 concentration (FIO_2), the difference between the alveolar and arterial oxygen tensions (A-aO_2 gradient) can be calculated (Appendix D). Another clinically useful parameter for determination of severity of hypoxemia is Pao_2/FIO_2 ratio. Because of the importance of these studies in respiratory disorders, the basic concepts on the transport of oxygen and carbon dioxide in blood as well as acid-base balance is briefly discussed.

Oxygen Transport

When a liquid is in equilibrium with a gas, the partial pressure of that gas will be the same in the liquid as in the gas form, re-

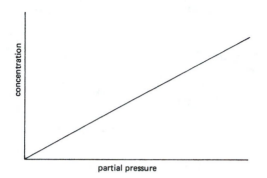

Figure 2–13. Relationship of concentration of a gas with its partial pressure in a simple solution.

gardless of its solubility or other factors. Water exposed to air, for example, will have the same *partial pressure* of oxygen and nitrogen as in the air, which is the product of barometric pressure and the fractional concentration of the respective gas. At sea level, the partial pressure of oxygen and nitrogen will be 760×0.2093 and 760×0.79, respectively. However, the *concentration* or the *amount* of gas in a liquid will be determined not only by its partial pressure, but also by its *solubility* in that liquid.

Concentration of a gas in simple solution has a linear relationship with its partial pressure at any particular temperature; that is, if partial pressure is doubled or tripled, the concentration will also double or triple (Fig. 2–13). In a liquid containing a gas in some other form in addition to simple solution, the relationship between the partial pressure of the gas and its concentration will not be linear. The presence of hemoglobin in blood makes it behave quite differently from other liquids in regard to the amount of certain gases that it can hold under various partial pressures. This is particularly applicable to oxygen, which is carried in the blood by both of the following mechanisms:

1. In simple solution, the amount of oxygen carried has a linear relationship with its partial pressure. Each 100 mL of blood carries about 0.003 mL of oxygen per mm Hg (torr) at body temperature in simple solution. At a partial pressure of 100 torr, the amount of oxygen in solution in 100 mL of blood at body temperature will be 0.3 mL.

2. Hemoglobin has the particular ability to carry oxygen as a chemical compound, oxyhemoglobin (HbO_2). Although the amount of oxygen carried this way is also dependent on its partial pressure, the relationship is not linear. This is due to the following two factors: (a) As in any chemical reaction, the amount of oxygen that can have chemical reaction with a finite amount of hemoglobin will be limited. (b) The affinity of hemoglobin for oxygen increases once it is partly combined with oxygen.

The particular characteristics of the chemical combination of oxygen with hemoglobin result in a special relationship between P_{O_2} and oxygen saturation of hemoglobin. This relationship is demonstrated by a curve referred to as the *oxygen–hemoglobin dissociation curve* (Fig. 2–14). It is evident from this curve that increasing the partial pressure of oxygen will have a different rate of increase in oxygen saturation depending on the area of the curve. The slope of the curve is small at the very beginning of the curve, then increases rapidly at the middle, and then progressively diminishes to an almost horizontal position toward the end.

The oxygen *content* of arterial blood is a function of the saturation of hemo-

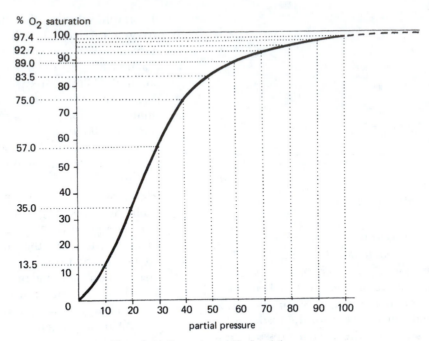

Figure 2–14. Oxygen–hemoglobin dissociation curve.

globin and the amount of hemoglobin. Each gram of hemoglobin, once fully saturated, contains 1.39 mL oxygen; therefore, 100 mL of blood with a hemoglobin content of 15 g will be able to combine and carry about 20 mL of oxygen when saturated. With an arterial partial pressure of 90 to 100 torr, the hemoglobin will be 96.5% to 97.5% saturated. The amount of oxygen carried in solution will be very small (0.3 mL) at this partial pressure.

The oxygen–hemoglobin dissociation curve has great importance in understanding various phenomena associated with oxygen transport and delivery. As can be seen from the upper part of the curve, reduction of partial pressure of arterial oxygen, as seen in many clinical situations, does not result in a proportional reduction of its oxygen content as happens with gases in simple solution. For ex-

ample, the reduction of arterial P_{O_2} from 100 torr to 60 torr will diminish its saturation from 97.5% to only 89% and, therefore, a significant amount of oxygen will still be available to the tissues. However, the steep portion of the curve will allow a larger amount of oxygen utilization without resulting in a dangerously low capillary blood P_{O_2}. Such a low P_{O_2} occurs in the capillary blood of the tissues with high oxygen extraction.

Under various physiologic and pathologic conditions, the oxygen–hemoglobin dissociation curve changes, shifting its position to the right or left. A right shift indicates a reduced hemoglobin affinity for oxygen; that is, the oxygen content of blood will be reduced with the same partial pressure. A left shift will result in an increased affinity and, therefore, a higher oxygen content with the same P_{O_2} (Fig. 2–15). A right shift facilitates release of

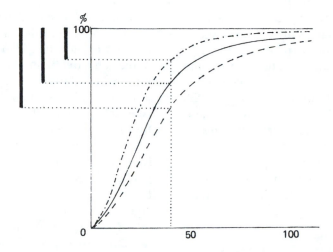

Figure 2–15. Right and left shift of oxygen–hemoglobin dissociation curve. Solid bars demonstrate the amounts of oxygen extracted from fully saturated arterial blood at the tissue sites: right shift facilitates release of oxygen (longest bar); left shift will have the opposite effect.

oxygen at the tissue site, and left shift will have the opposite effect.

Factors known to cause changes in the oxygen–hemoglobin dissociation curve include pH and temperature. Both high hydrogen ion concentration (low pH) and elevated temperature result in right shift of the curve; in contrast, alkalosis and low temperature shift it to the left. A special phosphorus compound present in red blood cells affects the oxygen affinity of hemoglobin. The substance is 2,3 diphosphoglycerate (2,3 DPG), which in high concentrations shifts the dissociation curve to the right and, therefore, facilitates oxygen delivery to tissues. Among the conditions known to increase red cell 2,3 DPG, prolonged hypoxemia as a result of residence at high altitudes or cardipulmonary disease and chronic anemia are well known. Storage of blood in a blood bank is a good example in which the red cell 2,3 DPG is reduced.

P_{50} refers to the partial pressure of oxygen at which the hemoglobin is 50%

saturated (Fig. 2–16). Normally, P_{50} is about 27 torr. It is evident that with the shift of the dissociation curve to the right, P_{50} will be increased, whereas it will be reduced with a shift of the curve to the left. Factors that result in the reduced affinity of hemoglobin for oxygen, such as acido-

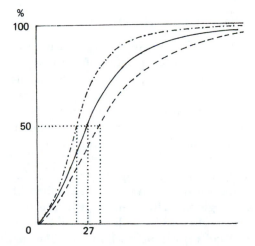

Figure 2–16. P_{50}. Right shift of oxygen–hemoglobin dissociation curve will increase the P_{50}; left shift will reduce the P_{50}.

sis, high temperature, or increased 2,3 DPG, cause a right shift of the oxygen–hemoglobin dissociation curve, and therefore the P_{50} will increase; factors resulting in increased oxygen affinity, such as alkalosis, low temperature, or reduced 2,3 DPG cause a left shift of the curve, and thus reduce the P_{50}. At the tissue sites, in addition to acidosis, which causes a right shift of the oxygen–hemoglobin dissociation curve, a high concentration of CO_2 also facilitates the unloading of oxygen **(Bohr effect).**

Carbon Dioxide Transport

Carbon dioxide, although a very soluble gas, is carried in blood mostly in chemical combination; only small amounts remain in simple solution. Once CO_2 diffuses to the capillary blood from its site of production, most of it moves inside the red blood cells, facilitated by O_2 unloading **(Haldane effect).** In plasma, very small amounts of carbon dioxide react with water to form carbonic acid, which then dissociates into bicarbonate and hydrogen ions:

$$CO_2 + H_2O \rightleftharpoons H_2CO_3 \rightleftharpoons HCO_3^- + H^+$$

Some of the dissolved CO_2 in plasma reacts with amino groups of plasma proteins, forming carbamino compounds. Hydrogen ions produced by these reactions are buffered by plasma buffering systems. Part of the carbon dioxide remains in simple solution in plasma.

In the red cells, a small amount of CO_2 remains in physical solution, and some forms carbamino compounds with hemoglobin. However, most of the CO_2 reacts chemically with water inside the red cells, forming carbonic acid, which immediately dissociates to HCO_3^- and H^+. The presence of an enzyme, carbonic

anhydrase, is essential for this reaction. Hydrogen ion is buffered by hemoglobin; this buffering effect is enhanced by loss of oxygen from hemoglobin. Bicarbonate ions, accumulated within red cells, create a concentration gradient between the red cells and plasma, which results in its diffusion into plasma.

The transfer of HCO_3^- (an anion) from the red cell to plasma is not accompanied by the transport of cation (positively charged ion). As a result, another anion, Cl^- (chloride), passes from plasma to red cells to maintain electrical neutrality. This process is known as the *chloride shift.*

At the pulmonary capillary, the reverse of the preceeding reactions takes place, and CO_2 is thus eliminated. As mentioned earlier, carbon dioxide loading and oxygen unloading in tissue capillaries are mutually helpful. Low O_2 improves CO_2 uptake, and high CO_2 facilitates unloading of oxygen. The reverse is true in pulmonary sites. At the pulmonary sites, addition of oxygen to capillary blood facilitates removal of carbon dioxide into the alveoli while lowering CO_2 tension in capillary blood enhances O_2 uptake from the alveoli.

Acid-Base Balance

Elimination of CO_2 by the lungs is of utmost importance in regulation of acid-base status of the body. The amount of hydrogen ion eliminated by the lungs far exceeds the amount excreted by the kidneys. Therefore, the respiratory system has a crucial role in acid-base balance.

An acid is defined as a molecular or ionic compound that is capable of donating a hydrogen ion (proton); a base is a substance capable of receiving a proton. Hydrogen chloride (HCl) is a strong acid because it is readily dissociated into H^+ and Cl^-, while H_2CO_3 is a weak acid (not as readily dissociated to its ionic components of HCO_3^- and H^+). HCO_3^- is a stronger base than Cl^- because the former readily takes up H^+ but the latter does not. When a weak acid is in solution in the presence of its salt, which is almost completely ionized, that solution will resist a change in pH when a strong acid or alkali is added. Such a mixture constitutes a buffer *pair* or *system*. From the law of mass action, the following equation of buffers is derived:

$$H^+ = K \, (\text{dissociation constant})$$
$$\times \frac{\text{acid}}{\text{salt (or base)}}$$

This equation was suggested by Henderson more than half a century ago.

Hydrogen ion in blood and some other body fluids has a very low concentration; in arterial blood it is about 40×10^{-9} Eq per liter. In dealing with extremely large or small numbers, use of a logarithm becomes very convenient. The negative logarithm of hydrogen ion concentration, termed as pH by Sorensen, is more commonly used to express this concentration. The normal arterial blood pH of 7.4 is the negative logarithm of 40×10^{-9}.

Hasselbalch converted the Henderson equation into the logarithmic terms, expressing H^+ in terms of pH as proposed by Sorensen. The equation was thus changed to

$$pH = pK + \log \left(\frac{\text{base}}{\text{acid}} \right)$$

which is known as the *Henderson-Hasselbalch* equation.

The CO_2–bicarbonate buffer pair, among other buffer systems in the blood,

is most convenient for studying the acid-base balance of the blood. With this buffer system, which has a pK of 6.1, the Henderson-Hasselbalch equation is written as follows:

$$pH = 6.1 + \log \frac{HCO_3^-}{(CO_2)}$$

In this equation, (CO_2) represents the total of physically dissolved CO_2 (99%) and hydrated CO_2 (1%). It is, therefore, directly dependent on the partial pressure of carbon dioxide (PCO_2). The equation may be rewritten as

$$pH = 6.1 + \frac{\log HCO_3^-}{\alpha (PCO_2)}$$

α is the solubility of carbon dioxide, which is 0.0301. From this equation, any of its three components can be calculated if the other two are known.

The equation demonstrates that it is the *ratio* of HCO_3^- to PCO_2 that determines the pH, rather than the absolute amount of each. The numerator is an indication of metabolic changes; the denominator is an indicator of ventilatory function. Normally, with a bicarbonate value of about 24 mEq per liter and (CO_2) of about 1.2, the ratio in arterial blood will be 20/1, or a pH of 7.4. Despite the continuous production of carbon dioxide and other metabolic end products, the respiratory system and the kidneys are normally able to keep the arterial PCO_2, bicarbonate, and pH within normal physiologic range. The protection of pH and its maintenance in a narrow range takes priority over the normalization of bicarbonate ion and PCO_2. Other protective mechanisms operative for this purpose include tissue and blood buffering activities and the exchange of ions between the plasma and the red cells. As long as the $HCO_3^-/\alpha(P_{CO_2})$ ratio remains at 20/1, regardless of absolute values of bicarbonate and P_{CO_2}, pH will stay normal. Only when this ratio is altered will the pH change. With a lower ratio, the pH will be reduced (acidemia), and with a higher ratio, it will be increased (alkalemia).

The arterial blood pH is considered normal when it is between 7.35 and 7.45. Thus, *acidemia* means an arterial blood pH of less than 7.35 and *alkalemia* signifies a pH higher than 7.45. **Acidosis** and **alkalosis,** by current convention, indicate the primary process that initiated an alteration in arterial blood pH. The term "respiratory" is used when the initial event is a change in carbon dioxide, and nonrespiratory or "metabolic" is applied when an acid-base disorder is initiated by an alteration in plasma bicarbonate. Each of these primary processes brings about *secondary* or *compensatory* changes in an attempt to minimize alterations in blood pH.

Primary metabolic operations result in a secondary ventilatory response that affects P_{CO_2}. Primary respiratory disturbances induce metabolic responses in two steps: an immediate effect through the buffering mechanism and the exchange of ions between the intracellular and extracellular fluid compartments, and a slow response (several hours to a few days) through the change in the renal excretion of H^+ and HCO_3^-. Therefore, there are six simple acid-base disorders (Fig. 2–17).

Secondary or compensatory responses in simple acid-base disturbances are to a certain limit predictable and are proportional to the magnitude of the primary changes. These relationships, which are the basis for designing various acid-base maps and nomograms, are shown in Appendix C.

Simple Acid-Base Disturbances

Metabolic Acid-Base Disorders. When the primary disturbance is in the concentration of bicarbonate, respiratory alteration reflected by a change in P_{CO_2}

SIMPLE ACID-BASE DISTURBANCE	pH	PRIMARY ABNORMALITY	SECONDARY CHANGE
Metabolic acidosis	↓	↓ HCO_3^-	↓↓ P_{CO_2}
Metabolic alkalosis	↑	↑ HCO_3^-	↑ P_{CO_2}
Respiratory acidosis, acute	↓	↑ P_{CO_2}	↑ HCO_3^-
Respiratory acidosis, chronic	↓	↑ P_{CO_2}	↑↑ HCO_3^-
Respiratory alkalosis, acute	↑	↓ P_{CO_2}	↓ HCO_3^-
Respiratory alkalosis, chronic	↑	↓ P_{CO_2}	↓↓ HCO_3^-

Figure 2–17. Six simple acid-base disorders. Primary abnormalities, changes in pH, and secondary responses are shown. Note that secondary changes are more marked (double arrows) with metabolic acidosis, chronic respiratory acidosis, and chronic respiratory alkalosis.

is the expected secondary response. In *metabolic acidosis* resulting from the increased production or the reduced excretion of H^+, the plasma HCO_3^- is lowered by its buffering function ($H^+ + HCO_3^- \rightarrow H_2O + CO_2$). Low plasma bicarbonate may also result from its excessive loss from the gastrointestinal tract or through the kidneys, or it may be due to its inadequate production by the kidneys. The respiratory response to simple metabolic acidosis is increased alveolar ventilation, which results in reduced arterial blood PCO_2. To a certain limit, patients with a normal respiratory system will be able to increase the alveolar ventilation to such a degree that for every mEq reduction in bicarbonate, PCO_2 will be lowered by about 1.2 torr. Significant deviation from this relationship indicates an additional primary acid-base disorder. The level of anion gap is commonly used for evaluation of metabolic acidosis. Anion gap is determined by subtracting the sum of concentration of serum bicarbonate and chloride from the serum sodium concentration. When the gap is more than the normal level of 12, the acidosis is known as anion-gap acidosis. The cause of widened gap is from an increase in unmeasured anions that may be organic as lactate in lactic acidosis or inorganic as phosphate or sulfate in renal failure. In nonanion gap acidosis, the reduced bicarbonate level is counterbalanced by increased chloride level. There are several causes of both anion gap and nonanion gap acidosis, which occur in various clinical settings.

Metabolic alkalosis usually results from the excessive loss of hydrogen ions through the gastrointestinal tract or the kidneys (increased production or reduced loss of bicarbonate by the kidneys). Sometimes it may be the result of the administration of alkali or the overcorrection of chronic respiratory acidosis by mechanical ventilation. The respiratory response to simple metabolic alkalosis is a reduction of alveolar ventilation (high PCO_2). The normal response is about 0.6 torr increase in PCO_2 for every mEq increase in plasma bicarbonate, up to a certain limit.

Respiratory Acid-Base Disorders. Simple respiratory *acidosis results* from increased arterial PCO_2, which in turn is due to inadequate alveolar ventilation. The causes of respiratory acidosis are discussed in Chapter 26. An acute increase in PCO_2 causes a more marked reduction in pH than if it develops chronically, as metabolic compensation for the former is meager. For each torr increment in PCO_2 acutely, the plasma bicarbonate level increases by about 0.1 mEq per liter. For example, an acute increase of PCO_2 to 70 torr from a normal level of 40 torr will result in 3 mEq increase in bicarbonate from the normal level of 24 to 27 mEq per liter. The pH will reduce to about 7.2. In chronic respiratory acidosis, renal compensation will be added, and the pH will be less acid. For every torr increase in PCO_2 in the chronic state, the plasma bicarbonate level will increase by about 0.35 mEq per liter. With the example of a PCO_2 of 70 torr in chronic respiratory acidosis, bicarbonate will increase to 34.5 mEq per liter with a pH of 7.31.

Respiratory alkalosis is due to increased alveolar ventilation. In the acute state, secondary (compensatory) change is small and averages about 0.2 mEq reduction in bicarbonate for every torr decrease in PCO_2. For example, acute hyperventilation resulting in an arterial PCO_2 of 20 will cause the plasma bicarbonate to reduce to 20 mEq, and the pH will be 7.62. In chronic respiratory alkalosis, there is additional renal compensation, which lowers the plasma bicarbonate further, with a reduction of about 0.5 mEq bicarbonate for each torr of decrease in P_{CO_2}. With a chronic hyperventilation to a P_{CO_2} level of 20 torr, the plasma bicarbonate will reach about 14 mEq with a pH of 7.46.

Mixed Acid-Base Disturbances

In practical settings, it is not unusual to encounter combinations of two, or occasionally more, simple acid-base disorders above and beyond compensatory changes. They are referred to as mixed acid-base disorders in which the arterial blood studies show changes of P_{CO_2} or HCO_3^- that are outside the range expected for the primary disturbance. Many times the mixed disturbance is strongly suspected from the clinical findings. Acid-base maps should be used in the context of clinical information for the interpretation of these disorders (Appendix C). Commonly encountered mixed acid-base disturbances are chronic respiratory acidosis with metabolic alkalosis, acute respiratory acidosis with chronic respiratory acidosis, acute respiratory acidosis with metabolic acidosis, and metabolic acidosis with chronic respiratory acidosis.

Measurement of Blood Gases

Arterial blood is most frequently used for blood gas and pH analysis. A blood sample is obtained by puncture of an accessible artery in the following order of preference: radial artery, brachial artery, and femoral artery. The blood is collected anaerobically (without air exposure) in a syringe, which has been prepared by rinsing its inside with a solution of heparin. Once the blood sample is obtained, it should be immediately cooled inside an ice-filled container and taken to the blood gas laboratory. Sometimes an indwelling cannula (arterial line) is used when frequent arterial blood sampling is necessary.

Occasionally, venous blood is studied for its gases and pH. A mixed venous blood sample obtained from a catheter in the pulmonary artery is used for determination of arteriovenous P_{O_2} difference, calculation of venoarterial shunt, and measurement of cardiac output.

Measurement of Blood Oxygen. Before the development of the oxygen electrode, oxygen content of blood was measured by cumbersome, time-consuming, and less accurate methods. At the present, partial pressure of oxygen is measured by the *Clark membrane electrode.* The introduction of such an electrode has markedly facilitated measurement of P_{O_2}, and most hospitals are equipped with it.

The Clark electrode (Fig. 2–18) consists of a very thin platinum wire sealed in glass except for its tip, which is covered with a membrane permeable to oxygen. Between the glass-platinum unit and membrane, there is a film of a weak electrolyte solution. A chloridated silver reference electrode (anode) is in contact with the solution. A potential of -0.7 volts (V) applied to the platinum results in the passage of a current that is directly proportional to the availability of O_2 *molecules* at the platinum surface. The availability of O_2 molecules is directly related to the P_{O_2} of solution (blood) to be tested, which is directly read from a calibrated galvanometer.

From the measured P_{O_2}, oxygen saturation and, if hemoglobin level is

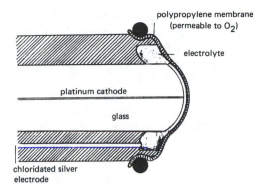

Figure 2–18. Clark electrode for measurement of blood oxygen tension.

known, oxygen content can be calculated.

Measurement of pH. The measurement of pH is done by a *glass electrode.* The principle of this method is based on the fact that hydrogen ions can pass through the silicate lattice of glass. If a bulb made of a thin glass containing hydrochloric acid is immersed in a solution containing H^+, a voltage develops between the hydrochloric acid in the bulb and the solution outside the bulb. This voltage is directly proportional to the logarithm of the ratio of the two hydrogen ion concentrations. The solution pH is thus read from a voltmeter.

Measurement of Carbon Dioxide. Among the methods available for determination of carbon dioxide, the direct measurement of P_{CO_2} by a special electrode is the most commonly used method, and is also the easiest and most accurate.

Known as the Severinghaus CO_2 electrode (Fig. 2–19), it consists of a glass pH electrode covered with a Teflon membrane. A thin layer of a solution of salt and sodium bicarbonate is held between the glass and teflon membrane by a "spacer" (cellophane or nylon stocking mesh). The Teflon membrane is permeable to CO_2, but not to H^+. A reference electrode in contact with the solution film permits measurement of the resulting pH, which is directly related to the P_{CO_2} of the sample to be studied. With proper calibration, P_{CO_2} is read directly.

Plasma bicarbonate is readily calculated from the Henderson-Hasselbalch equation, or read from a nomogram, once pH and P_{CO_2} are known.

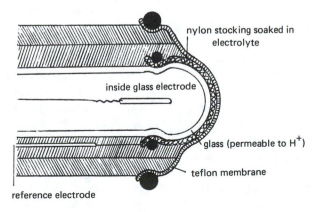

Figure 2–19. Severinghaus CO_2 electrode.

Other Methods of Monitoring Blood Gases

In addition to intermittent measurements of P_{O_2} and P_{CO_2} of arterial blood samples, recent technological development has enabled clinicians to monitor arterial blood gases continuously without subjecting patients to the discomfort and risk of arterial punctures. The knowledge that P_{O_2} and P_{CO_2} immediately over a well-perfused and properly heated skin surface (about 42°C) approach those of arterial blood has allowed the use of special transcutaneous electrodes that measure the oxygen and sometimes carbon dioxide tensions of "arterialized" capillary blood. Because of their closer approximation with arterial gas tensions in newborn infants, transcutaneous technique has gained popularity in neonatal intensive care units. As the accuracy of correlation of transcutaneous gas tensions with those of arterial blood depends on cardiac output and cutaneous blood flow, low readings in hemodynamically unstable patients should be interpreted with caution and should be confirmed by other methods. Because with increasing age the difference between transcutaneous and arterial blood gas tensions widens, this technique has not been very useful for noninvasive monitoring of adult patients.

Carbon dioxide tension at the end of each expired tidal volume, known as *end-tidal P_{CO_2}*, can be measured by spectrometry or infrared analyzer as an estimate of arterial P_{CO_2}, provided that there is no significant ventilation-perfusion mismatching. This method, known as capnography, has the advantage of monitoring the ventilatory status of patients on respirator on a continuous basis. Although end-tidal P_{CO_2} measurement un-derestimates the arterial P_{CO_2} when dead-space ventilation is increased, it may still be relied on for following the trend of changes in ventilation if the physiologic dead space remains constant.

Pulse Oximetry. Among the noninvasive innovations for monitoring changes of arterial blood oxygen, *transmission oximetry* is having a significant impact on the practice of pulmonary medicine in increasing numbers of clinical applications. Using the spectrophotometric principle, which differentiates light absorption by oxyhemoglobin and deoxygenated hemoglobin, percentage of O_2 saturation of capillary blood is transcutaneously determined. The nonpulse oximeter, introduced earlier, has been almost completely replaced by much more practical and smaller pulse oximeters. The probe of a pulse oximeter is made of two light-emitting elements that send two different wavelengths across a fingertip or an earlobe. A photodetector on the other side senses the transmitted light, which changes with the pulsating arterial blood. The oxygen saturation of the arterial blood is calculated automatically from changes in transmission with each pulse. It should be noted that the result of pulse oximetry overestimates O_2 saturation in patients exposed to carbon monoxide. As the absorption of light by other tissue factors and baseline blood is automatically canceled out, a pulse oximeter senses only the arterial blood flowing to the tissues with each pulse. Individual variability in skin color therefore has little effect on measurements. Because pulse oximetry is becoming almost a routine monitoring method and its wide clinical applications are involving many health professionals in its use, they should become familiar with its indications and limitations. Most pulse oximeters in clinical use show a reasonable accuracy with O_2 saturations between 70% and 100%. When O_2 saturation is less than 70%, its accuracy diminishes. Moreover, in patients receiving supplemental oxygen, as during general anesthesia, when PaO_2 levels are high, pulse oximetry cannot be relied on to show significant alteration in oxygen tension if changes in saturation are small. This is related to the shape of the oxygen–hemoglobin dissociation curve. Changes in arterial O_2 tensions at the horizontal portion of the curve cause only minimal changes in O_2 saturation (see page 48). Monitoring O_2 saturation by oximetry, even in these situations, is useful for warning the clinicians when the impairment of oxygenation becomes severe enough to result in O_2 desaturation. The clinical use of pulse oximetry continues to increase. Currently, it is routinely used in critical care units; during bronchoscopy, sleep studies, and exercise tests; and with general anesthesia.

Intravascular monitoring of oxygen saturation is feasible with the help of fiberoptic filaments and an oximeter using the principle of reflection spectrophotometry. This technology has helped in developing a special form of balloon-flotation catheter, which can be used for the continuous monitoring of mixed-venous blood saturation in the pulmonary artery.

■ HEMODYNAMIC MEASUREMENTS AND MONITORING

Although the study of pulmonary hemodynamics is part of a thorough evaluation of respiratory function, in practice it is limited to situations in which important therapeutic measures are based on the information derived from such a study. As the hemodynamic measurements necessitate cardiovascular catheterization, they are done in critical care units or in catheterization laboratories. Three basic variables studied are pressure, flow, and resistance. Pressures inside the central veins, right heart chambers, and pulmonary artery are determined by passing a special catheter connected to pressure-sensing and measuring device.

Central systemic venous pressure (CVP) is the most common parameter measured in clinical situations. It not only gives information on the adequacy or deficit of circulating volume, but also reflects the function of the right side of the heart. CVP is the filling pressure or preload of the right ventricle. It is always elevated in right ventricular heart failure. For measurements of pressures inside the right heart chambers and beyond, a specially designed catheter with a small balloon at its end (Swan-Ganz) is commonly used. This type of catheterization is usually done at the bedside with or without fluoroscopic guidance. The catheter, which has usually 3 or 4 lumens and a small thermistor near its tip, is inserted through a peripheral or central vein while connected to a pressure monitoring device. The balloon at the end of the catheter is inflated with air that is injected through the lumen connected to it. The catheter is advanced into the right atrium, right ventricle, and pulmonary artery, directed by the blood flow carrying the inflated balloon (Fig. 2–20). Pressure waveforms displayed on the oscilloscope indicate the position of the catheter tip, and the pressures are directly displayed or recorded. Once in the pulmonary artery, further advancement of the catheter re-

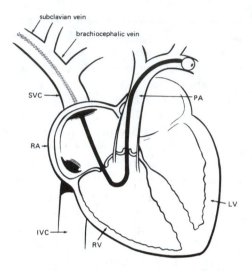

Figure 2–20. Balloon-tipped pulmonary artery catheter that has passed through the right subclavian vein, right brachiocephalic vein, superior vena cava (SVC), right atrium (RA), right ventricle (RV), pulmonary artery trunk (PA), and left pulmonary artery. It is wedged, with the balloon inflated, in a branch of the left pulmonary artery.

sults in "wedging" of the balloon tip when the pressure waveform similar to one of the right atrium is formed (Fig. 2–21). The pressure recorded at this point is the pulmonary artery occlusion or wedge pressure, also known as pulmonary-capillary pressure, which is a reflection of left atrial pressure (left ventricular filling pressure). With deflation of the balloon, pulmonary artery pulsations reappear. For continuous monitoring, the catheter is left in this position with the balloon deflated. Blood sampled from the distal opening of the catheter in the pulmonary artery is the mixed venous blood that is used for measuring arteriovenous oxygen content difference and cardiac output. The proximal lumen opening located 30 cm from the tip of the catheter is usually located at the right atrium. It is used for measurement of right atrial pressure (central venous pressure) and also for infusion of fluids.

Although cardiac output can be calculated from arterial and mixed venous oxygen contents and oxygen consumption (Fick's method), it can more easily be measured by the thermodilution variant of the Swan-Ganz catheter. Using the proximal lumen, a bolus of cold glucose solution is injected rapidly. The thermistor, near the tip of the catheter, senses the temperature change and transfers it via a

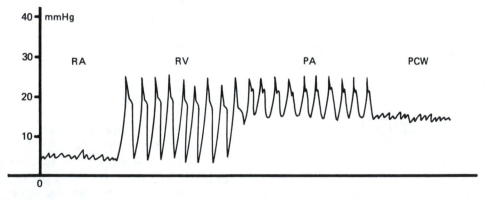

Figure 2–21. Pressure recordings from a balloon-tipped pulmonary artery catheter as it passes through the right atrium (RA), right ventricle (RV), and pulmonary artery (PA) to pulmonary capillary wedge (PCW) position.

thin wire embedded in the catheter to a special cardiac output computer. By integrating the time-temperature curve, the computer displays the cardiac output.

As vascular resistance is the pressure change across a vascular bed divided by the flow:

Resistance = driving pressure/blood flow

pulmonary vascular resistance can be calculated from the pressure difference between two areas of the pulmonary vascular bed (driving pressure) and cardiac output. Total pulmonary vascular resistance equals the difference between the mean pulmonary artery and wedge pressures divided by cardiac output. Normal hemodynamic values are shown in Appendix G.

■ SLEEP STUDY

In recent years, with better recognition and definition of sleep-related alteration of respiration, especially sleep apnea, evaluation of ventilatory events during sleep has become a common practice. Such a study not only identifies the presence of sleep apnea and other breathing disorders, but also determines their mechanism, magnitude, and pathophysiologic effects. Proper therapeutic decisions are based on the analysis of the information thus obtained.

As the sleep study comprises several simultaneously recorded events on a polygraphic paper, it is also referred to as **polysomnography.** It usually includes continuous recordings of the following during a night's sleep:

1. Brain waves (electroencephalogram) and eye movements (electrooculogram) for the purpose of determining the stages of sleep.
2. Airflow for detection of apneic episodes, which may be monitored by a thermistor, CO_2 analyzer, pneumotachograph, or tracheal sound recorder.
3. Motion of the abdomen and the rib cage for determination of their mechanical activities and their paradoxical movements.
4. Pulse oximetry for displaying the changes in O_2 saturation and its correlation with ventilatory alterations.
5. Electrocardiogram for monitoring the heart rate and rhythm.

Proper analysis and interpretation of these recordings, above all, will allow the diagnosis (or exclusion) of sleep apnea, frequency and duration of apneic episodes, and determination of their cause as well as their effect on the arterial blood oxygenation. Sleep apnea syndrome is discussed in Chapter 25.

■ BRONCHIAL PROVOCATION TEST

This test measures the bronchial responsiveness to certain agents. It is based on the knowledge that individuals with asthma demonstrate a distinct feature of bronchial reactivity characterized by an exaggerated sensitivity of the airways to the bronchoconstrictive effect of a variety of physical, chemical, and biological agents. Most of these stimuli are nonspecific and affect all asthmatics, while specific response to known allergens can be demonstrated only in asthmatics allergic to them. For demonstration of nonspecific bronchial hyperreactivity, inhalational challenge tests can be performed by a number of techniques, including cold air, hyperventilation, osmotic challenge, and inhalation of a cholinergic agent. The most commonly used method is inhalation challenge with the cholinergic agent *methacholine*. After determining the baseline FEV_1 and establishing the control value by inhalation of the diluent, gradually increasing concentrations of methacholine are administered by inhalation. Trial with each concentration consists of inhalation of five breaths from FRC position followed by measurement of FEV_1 within 1 to 2 minutes. Once a 20% reduction of FEV_1 is achieved, the test is terminated; otherwise it is continued until the inhalation of the last concentration. An inhaled bronchodilator should be given whenever there is an excessive bronchoconstrictive response. The lowest concentration of methacholine that results in a FEV_1 reduction of 20% is known as PC_{20} (provocative concentration to reduce flow rates by 20%). The lower the PC_{20}, the higher the airway responsiveness is to the agent. The bronchial provocation test is most useful in situations in which the history, physical findings, and simpler pulmonary function tests for bronchial asthma are atypical and equivocal, or when the diagnosis of a chronic cough is in question.

■ EXERCISE TEST

Although the information obtained by history, physical examination, and routine pulmonary function and other laboratory tests is often adequate for detecting the presence of cardiorespiratory impairment and for estimating the degree of disability from it, in some clinical situations a more objective and quantita-tive functional assessment will be necessary. This is usually accomplished with the help of exercise testing, by which cardiovascular and respiratory responses to varying external workloads are assessed. As increased muscle contractions during exercise stress both ventilatory and cardiovascular systems, their response determines whether they can meet the additional workload of respiration and circulation. Dependent on the clinical and physiologic information inquired, exercise testing varies from simple and noninvasive to complex and invasive types.

Simple tests such as climbing stairs (number of stairs climbed without difficulty) or walk test (the distance walked in 6–12 minutes) may give significant information about exercise tolerance. For a more formal testing, either a treadmill or cycle ergometer is used for exercise testing. The latter allows for easy determination of power (watts) used and assessment of its effect on other variables. A noninvasive test consists of observing the subject perform increasing levels of standardized exercise loads, while measuring pulse rate, respiratory rate, and blood pressure; assessing the subject's appearance; looking for signs of distress; and noting subjective complaints of dyspnea and muscle fatigue. This simple study usually provides an adequate guide to the maximum level of exercise that the subject is able to perform and maintain. Additional useful information can be obtained by pulse oximetry, electrocardiography, and measurement of minute ventilation. If not measured directly, oxygen uptake ($\dot{V}O_2$) with various workload on a cycle ergometer can be estimated by the formula based on mechanical power output and the subject's body weight (see Appendix B).

In more complex and sophisticated exercise testing, which necessitates invasive procedures, several other metabolic, cardiovascular, and respiratory parameters are also measured. They include monitoring of arterial and venous blood gases, measurement of diffusing capacity, actual oxygen uptake and carbon dioxide elimination, determination of maximum oxygen consumption ($\dot{V}O_2$ max) and anaerobic threshold, and measurement of cardiac output and pulmonary artery pressures.

The major practical and most common indication of exercise testing in pulmonary medicine is for demonstration and quantification of hypoxemia during exercise in two common clinical situations: (1) in patients with restrictive lung disease with a normal or near normal arterial PO_2 and alveolar-arterial oxygen gradient, and (2) in patients with chronic obstructive lung disease who appear to have disabling symptoms with only a mild to moderate resting hypoxemia. The result of exercise testing would help to determine a need for oxygen therapy with exertion. Other indications for cardiopulmonary exercise tests include determination of disability, evaluation for unexplained dyspnea, estimation of operative risk in major thoracic and pulmonary resectional surgery, and determination of suitability for lung transplantation.

BIBLIOGRAPHY

Acres JC, Kryger MH. Clinical significance of pulmonary function tests: Upper airway obstruction. *Chest.* 1981; 80:207–211.

American Thoracic Society. Clinical role of bronchoalveolar lavage in adults with pulmonary disease. *Am Rev Respir Dis.* 1990; 142:481–486.

American Thoracic Society. Indications and standards for cardiopulmonary sleep studies. *Am Rev Respir Dis.* 1989; 139:559–568.

American Thoracic Society. Lung function testing: selection of reference values and interpretative strategies. *Am Rev Respir Dis.* 1991; 144:1202–1218.

American Thoracic Society. Standardization of spirometry. *Am J Respir Crit Care Med.* 1995; 152:1107–1136.

Braman SS, Corrao WM. Bronchoprovocation testing. *Clin Chest Med.* 1989; 10:165–176.

Briscoe WA. Lung volumes. In: Fenn WO, Rahn H, eds. *Handbook of Physiology, II.* Washington, DC, American Physiological Society; 1965; 1345–1379.

Buist AS. Tests of small airways function. *Respir Care.* 1989; 34:446–452.

Celli BR. Clinical and physologic evaluation of respiratory muscle function. *Clin Chest Med.* 1989; 10:199–214.

Clark JS, Votteri B, Ariagno RL, et al. Noninvasive assessment of blood gases. *Am Rev Respir Dis.* 1992; 145:220–232.

Clausen JL. Clinical interpretation of pulmonary function tests. *Respir Care.* 1989; 34:638–645.

Crapo RO. Pulmonary function testing. *N Engl J Med.* 1994; 331:25–30.

Crapo RO, Foster RE II. Carbon monoxide diffusing capacity. *Clin Chest Med.* 1989; 10:187–198.

Dellinger RR. Fiberoptic bronchoscopy in adult airway management. *Crit Care Med.* 1990; 18:882–887.

Felson B. *Chest Roentgenology.* Philadelphia: Saunders; 1973.

Fulkerson WJ. Fiberoptic bronchoscopy. *N Engl J Med.* 1984; 311:511–515.

Funsten AW, Suratt PM. Evaluation of respiratory disorders during sleep. *Clin Chest Med.* 1989; 10:265–276.

Gardner RM, Crapo RO, Nelson SB. Spirometry and flow-volume curves. *Clin Chest Med.* 1989; 10:145–164.

Gilbert HC, Vender JS. Arterial blood gas monitoring. *Crit Care Clin.* 1995; 11: 233–248.

Goldberg M, Green SB, Moss ML, et al. Computer-based instruction and diagnosis of acid-base disorders. *JAMA.* 1973; 223: 269–275.

Hansen JE. Arterial blood gases. *Clin Chest Med.* 1989; 10:227–237.

Kacmarek RM, Cycyk-Chapman MC, Young-Palazzo PJ, Romagnoli DM. Determination of maximal inspiratory pressure. *Respir Care.* 1989; 34:868–878.

Kramer EL, Divgi CR. Pulmonary applications of nuclear medicine. *Clin Chest Med.* 1991; 12:55–75.

Laski ME, Kurtzman NA. Acid-base disorders in medicine. *Dis Mon.* 1996; 42:61–125.

Leitman BS, Naiclich DP. Computerized tomography of the chest: indications and basic interpretation. *Hosp Med.* 1990 (August); 114–128; (September); 75–88.

Marini JJ. Lung mechanics determinations at the bedside: instrumentation and clinical application. *Respir Care.* 1990; 35:669–693.

McKelvie RS, Jones NL. Cardiopulmonary exercise testing. *Clin Chest Med.* 1989; 10:277–291.

Ries AL. Measurement of lung volumes. *Clin Chest Med.* 1989; 10:177–186.

Schnapp LM, Cohen NH. Pulse oximetry: uses and abuses. *Chest.* 1990; 98:1244–1250.

Swan HJC. The pulmonary artery catheter. *Dis Mon.* 1991; 37:478–543.

Thomas HM, Lefrak SS, Irwin RS, et al. The oxyhemoglobin dissociation curve in health and disease. *Am J Med.* 1974; 57:331–348.

Tobin MJ. Respiratory monitoring. *JAMA.* 1990; 264:244–251.

Weinreb JC, Naidich DP. Thoracic magnetic resonance imaging. *Clin Chest Med.* 1991; 12:33–54.

Weisman IM, Zeballos RJ, eds. Clinical exercise testing. *Clin Chest Med.* 1994; 15(2): 173–445.

Zerhouni E. Computed tomography of the pulmonary parenchyma: an overview. *Chest.* 1989; 95:901–907.

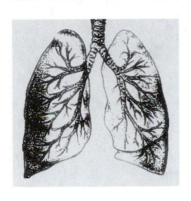

INFECTIOUS DISEASES
OF THE LUNG

3.

Acute Lower Respiratory Tract Infections

The lower respiratory tract begins at the main carina and comprises the bronchi, bronchioles, alveolar ducts, alveolar sacs, and alveoli. With rare exceptions, bacteria, mycoplasmas, and viruses are the causes of acute infections of the lower respiratory tract in immunocompetent persons. In immunocompromised hosts, however, opportunistic organisms may also be involved. Mycobacteria and fungi usually result in chronic infection. In most instances, the infective agents enter the lower respiratory tract through the airways by inhalation or aspiration. Occasionally, the infection occurs via the bloodstream. Although the inhalation of airborne organisms and the aspiration of contaminated upper airway secretions occur even in healthy individuals, the airways distal to the larynx are normally sterile. Several defense mechanisms prevent the contamination of the lower respiratory tract in the normal host. The filtration action of upper airways, reflexes resulting in the timely closure of laryngeal entry by the epiglottis and the glottis by the vocal cords, coughing, and the mucociliary escalator constitute the primary line of defense. After that, the offending organisms encounter various antibodies present in the mucus and available from the blood, the scavenging alveolar macrophages, and the white blood cells. When the defense mechanisms of the respiratory tract and immune system are weakened or inoperative, or when, because of the number and aggressiveness of the organisms the normal defenses are overwhelmed, infection will result.

Depending on the region of the lower respiratory tract predominantly involved with inflammation, the terms bronchitis, bronchiolitis, and pneumonia are applied.

■ ACUTE BRONCHITIS

Acute infectious bronchitis is an acute inflammation of the bronchial mucous membrane resulting from infectious agents. Because of frequent involvement of the trachea, the term acute tracheobronchitis may be more appropriate. Bronchitis due to noninfectious causes, such as physical or chemical irritants or allergy, is discussed in Chapters 8, 9, and 15.

Etiology. The most common infectious causes of acute bronchitis are viruses. These viruses are also causative agents of the upper respiratory infections that usually precede acute bronchitis. They include influenza viruses, parainfluenza viruses, adenoviruses, rhinoviruses, and a variety of other viruses. *Mycoplasma pneumoniae* is also a common cause of acute bronchitis. The role of bacterial infection in acute bronchitis, however, is more difficult to define. Primary acute bacterial bronchitis is very uncommon. Whether secondary bacterial infection plays a significant part in previously healthy individuals with viral bronchitis is not clear. Frequent isolation of organisms such as pneumococci, streptococci, and *Haemophilus influenzae* from the sputum does not necessarily indicate that they are acting as pathogenic agents in acute bronchitis. These bacteria are usually cleared without specific therapy. However, in patients with underlying chronic obstructive pulmonary disease (COPD), such as emphysema, chronic bronchitis, and bronchiectasis, the role of bacterial infection of the bronchi is more important. Similarly, in elderly and debilitated individuals and patients with cardiac failure or certain other chronic disorders, bacterial superinfection may have more significance.

Acute bronchitis is seen in all age groups. Its incidence is higher during cold seasons.

Clinical Manifestations. Acute tracheobronchitis is usually preceded by signs of upper respiratory tract infection, such as stuffy and runny nose and sore throat. Cough is always present and varies in severity. It is initially dry and very annoying. Cough is more troublesome at night. Exposure to cold, deep breathing, talking, and even laughing may precipitate coughing bouts. The patient may complain of a retrosternal, uncomfortable, scratchy feeling. In a few days, when bronchial secretions are established, cough becomes productive of mucus or mucopurulent sputum. Dyspnea is usually not present, except when there is underlying chronic cardiopulmonary disease. Inflammation of bronchial mucosa is known to result in hyperreactivity of the airways and thus may result in bronchospasm. It is a common precipitating cause of bronchospasm in patients with bronchial asthma.

The physical examination may show evidence of inflammation of the upper respiratory tract. The examination of the chest may be entirely normal. Sometimes scattered wheezing may be heard. A few rales may also be present at the time of increased bronchial secretions. Fever, if present, is usually mild, except in young children, who may have high temperatures.

A chest x-ray, which is normal in uncomplicated acute bronchitis, will be necessary to rule out pneumonia in questionable cases.

Management. The treatment of acute bronchitis is generally symptomatic. Bed rest may be advisable in more severe cases to avoid cold and dry air. The patient's room should be well humidified. Sometimes steam inhalation is beneficial. The role of cough syrups and expectorants is not clearly established in the treatment of acute bronchitis. In cases where the cough is very distressing and interferes with rest and sleep, certain preparations containing codeine or dextromethorphan may be prescribed. Antibiotics are not usually indicated in management of uncomplicated acute bronchitis. They do, however, have an important role in treating acute bronchitis superimposed on chronic obstructive lung disease as discussed in Chapter 7.

Prognosis. Acute bronchitis without accompanying chronic illness is a self-limited disease and has a good prognosis. In a few patients it may progress to pneumonia or bronchopneumonia. The role of recurrent acute bronchitis in the pathogenesis of COPD has not been unequivocally established. However, it is known to play a significant part in exacerbation and progression of COPD.

■ ACUTE INFECTIOUS BRONCHIOLITIS

Acute infectious bronchiolitis (inflammation of the bronchioles) is a serious respiratory infection that is almost exclusively seen in young children, particularly in the first 2 years of life. Inflammation involves the bronchioles, resulting in their obstruction. Although occasionally bacteria may be the cause, it is most commonly a viral infection. Respiratory syncytial virus (RSV) is the most important offending organism in causing bronchiolitis in children. RSV respiratory infection may be hospital acquired. Other microorganisms such as parainfluenza virus and *Mycoplasma pneumoniae* may also cause bronchiolitis in infants and young children.

As in acute bronchitis, upper respiratory tract infections frequently precede the onset of bronchiolitis. The onset of disease is heralded by cough and varying degrees of dyspnea. At its early stage, respiratory symptoms are suggestive of an asthma attack. Systemic manifestations of progressive fever and prostration indicate an infectious process.

On *physical examination,* the child appears apprehensive and irritable; respiration is rapid and shallow, often accompanied by expiratory grunt. The child uses his or her accessory respiratory muscles. In more severe cases, there is marked cyanosis, as well as some pallor. The chest is hyperresonant to percussion; scattered wheezes are heard in both lung fields. When the airway obstruction is more severe, breath sounds are barely audible. Untreated, the child may succumb to respiratory or cardiac failure.

The chest x-ray shows marked hyperradiolucency with or without parenchymal infiltration. Arterial blood shows significant hypoxemia. Acute bronchiolitis is sometimes very difficult to differentiate from bronchial asthma.

Management. The treatment of acute bronchiolitis is mainly supportive. The child should be placed in an atmosphere high in humidity and oxygen (children's tent) with precautions of respiratory isolation. Adequate fluid by parenteral route should be administered. Bronchodilators may be beneficial; they should be given whenever there is significant bronchospasm or if asthma cannot be excluded. The antiviral drug ribavirin in aerosolized form is effective in the treatment of respiratory syncytial viral disease. It is given for 12–18 hours daily and delivered to an infant oxygen hood by a special small-particle aerosol generator (SPAG). Duration of treatment is between 3 and 7 days. Severely ill patients, not responding to the above regimen, may require mechanical ventilatory support. Antibiotics are frequently administered, despite the fact that bronchiolitis is most often a viral infection and, therefore, not responsive to these therapeutic agents.

■ PNEUMONIA

Pneumonia is defined as an acute inflammation of the gas-exchanging units of the lungs, which include respiratory bronchioles, alveolar ducts, alveolar sacs, and alveoli. Although it may also result from noninfectious causes, the term *pneumonia* usually applies to acute infection unless otherwise specified. Pneumonia is the most common cause of death from infection in the United States. Despite availability of effective antimicrobial agents, mortality from pneumonia continues to increase especially in the elderly.

Etiology. The direct causes of infectious pneumonia are various microorganisms; however, the host factors are most important in its pathogenesis. Pneumonia occasionally occurs in apparently healthy people, but in the majority of cases it is associated with conditions in which there is significant impairment of the lung defense mechanisms as depicted in Table 3–1. Contamination of distal airways and

TABLE 3–1. CAUSES OF IMPAIRED PULMONARY DEFENSES

Altered protective effects of epiglottis and glottis
Suppressed or ineffective cough
Impaired consciousness
Obstructing airway lesions
Abnormal mucus
Defective cellular immunity
Impaired humoral immunity
Recent viral infection

alveoli by potentially pathogenic organisms is a prerequisite for the development of pneumonia. Prior colonization of the upper airway usually precedes infection of the lower respiratory tract. A break in the defense mechanisms that normally prevent such a contamination is the major cause. Altered protective reflexes of the epiglottis and the glottis, a suppressed or ineffective cough mechanism, impaired mucociliary transport, and obstructed airways are important contributory factors. Impairment of blood supply, abnormal number or function of phagocytic cells and other cells involved in cellular immunity, lack of proper antibodies, and alteration of other elements of the immunologic system deprive the lungs of their second line of defense. In conditions known to predispose to pneumonia, one or often several of these physical and biological defenses are defective. These conditions include chronic lung disease, alcoholism, seizure disorder and other causes of altered consciousness, malnutrition, neuromuscular diseases, chronic debilitating illnesses, immunologic disorders, malignant conditions and their treatment, major surgical operations, and old age.

Pathogenesis and Pathology. Pathogenic organisms reaching the distal airways and alveoli incite an intense tissue reaction resulting in the outpouring of inflammatory exudates and cells. Interstitial tissue and alveolar spaces are variably involved in the inflammatory process and infiltrated or filled with exudative fluid and migrating cells. White blood cells, particularly neutrophilic granulocytes, and indigenous cells actively phagocytize the organisms and release their enzymes and immunologic mediators, which in turn cause further inflammation and recruitment of more inflammatory cells. Depending on the number and the virulence of the organisms and the body's ability to ward off their onslaught, further progression of the infection may be halted, or it may continue to involve adjacent lung tissue through the airways and/or interalveolar openings. Once a significant portion of the lung is filled with inflammatory cells and exudate, it becomes consolidated. Bacteria capable of causing significant destruction or loss of lung tissue result in necrotizing pneumonia. Adjacent pleura may also be involved with inflammation resulting in pleural effusion, which may be invaded by the organisms. The microorganisms may enter the bloodstream resulting in septicemia (bacteremic pneumonia). *Bronchopneumonia* is a term used to indicate simultaneous involvement of the airways and the lung parenchyma with infection. Inflammation due to viruses and mycoplasmas is predominantly in the interstitial tissue.

Once the infection is brought under control, either spontaneously or by antimicrobial therapy, the resolution of inflammation and healing take place. In situations in which there is no significant tissue necrosis, the resolution without sequelae is expected to be complete, and the normal lung function will be restored; whereas when there are significant destructive changes, healing proceeds slowly by deposition of fibrous scar tissue, and there will be measurable loss of lung function.

Pathophysiologic changes with pneumonia are the result of reduced functioning lung volume and alteration of ventilation and blood flow. Mismatching of ventilation with perfusion and intrapulmonary shunting are the causes of arterial hypoxemia commonly seen in pneumonia.

Clinical Manifestations. The onset of pneumonia, which may be abrupt or gradual, is usually heralded by systemic manifestations of infection, such as general malaise, chills, and fever, as well as local symptoms of cough, chest pain, and dyspnea. Upper respiratory symptoms often precede the onset of pneumonia. Expectoration varies depending on the causative organisms, stage of disease, and other factors. It may be scant or totally absent at the beginning but increases with the progression of the disease; at which time it is usually purulent but may also be bloody or rusty in color. Extrapulmonary features, such as mental confusion or disorientation, sometimes overshadow the respiratory symptoms, particularly in the elderly and the alcoholic. In patients with involvement of multiple lobes, either at the presentation or with the progression of disease, dyspnea and cyanosis predominate.

On physical examination, the patient with pneumonia usually appears quite ill. The common findings are fever, tachycardia, rapid breathing, and abnormalities on the examination of the chest. The latter are variable and may include poor respiratory excursion, dullness to percussion, reduced breath sounds, and inspiratory crackles. Bronchial breath sounds and tactile fremitus, if present, are indicative of a significant area of consolidation. In some patients, particularly with viral or mycoplasmal pneumonia, the physical examination of the chest may be normal despite significant radiographic abnormalities.

Common abnormal laboratory findings are low arterial blood Po_2 and Pco_2 and frequent elevation of the white blood cell count. Blood cultures may be positive for the offending organism.

Radiographic Findings. The radiographic examination of the chest is usually the clue for the diagnosis of pneumonia. A normal chest x-ray study with at least two properly taken posteroanterior (PA) and lateral projections usually excludes the diagnosis of pneumonia. Radiographic patterns reflect the pathologic changes of the lungs. A homogeneous density involving a large area and showing an air bronchogram is indicative of consolidation (Fig. 3–1). Patches of density along the airways with segmental distribution signify bronchopneumonia. A diffuse reticular density indicates thickening of the interstitial tissue, which is seen in interstitial pneumonia resulting from viral or mycoplasmal infection. In necrotizing pneumonia, radiolucent areas inside the airspace densities are usually seen (Fig. 3–2). Pleural effusion may

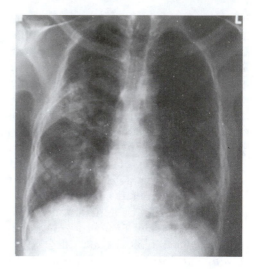

Figure 3–2. Chest radiograph of a patient with bilateral necrotizing pneumonia.

be detected by standard radiographic examination or other imaging techniques such as lateral decubitus film, ultrasound, or CT scan. If it occurs at the time of development of pneumonia, it is known as parapneumonic effusion.

■ DIAGNOSIS AND CLASSIFICATION OF PNEUMONIAS

A diagnosis of pneumonia is often established with consistent radiographic findings in a proper clinical setting of history and physical examination. The difficulty in clinical practice is the accurate identification of the bacteriologic cause of a pneumonia. Although sputum examination seems to be the most important study for this purpose, it is often fraught with problems arising from improper sampling and interpretation of its results. Moreover, the identification of organisms

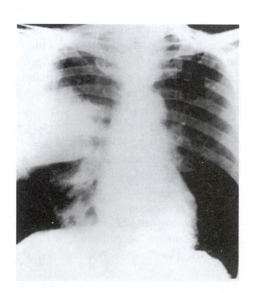

Figure 3–1. Consolidation of the right upper lobe due to pneumococcal pneumonia.

essential for early therapeutic decision making may be delayed and, in almost 50% of cases, the causative pathogen cannot be identified. For these reasons, host factors and other circumstances under which pneumonia develops are usually considered in deciding which microorganisms are likely to be involved so that proper initial antimicrobial therapy can be selected. This concept is the basis for classifying pneumonias for practical purposes into three broad categories of community-acquired pneumonia; hospital-acquired (nosocomial) pneumonia, including ventilator-associated pneumonia (VAP); and pneumonia in an immunocompromised host.

Community-Acquired Pneumonias

Community-acquired pneumonias are, by definition, contracted outside the hospital environment. Each year in the United States 4.5 million cases of community-acquired pneumonia are diagnosed, of which 1 million are hospitalized. In bacterial pneumonia, the organism most commonly involved is *Streptococcus pneumoniae* (pneumococcus), which characteristically results in *lobar pneumonia*. The onset of pneumococcal pneumonia is acute and often ushered in by a severe shaking chill followed by a high fever. Signs of consolidation on the physical examination and the chest x-ray film are more commonly observed in pneumococcal pneumonia. The sputum is often purulent and may be rusty in color. On a smear with gram stain, characteristic gram-positive diplococci are often seen inside or along with numerous polymorphonuclear leukocytes. Sputum culture may be positive for *S pneumoniae*, but a negative culture does not exclude the diagnosis. As these or-

ganisms may enter the bloodstream, blood cultures are positive in about a quarter of the cases.

Other bacteria cause pneumonia less commonly but are important to be considered in various clinical situations. Frequently, the identification of these conditions and other predisposing factors may help to consider the most likely bacteria involved. *Haemophilus influenzae,* a gram-negative bacterium, is a fairly common cause of pneumonia in patients with COPD. Pneumonia from *Moraxella catarrhalis* (a gram-negative diplococcus) is also more commonly seen in patients with COPD. *Klebsiella pneumoniae* should be suspected in alcoholics. Although staphylococcus causes pneumonia in otherwise healthy adults, it is not an uncommon cause of pulmonary infection in infants and, during influenza epidemics and in association with intravenous drug abuse, in adults. *Escherichia coli* pneumonia may occur in alcoholics and diabetics. Pseudomonas and staphylococcus are common causes of respiratory infection in cystic fibrosis. Anaerobic organisms as a cause of bacterial pneumonia should be seriously considered in a setting of aspiration resulting from alcohol intoxication, seizure disorders, and other causes of altered consciousness. Lung abscess, discussed later in this chapter, is often a consequence of aspiration-induced lower respiratory infection.

The onset of pneumonias caused by gram-negative bacteria, anaerobic organisms, and staphylococci are less abrupt and the clinical picture is less distinct because of frequent association with other debilitating medical conditions. Radiographic findings suggesting a necrotizing process and the presence of a significant amount of pleural reaction are strongly suggestive of pneumonia from these organisms. Sputum examination, as in hospital-acquired pneumonias, is important for diagnosis. Unfortunately, a specific diagnosis based solely on sputum examination cannot be made because of the likelihood of its contamination by oral or pharyngeal flora, especially with anaerobic bacteria. However, the demonstration of large numbers of morphologically distinct bacteria on a properly obtained sputum sample or their predominant growth on culture is highly suggestive of their role in pulmonary infection. Bacteriologic studies from other sources and by various methods discussed earlier (page 25) may be needed. If pleural effusion is present, its removal by thoracentesis is indicated. Blood cultures, if positive, will be very helpful.

Conventionally, pneumonia from above pyogenic bacteria in immunocompetent patients is characterized as "typical" to differentiate them from "atypical pneumonias," caused by organisms discussed as follows. This classification is somewhat artificial and not very helpful in diagnostic or therapeutic decision making as the distinction between typical and atypical pneumonias is often made retrospectively.

Pneumonia resulting from *Legionella* organisms, especially *Legionella pneumophila,* develops mostly from inhalation of aerosolized droplets containing these organisms. These small gram-negative bacilli are ubiquitous with an affinity for warm water. Drinking contaminated water has also been implicated in its transmission. The outbreaks of this disease occur mostly during late summer and early fall. Legionnaires' disease starts as an acute pneumonia with high fever and a nonproductive cough, which may rapidly progress, causing hypoxemia and respiratory failure. Extrapulmonary manifestations may suggest the diagnosis. Headache, muscle ache,

general malaise, mental confusion, prostration, diarrhea and other gastrointestinal symptoms, and abnormal liver function are commonly present. Radiographic changes have no characteristic features, but they are known to progress rapidly. Once this disease is suspected, the examination of materials such as sputum; bronchial washings or brushings, especially BAL; and pleural fluid will help the diagnosis. Direct immunofluorescent antibody (DFA) staining of these materials is more rapid and considered to be specific, whereas culturing in special media, as well as serologic tests, require more time and are useful for retrospective confirmation. Legionella antigen may also be detected in urine.

The most common cause of community-acquired pneumonia in young adults, especially in military recruits, is *M pneumoniae.* It should be noted that an increasing number of older people also are being affected. The organism is smaller than bacteria, but larger than viruses, and is only identifiable by its cultural characteristics. *Mycoplasma pneumoniae* is commonly associated with mild respiratory infection in children. The infection occurs in several family members and, as small epidemics, among military recruits. Mycoplasma pneumonia is usually preceded by an upper respiratory infection, and its manifestations are cough (often nonproductive), headache, and fever. Persistent cough after mycoplasma infection is common. The examination of the chest usually is normal, or findings are few and less striking than expected from radiographic changes. In an occasional patient, a characteristic bullous lesion on the eardrum may be seen. X-ray findings vary widely in their character and distribution. An interstitial, ill-defined pattern suggestive of viral pneumonia is most common. At times the findings may mimic bacterial pneumonia. The diagnosis is often suspected on clinical grounds and further supported by excluding bacterial infection. The presence of a serum antibody that agglutinates the red cells at a low temperature is the basis for cold agglutination test, which may become positive in many patients; however, it is not specific for this disease. More specific tests of complement fixation or culture of the organisms from the sputum will confirm the diagnosis in retrospect. *Chlamydia pneumoniae* is being recognized as a cause of "atypical pneumonia." It often starts with pharyngitis and hoarseness about a week prior to onset of pneumonia.

Viral pneumonias are uncommon in the civilian population with normal immunologic states. A variety of viruses can sporadically cause pneumonia among the general population; however, influenza, chickenpox, and adenovirus infection are better known for their association with pneumonia.

Influenza, generally a self-limited disease, usually affects the cell lining of the respiratory tract, causing local and systemic symptoms of flu. Occasionally a minimal and transient infiltration may be noted in the chest roentgenogram coinciding with flu symptoms. A more severe form of pneumonia that typically presents several days after the onset of influenza is characterized by increasing dyspnea, anxiety, and cyanosis. These symptoms usually begin when flu symptoms seem to be improving. Cough that is often nonproductive may be associated with hemoptysis. Severe influenza virus pneumonia is more commonly seen in patients with heart disease, chronic lung disease, old age, and general debility. It may be complicated by bacterial superinfection.

Chickenpox (varicella), although generally a mild disease in children, may be complicated by primary viral pneumonia in adults. It may be quite severe and life threatening. The diagnosis is often established by a chest roentgenogram associated with the characteristic skin rash of chickenpox, which is always present.

Adenovirus is probably the most common cause of viral pneumonia outside of influenza epidemics. It may be seen sporadically, but often in small epidemic form especially among military recruits. This virus is the most common etiologic agent of acute respiratory disease (ARD), a syndrome characterized by fever, sore throat, cough, hoarseness, and conjunctivitis. Adenovirus pneumonia is usually mild and is always associated with upper respiratory symptoms.

Viral pneumonias like mycoplasma pneumonia have the clinical features of scant physical findings on the examination of the chest despite obvious abnormality on radiographic study. The latter usually shows patchy interstitial density, which in severe form is diffuse and may involve the entire lung fields. In advanced cases with respiratory failure, diffuse airspace densities resembling pulmonary edema may be present. Viral pneumonia is one of the causes of the acute respiratory distress syndrome (ARDS) discussed in Chapter 27.

Hospital-Acquired Pneumonias

Hospital-acquired or nosocomial pneumonia by definition is contracted after a minimum of 3 days of hospitalization. It is a major cause of morbidity and mortality in hospitalized patients. Unlike community-acquired respiratory tract infections, nosocomial pneumonias are frequently due to gram-negative bacteria and staphylococci. Advancement in medical technology; progress in the care of critically ill patients; prolongation of survival of seriously ill and "terminal cases";

extended hospitalization; subjection to a variety of diagnostic and therapeutic instrumentations; and increasing use of antimicrobials, cytotoxic drugs, and immunosuppressants are some of the causes of predisposition to pneumonia from these organisms. In contradistinction to the healthy population who rarely harbor aerobic gram-negative bacteria in their upper airways, hospitalized patients, particularly when chronically and seriously ill and/or confined to critical care units, are readily colonized with these organisms. A combination of presence of these pathogenic bacteria and defective pulmonary or systemic defense mechanisms—so common in these patients—markedly increases the risk of developing hospital-acquired pneumonia (Fig. 3–3). Poor state of consciousness, aspiration of upper airway secretions, presence of an artificial airway and nasogastric tube, and laxity in the use of sterile technique for airway suctioning are important precipitating events. Elderly hospitalized patients are particularly prone to nosocomial respiratory tract infection.

Although any pathogenic organism may cause pneumonia in hospitalized patients, the most common agents are enteric gram-negative organisms (*Klebsiella, E coli,*

Enterobactor, Proteus, and *Serratia*), *H influenzae, Pseudomonas, Acinetobacter,* staphylococci, and *S pneumoniae.* Although anaerobic bacteria also may be involved in hospital-acquired pneumonia resulting from aspiration, one or several of the above organisms is more often the cause of lower respiratory infection in this setting. Prior antibiotic therapy increases the likelihood of developing infection with antibiotic resistant organisms such as *Pseudomonas, Acinetobacter,* and methicillin-resistant *Staphylococcus aureus* (MRSA). Infection with these organisms should always be suspected in pneumonia that develops after extended hospitalization, in patients on mechanical ventilation for a prolonged period of time, and following or during the extended use of antimicrobials. Patients who are from nursing homes are likely to be colonized by MRSA, making them susceptible to respiratory infection by this organism.

Clinical manifestations of pneumonia developing while the patient is in the hospital are often less clear and overshadowed by the underlying illness. Nevertheless, it is usually suspected with the occurrence of or increase in fever and the onset of or a change in respiratory symptoms, and confirmed by chest roentgenography. Its bacteriologic diagnosis, however, remains a difficult clinical challenge. In the elderly, hospital-acquired pneumonia develops more insidiously with atypical symptoms, such as change in mental status and failure to thrive. They may have no fever, cough, or expectoration. In such patients, high index of suspicion and radiographic studies will be necessary for diagnosis.

Bacteriologic diagnosis of nosocomial pneumonia from the result of examination of expectorated sputum may be very difficult, because of the frequent colonization of upper respiratory tract with

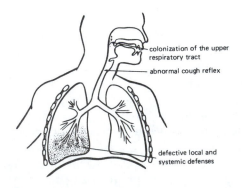

Figure 3–3. Pathogenesis of gram-negative pneumonia.

various pathogenic organisms. As in community-acquired pneumonia, sputum gram stain will be more useful than its culture. Blood culture and, if present, pleural fluid culture should be obtained. Sometimes, more invasive diagnostic studies such as bronchoscopy, bronchoalveolar lavage (BAL), percutaneous lung aspiration biopsy, and, rarely, open-lung biopsy may be necessary, especially when empiric therapy is unsuccessful.

Postoperative pneumonia is discussed in Chapter 19. Ventilator-associated pneumonia (VAP) as a complication of mechanical ventilation is discussed in Chapter 28.

Pneumonia in Immunocompromised Host

Although many patients who develop pneumonia have some unknown defect in their immunologic defense, this section addresses pneumonia in patients with known immunologic disorders. As the body's immune system is essential in defending it against ever-present infecting agents, it should not be surprising that infection by a variety of organisms is so prevalent in individuals with immunologic deficiency. Either or both limbs of immunity, known as humoral and cellular, may be deficient (see Chapter 14). Lymphocytes mediate both humoral and cellular immunities through their B-cell and T-cell lines, respectively. The activities of T and B lymphocytes in host defense against infection also involve other cells important in fighting infection. Antibodies produced by the B lymphocytes enhance the phagocytic activities of polymorphonuclear leukocytes, and the products of T lymphocytes activate macrophages, which in turn are important in trapping and processing the antigens.

Although both types of immunodeficiency predispose to infection, certain characteristics differentiate the two. Patients with a defect in humoral immunity lack antibodies and are more susceptible to infection with certain bacteria that are usually extracellular and encapsulated, such as pneumococci, *H influenzae,* and *Klebsiella;* while the individuals with cellular immunodeficiency have recurrent infection with low-virulence or opportunistic organisms, such as fungi, mycobacteria, certain viruses, and *Pneumocystis carinii.*

Immune deficiency may be primary or secondary to a variety of causes. Primary immunodeficiency states are usually congenital, and their manifestations occur early in childhood. There are increasing numbers of patients with secondary immune deficiency as a result of advances in the fields of cancer chemotherapy and organ transplantation. Many malignant diseases such as multiple myeloma and chronic lymphocytic leukemia result in impaired antibody production, whereas others such as Hodgkin's disease cause cellular immune deficiency. Treatment with cytotoxic drugs or immunosuppressants may depress both humoral and cellular immunity. The production of granulocytic white blood cells is also known to be suppressed by cancer chemotherapy. Chronic debilitating diseases, especially renal failure, and long-term treatment with corticosteroids impair cell-mediated responses. Because of the importance and unique features of *acquired immunodeficiency syndrome* (AIDS), its pulmonary complications, including pneumonia, are discussed separately in this text (see Chapter 6).

Pulmonary infection in the immunocompromised host may result not only from common pathogens but also from unusual and so-called opportunistic organisms. This is the major difference between pneumonia in these patients and that of persons with a normal immunologic state. The unusual microorganisms involved in infection among these patients include, but are not limited to, nocardia, aspergillus, cryptococcus, atypical mycobacteria, legionella, pneumocystis, and cytomegalovirus. Pneumonias from these organisms and common bacteria in immunocompromised patients have no distinguishing clinical or radiographic features; and, therefore, specific diagnosis will depend on demonstration or isolation of the causative agent. As these patients, by nature of their underlying immune deficiency, are unable to ward off their infection, it may be rapidly progressive and fatal. Therefore, an accurate diagnosis in a most expeditious way is essential for instituting early effective treatment. Most patients with common bacterial pneumonia have productive sputum, which should help in bacteriologic diagnosis. However, many patients, particularly when unusual organisms are involved, have no significant expectoration, or their sputum examination is inconclusive. In this situation, invasive methods will be necessary to obtain material for bacteriologic studies. Blood culture and bacteriologic examination of pleural fluid, if present, should always be done. Bronchoscopy with brushing and transbronchial biopsy, bronchoalveolar lavage, transthoracic needle aspiration of the lung, and open lung biopsy are the procedures that may have to be resorted to for specific diagnosis. Because of its high yield, some prefer open lung biopsy as the procedure of choice. However, the information obtained from simpler methods may suffice in most instances, especially when the organisms can be readily demonstrated with a special staining method as in infection with *pneumocystis*.

■ MANAGEMENT OF PATIENTS WITH PNEUMONIA

In view of the many causes of pneumonia, significant variations in its presentation, and widely different respiratory consequences, only a brief discussion of the principles and the objectives of management applicable to pneumonias in general is presented here. Although treatment of the patient with pneumonia should be individualized, the basic therapeutic principles of eradication of infection and supportive, as well as symptomatic, measures are appropriate in every case.

Patients with mild or moderate disease who are not immunocompromised and do not have serious underlying medical conditions are treated as outpatients with proper follow-up. Considering the fact that pneumonias in such patients are often from infection with organisms sensitive to macrolide antibiotics, erythromycin is considered the drug of choice. When *H influenzae* is suspected, as in patients with COPD, clarithromycin or azithromycin is preferred. With more severe pneumonia and when they are immunocompromised, or there is evidence of significant comorbid conditions, the patients are hospitalized. Adequate hydration, proper nutrition, supplemental oxygen, analgesics, and encouragement of effective coughing are the measures that help in alleviating symptoms and enhancing recovery. There is no therapeutic benefit of intermittent positive pressure (IPPB) treatment, and the indication for postural drainage is limited to situations in which there is a significant collection of secretions difficult to be expectorated by cough alone. In poorly responsive patients, tracheal suctioning may be necessary. In patients who have severe respiratory difficulty and intractable hypoxemia, tracheal intubation and mechanical ventilation will be required.

In choosing the proper antibiotic for hospitalized community-acquired pneumonia, it should be kept in mind that: 1) in most instances definitive bacteriologic diagnosis is impossible; 2) antibiotics should be initiated in a timely fashion; and 3) in selection of antibiotic regimen, the likely pathogenic organisms to be considered. For these reasons, initial antibiotic therapy is empiric with rather a broad-spectrum effect pending the result of diagnostic testing. In most instances, the same regimen will be continued because of adequate therapeutic response, without identification of a specific pathogen. Most clinicians follow the guidelines recommended by ATS and start patients on a third-generation cephalosporin plus a macrolide antibiotic, most often erythromycin. There are other antibiotic regimens that may be equally effective for treatment of community-acquired pneumonia in hospitalized patients. If the causative organism is identified, antimicrobial coverage is properly revised to include only the antibiotic with narrower spectrum of activity against the specific organism. Penicillin is adequate for pneumococcal infection in most instances. Cephalosporins are also generally effective. If there is a history of penicillin allergy, erythromycin is a good alternative to penicillin. This drug, as well as newer macrolides, are effective against pneumococci, *Legionella*, *Mycoplasma*, and *Chlamydia*. For anaerobic pneumonia, clindamycin is preferred, although certain other antibiotics are also effective. Staphylococcal pneumonia is best treated with a penicillinase-resistant penicillin such as nafcillin or oxacillin except when the organism is methicillin resistant (MRSA). Vancomycin is the antibiotic of choice against pneumonia resulting from MRSA. *Haemophilus influenzae* pneumonia responds well to ampicillin, cephalosporins, and trimethoprim-sulfamethoxazole (TMP-SMX). Other gram-negative pneumonias are treated with a third-generation cephalosporin with or without an aminoglycoside. Most community-acquired viral pneumonias have no specific therapy, except varicella pneumonia, which is treated with acylovir, and RSV pneumonia in children, which responds to inhaled ribavirin.

In nosocomial pneumonia, the initial antibiotic regimen should be according to severity of illness, the duration of hospitalization prior to onset of pneumonia, and prevalence of nosocomial pathogen and antibiotic resistance pattern in a given hospital. A second- or third-generation cephalosporin or ampicillin-sulbactam (Unasyn) is often chosen for mild-to-moderate illness without significant risk factors for occurrence of drug-resistant infections. When pneumonia is severe, or occurs after prolonged hospitalization with prior antibiotic therapy, an antibacterial regimen effective against the organisms likely to be resistant to common antibiotics should be selected. These organisms include pseudomonas, acinetobacter, and MRSA. As in community-acquired pneumonia, the therapeutic regime will be revised if diagnostic test results necessitate it.

Because pneumonia in immunocompromised hosts is often from unusual organisms, empiric therapy will be less useful. Therefore, every effort should be made for a specific diagnosis in order to choose an effective treatment.

Preventive Measures. Despite the availability of very effective antimicrobials for the treatment of respiratory tract infections, pneumonia remains one of the most common causes of hospitalization and death. Therefore, every attempt should be made to prevent its occurrence. Unfortunately, the factors that play major roles in the etiology of pneumonia are host factors that are difficult to alter. An increasing population of elderly, chronically ill, and immunocompromised people is an example that demonstrates the complexity of the problem. However, good public and personal health habits, including proper nutrition and the avoidance or cessation of smoking and excessive alcohol consumption would reduce the incidence of pneumonia, as well as many chronic illnesses that predispose to it. In dealing with hospitalized patients, particularly in critical care units, the role of hospital infection control cannot be overstressed. Proper care of respiratory therapy equipment, handwashing after patient contact, prevention of aspiration by proper positioning, more judicious use of antimicrobials, and maintenance of gastric acidity are some of the important preventive measures against hospital-acquired pneumonia.

Influenza vaccine is an effective measure against developing pneumonia as a complication of influenza. A vaccine made of pneumococcal capsular antigen is intended to enhance antibody production against 23 capsular serotypes of pneumococci known to cause significant illness in humans. Pneumococcal vaccination is recommended to be given once for individuals with sickle cell anemia; persons whose spleen has been removed; elderly persons; and patients with chronic lung, heart, or kidney disease. Although patients with altered humoral responses are at a higher risk for developing serious pneumococcal infection, they are unable to mount an adequate antibody response to the vaccine and thus may not benefit from it.

■ LUNG ABSCESS

Pulmonary abscess is a localized area of suppurative lesion associated with necrosis of lung tissue. Although small areas of necrosis and microscopic evidence of abscess formation may be present in many pulmonary infections, only those in which abscess is the predominant pathologic process are considered here. Because of its ready communication with an airway, lung abscess will usually present as an air-containing cavitary lesion.

Etiology and Pathogenesis. Almost any pyogenic organism may cause lung abscess; however, the most common causes of community-acquired lung abscess are anaerobic bacteria. They commonly include peptostreptococci, peptococci, fusobacteria, and bacteroides. Staphylococci, streptococci, and most aerobic gram-negative organisms are also fairly common etiologic agents. Aspiration is a frequent preceding event, and most patients present with a history of impaired consciousness or swallowing problems. Bronchial obstruction due to bronchogenic carcinoma, foreign body, or other causes is an important local predisposing factor. In cigarette smokers older than 50 years of age, the underlying predisposing factor for lung abscess may be bronchogenic carcinoma. Occasionally, abscess formation in the lung may be the result of septic embolism from a remote infected site, especially in IV drug users. Other rare causes include penetrating chest wound and suppurative lesion below the diaphragm with extension into the lung.

An area of pneumonitis always precedes the formation of an abscess. The time interval between known aspiration and abscess formation averages about 2 weeks. In production of a lung abscess, usually more than one type of organism is involved that often includes anaerobic bacteria.

Clinical Manifestations. The onset may be acute or insidious. The common presenting symptoms of lung abscess include cough, expectoration, fever, chest pain, hemoptysis, and weight loss. The mode of presentation and duration of symptoms prior to hospitalization will determine acuteness or chronicity of illness.

An initially dry or minimally productive cough is soon followed by sudden increase in the amount of expectoration of purulent and often foul-smelling sputum. This coincides with communication of the abscess with the bronchial tree. Fever, which may decrease at this time, continues at a variable level. Hemoptysis, although uncommon, may be sometimes massive and life threatening. Weight loss is common in patients with chronic lung abscess.

In acute lung abscess, there is high temperature, tachycardia, and tachypnea; dullness and impaired breath sounds may be detected over the diseased area; and a few rales may also be heard. Patients with protracted lung abscess appear chroni-

cally ill, fever is variable and may even be absent, and digital clubbing is common.

Radiographic Findings. Prior to cavity formation, the chest x-ray shows a localized area of consolidation. Only after communication with a bronchus and evacuation of part of its purulent contents will the lung abscess manifest its characteristic radiographic picture, which is an area of radiolucency surrounded by variable parenchymal density and containing an air-fluid level (Fig. 3–4). The most common sites for lung abscess are the superior segments of lower lobes and the posterior segments of upper lobes. Abscess in basilar segments is less common; other segments are rarely involved. This predilection is due to the effect of gravity and the direction of the bronchi at the time of aspiration, which commonly takes place in the supine position. The right lung is involved more often than the left.

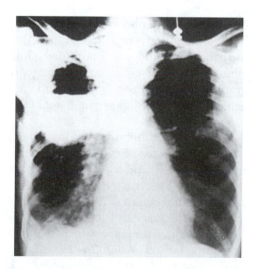

Figure 3–4. Radiographic demonstration of a large lung abscess involving the right upper lobe.

Laboratory Findings. Leukocytosis and mild to moderate anemia are frequently present. Sputum examination shows numerous pus cells and necrotic materials. Both gram-positive and gram-negative organisms are seen, which may or may not be representative of bacterial population of the abscess. Because of the significance of anaerobic bacteria in lung abscess and contamination of sputum by the normal anaerobic oral flora, material for bacteriologic study should be obtained by methods bypassing the oropharynx. Transtracheal aspiration is one such method. If pleural fluid is present, it should be tapped for bacteriologic study and for the exclusion of empyema.

Management. Ever since the advent of antibiotics and their proper use, treatment of lung abscess has been primarily medical. Surgical intervention has been very infrequently necessary. Although penicillin is often effective in lung abscess, because of resistance to this antibiotic alone in some cases, either clindamycin or penicillin with metronidazole is recommended empiric therapy. Antimicrobials should be continued until clinical improvement and roentgenographic clearing or stabilization are achieved. This may take from 3 weeks to a few months.

Adjunctive therapy should include adequate nutrition, treatment of underlying conditions, and *effective drainage* of the abscess. The latter is essential in successful management of pulmonary abscess, and is usually accomplished by proper *postural drainage* with or without other maneuvers. When abscess is large, this procedure should be performed with great caution as the patient may be unable to expectorate the volume of pus

that may drain. Postural drainage should be done several times a day, at least initially. As proper positioning is crucial for effective drainage, exact location of the abscess in relation to the bronchopulmonary segments should be ascertained by radiographic studies.

Bronchoscopy is sometimes indicated for diagnostic and therapeutic purposes, mostly in older smokers in whom lung cancer may be the underlying cause of the abscess. Surgical procedures for drainage or resection are resorted to when the patient does not respond to appropriate medical therapy. In very ill and weak patients, tracheostomy may be needed for adequate tracheobronchial toilet or for mechanical ventilatory support. Complicating pleural empyema should be drained.

Course and Prognosis. With proper management, lung abscess will show clinical and radiographic improvement in a majority of cases. In acute abscess, the size of the cavity diminishes rapidly and closes in a short period of time. However, in the chronic form, and when there are complicating underlying conditions, response to therapy will be slow or insignificant. Prolonged antibiotic therapy will be necessary to reduce the risk of relapse. Massive hemoptysis with lung abscess has a poor prognosis.

BIBLIOGRAPHY

American Thoracic Society. Guidelines for the initial management of adults with community-acquired pneumonia: diagnosis, assessment of severity, and initial antimicrobial therapy. *Am Rev Resp Dis.* 1993; 148:1418–1426.

American Thoracic Society. Hospital-acquired

pneumonia in adults: diagnosis, assessment of severity, initial antimicrobial therapy, and preventive strategies. *Am J Respir Crit Care Med.* 1996; 153:1711–1725.

Bartlett JG. Anaerobic bacterial infections of the lung. *Chest.* 1987; 91:901–909.

Campbell GD. Overview of community-acquired pneumonia: prognosis and clinical features. *Med Clin North Am.* 1994; 78:1035–1048.

Chastre J, Trouillet JL, Fagon JY. Diagnosis of pulmonary infections in mechanically ventilated patients. *Semin Respir Inf.* 1996; 11:65–76.

Fang GD, Fine M, Orloff J, et al. New and emerging etiologies for community-acquired pneumonia with implications for therapy. *Medicine.* 1990; 69:307–316.

Fein AM. Treatment of community-acquired pneumonia. *Semin Respir Crit Care Med.* 1996; 17:237–242.

Fine MJ, Smith MA, Carson CA, et al. Prognosis and outcomes of patients with community-acquired pneumonia. *JAMA.* 1996; 275:134–141.

Finland M. Pneumonia and pneumococcal infection, with special reference to pneumococcal pneumonia. *Am Rev Respir Dis.* 1979; 120:481–502.

Hammond JM, Potgieter PD, Hanslo D, et al. The etiology and antimicrobial susceptibility pattern of microorganisms in acute community-acquired lung abscess. *Chest.* 1995; 108:937–941.

Luby JP. Pneumonia caused by *Mycoplasma pneumoniae* infection. *Clin Chest Med.* 1991; 12:237–244.

Mandell LA. Community-acquired pneumonia: etiology, epidemiology, and treatment. *Chest.* 1995; 108(suppl):35S–42S.

Marie TJ. Atypical pneumonia revisited. *Semin Respir Crit Care Med.* 1996; 17:221–229.

McIntosh K. Respiratory syncytial virus infection in infants and children: diagnosis and treatment. *Pediatr Rev.* 1987; 9:191–196.

Muder RR, Yu VL, Fang GD. Community-acquired Legionnaires' disease. *Semin Respir Infect.* 1989; 4:32–39.

Murray HW, Tuazon CU. Atypical pneumonias. *Med Clin North Am.* 1980; 64:507–527.

Niederman MS. An approach to empiric therapy of nosocomial pneumonia. *Med Clin North Am.* 1994; 78:1123–1141.

Nguyen MLT, Yu VL. Legionella infection. *Clin Chest Med.* 1991; 12:257–268.

Ortiz CR, La Force FM. Prevention of community-acquired pneumonia. *Med Clin North Am.* 1994; 78:1173–1183.

Panitch HB, Callahn CW, Schidlow DV. Bronchiolitis in children. *Clin Chest Med.* 1993; 14:715–731.

Reynolds HY. Pulmonary host defenses. State of the art. *Chest.* 1989; 95(suppl): 223S–230S.

Ruben FL, Nguyen MLT. Viral pneumonitis. *Clin Chest Med.* 1991; 12:223–235.

Skerrett SJ. Host defenses against respiratory infection. *Med Clin North Am.* 1994; 78:941–966.

Stover, DE, Zaman MB, Hadju SI, et al. Bronchoalveolar lavage in the diagnosis of diffuse pulmonary infiltrates in the immunosuppressed host. *Ann Intern Med.* 1984; 101:1–7.

Thompson R. Prevention of nosocomial pneumonia. *Med Clin North Am.* 1994; 78: 1185–1198.

Wiedemann HP, Rice TW. Lung abscess and empyema. *Semin Thorac Cardiovasc Surg.* 1995; 7:119–128.

4.

Pulmonary Tuberculosis

Mycobacteria are rod shaped bacteria (bacilli) with a characteristic staining property related to their unusual cell wall, which has a high lipid and wax content. Once stained, they resist decolorization by a mixture of ethanol and hydrochloric acid, and are therefore called *acid-fast bacilli*. These organisms require special culture media for their growth. They have a slow replication time of about 24 hours (replication time of streptococci is about 20 minutes). Of the several groups of mycobacteria, mammalian tubercle bacilli, *Mycobacterium tuberculosis* and *Mycobacterium bovis,* are the agents of tuberculosis in humans and cattle. In addition, certain other mycobacteria may cause pulmonary infection in humans. They are known as *atypical mycobacteria.*

Tuberculosis (TB) is one of the oldest diseases known to afflict the human race and still remains one of the most widespread maladies in the world. Worldwide, nearly 3 million deaths occur yearly as a result of tuberculosis. Many organs may be affected; however, the most common site of tuberculosis is the lung, which is also the major port of entry and primary source of dissemination of tubercle bacilli. Tuberculosis is usually a chronic infection with variable manifestations, depending on the stage and duration of the disease, host response, organs involved, and many other known and unknown factors.

Epidemiology and Transmission of Tuberculosis. Although tuberculosis is still an important worldwide health problem, there is significant variation in its incidence and prevalence in different parts of the world. Among the factors responsible for its high prevalence in certain countries, poverty, overpopulation, inadequate nutrition, and lack of proper health care are most noticeable. Improved living conditions, social awareness, early diagnosis, and appropriate treatment have been important reasons for steady decline of tuberculosis in most developed countries. In the United States, this trend was halted in 1985. Since then, the incidence of tuberculosis began to rise until recent years. Factors responsible for the increase include human immunodeficiency virus

(HIV) epidemics; a rise in the number of immigrants and refugees, IV drug users, homeless persons, and persons who are incarcerated; and the emergence of multidrug-resistant (MDR) strains of *M tuberculosis.* The increase in tuberculosis cases has occurred mainly in large metropolitan centers with high populations of minorities and foreign-born inhabitants, where most of the cases of HIV infection and MDR tuberculosis have also been reported. Among persons infected with HIV, IV drug users are especially prone to develop tuberculosis (both drug sensitive and MDR).

In many nations, in addition to high incidence of tuberculosis due to human mycobacteria, bovine bacilli play an important role in human infection, usually acquired through ingestion of contaminated milk from tuberculous cattle. In more developed countries, this source of infection is almost totally eradicated, and humans remain the only source of new infections.

The transmission of tuberculosis occurs by way of infected materials, particularly sputum from a patient with untreated pulmonary tuberculosis. It is spread in the form of aerosolized droplets that are produced during coughing, sneezing, talking, or singing. Rapid evaporation of the aerosolized droplets from the respiratory secretions results in smaller residual particles known as droplet nuclei, which are small enough to remain suspended in air for a long period of time and breathed in by exposed persons. Droplet nuclei with sizes of 1–5μ in diameter will reach and settle in the alveoli, where the tuberculosis infection occurs. Individuals with undiagnosed and, therefore, untreated tuberculosis are particularly dangerous in disseminating the organisms and infecting the people around them. Once the patient with tuberculosis is on proper antituberculosis drugs, the infectiveness diminishes

rapidly and ceases within a few weeks. There is no evidence that tuberculosis can be transmitted from contaminated surfaces, either by contact or by breathing dust emanating from such surfaces.

Pathogenesis and Pathology. After reaching the distal airways beyond the protective mucous blanket, aerosolized tubercle bacilli in the droplet nuclei are met by the resident (alveolar) macrophages. These cells ingest the bacilli and, in most instances, kill them, thus preventing the development of infection. However, because of increased host susceptibility and heavier exposure, the tubercle bacilli may remain alive and begin to multiply freely. When this occurs, infection develops and the body tries to limit its progression to disease. This occurs with the help of macrophages and their interaction with lymphocytes through various cytokines. Involvement of these cells and cytokines is the basis of cell-mediated immunity. This protective mechanism occurs within 2 to 10 weeks following infection, which coincides with development of positive tuberculin reaction. In the infected area, a characteristic arrangement of lymphocytes and transformed macrophages (epithelioid cells and giant cells) results in formation of granuloma, which may show necrosis at its center. These lesions usually occur in a lower lobe or the anterior segment of an upper lobe. The draining regional lymph nodes, usually hilar, also become infected and enlarged. The infection is often confined to these areas and walled off by fibrosis. This stage of tuberculosis is known as *primary infection,* and the combination of the initial lung lesion and lymph node involvement is recognized as the *Ghon complex.* In a majority of individuals, the primary tuberculosis completely heals, leaving only a small scar, which may calcify later. Occasionally, primary infection progresses and causes a significant pulmonary or pleural disease.

During the early stage of primary infection, some of the tubercle bacilli escape and are carried by the bloodstream to different organs, where they settle. The areas that have high tissue oxygen tensions are particularly predisposed to secondary involvement by tubercle bacilli. These areas include the apexes of the lungs, the kidneys, the ends of long bones, and the brain. Among these, the most common site for secondary settlement of tubercle bacilli is the lung. With the development of immunity, infection in these foci, as well as in the primary focus, is usually brought under control. However, they may continue to harbor the organisms without evidence of disease activity except for a positive tuberculin test. Occasionally, the infection progresses either in the primary site or the metastatic foci, producing clinical tuberculosis in lungs, pleural effusion, meningitis, or other extrapulmonary lesions. A disseminated form may also develop in a few patients, which is referred to as miliary tuberculosis. Local progression during the primary infection and disseminated tuberculosis usually occur in immunocompromised patients, especially in persons with HIV infection.

The patients with clinical evidence of tuberculosis are said to have *tuberculous disease*. *Tuberculous infection without disease* refers to the stage following primary infection when there is no clinical evidence of disease, except for a positive tuberculin test. It is assumed that a positive reaction to tuberculin indicates the presence of live bacilli in the body.

Postprimary or *reactivation tuberculosis* is the result of reactivation of tuberculous infection in one of the dormant foci at a later date (usually several years later). The factors responsible for reactivation are not entirely understood, but it seems that impairment of local and systemic body defense, due to old age, alcoholism, nutritional deficiency, diabetes, or other chronic debilitating disorders, plays a major role. Impairment of cellular immunity is considered to be a most important factor in the reactivation process. Infection with HIV is a good example in which impaired cellular immunity predisposes to reactivation of a dormant tuberculosis infection. In HIV-negative persons, the risk of reactivation from a primary infection is estimated to be 5% to 10% for a lifetime; in HIV-positive patients, this risk is increased to 5% to 10% per year. As is discussed in Chapter 6, tuberculosis should be suspected in HIV-infected persons and HIV infection should be suspected in patients with tuberculosis.

The pathologic hallmark of reactivation tuberculosis is the presence of characteristic granulomas or tubercles around areas of caseous necrosis. Healing with fibrosis is part of the pathologic picture, even while there is active disease. Cavitation, which is one of the distinctive features of pulmonary tuberculosis, is the result of lung tissue necrosis and sloughing. With the control of infection, the healing process continues, and eventually fibrosis replaces the granulomatous lesions. The involved lung tissue becomes retracted and calcium may deposit. Distortion and dilatation of bronchi are common sequelae of pulmonary tuberculosis. *Reinfection tuberculosis* is referred to as acquisition of tuberculosis from an exogenous source by a patient known to have been infected from another source.

Clinical Manifestations. The vast majority of patients with *primary pulmonary infection* have no *clinical* evidence of disease, and in most instances conversion of tuberculin sensitivity from negative to positive takes place with no symptoms whatsoever. When present, symptoms are generally mild: low-grade fever, listlessness, loss of appetite, and occasional cough may be noted. More severe symptoms may develop as a result of complications or progressive primary disease. Significant hilar node enlargement may cause more severe cough or signs of airway obstruction. Pleural involvement causes chest pain. In the disseminated form, systemic symptoms with high fever and prostration predominate. Extrathoracic involvement of meninges, kidneys, joints, bones, or lymph nodes will result in symptoms and signs referable to these structures. In tuberculous infection without disease, the only finding in relation to tuberculosis is a positive skin test.

In *postprimary* (*reactivation* or *reinfection*) *tuberculosis* of the lung, symptoms will depend on location, extent, and duration of disease. Classic presentation with hectic fever, drenching night sweat, cachexia, chronic cough, and hemoptysis characteristic of "consumption" is rarely seen currently in the United States. The diagnosis of tuberculosis in most cases is suggested by a chest x-ray taken in the process of case findings or for other reasons. Some patients will volunteer having certain symptoms such as lack of pep, generalized weakness, or mild to moderate cough. Some may seek medical advice for unremitting cough, bloody sputum, chest pain, or unexplained systemic symptoms, especially fever. Rarely, pulmonary tuberculosis manifests with an acute onset suggesting pneumonia.

The *physical examination* is usually normal in patients with primary infection unless it is severe, progressive, or complicated. Signs of pleural effusion may be present in some patients. With minimal lesion in reactivation tuberculosis, there are usually no significant physical findings. In more advanced cases, dullness to percussion, impaired breath sounds, and rales may be heard over the diseased area. The severity of fever and tachycardia is quite variable. Body temperature may range from normal to as high as 40°C. Fever is more pronounced in the evenings. Evidence of weight loss and debility usually indicates protracted disease. It is not uncommon to find signs of various predisposing conditions. In HIV-infected patients, because of other commonly occurring infections, clinical manifestations may be less clear. Tuberculosis should always be seriously considered in HIV-infected patients with pulmonary or unexplained systemic symptoms.

Radiographic Findings. Physical examination is often unreliable in screening for pulmonary tuberculosis, but radiographic examination of the chest is indispensable not only for its diagnosis, but also for its follow up. Chest x-ray examination, along with tuberculin testing, has become the most important means for tuberculosis screening.

Roentgenographic changes in *primary intrathoracic tuberculosis* are due to involvement of lung parenchyma, hilar and/or mediastinal lymph nodes, and pleura (Fig. 4–1). Parenchymal lesion is a small area of airspace consolidation, usually located in the upper part of a lower lobe or lower part of an upper lobe at the lung periphery. Hilar and/or mediastinal lymph node enlargement is one of the important features of primary infection. It is more prominent in primary tuberculosis of children on the side of parenchymal lesion (primary complex). Sometimes lymph node enlargement is the only radiographic manifestation of primary infection. Certain children with significant

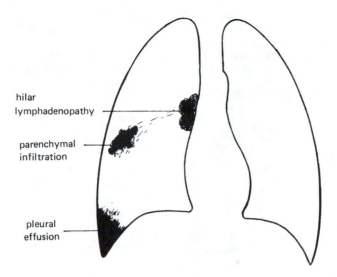

hilar
lymphadenopathy

parenchymal
infiltration

pleural
effusion

Figure 4–1. Diagrammatic drawing showing patterns of primary intrathoracic tuberculosis.

lymph node enlargement may develop atelectasis of a segment or a lobe. Tuberculous lymphadenopathy is one of the causes of "middle-lobe syndrome," which is atelectasis of the right middle lobe.

Pleural involvement with tuberculosis usually manifests by pleural effusion. A small area of parenchymal and/or hilar calcification in adults frequently is due to healed primary tuberculosis of childhood. In many cases, particularly in adults, primary infection will have no demonstrable x-ray change.

In reactivation tuberculosis of the lungs, chest radiograph is almost always abnormal. There is a characteristic tendency for reactivation tuberculosis to involve the apical and posterior segments of the upper lobes. In the early stage, x-ray change is limited to patchy airspace density of small to moderate size. With the progression of the disease, the addition of fibrosis may result in irregularly shaped densities and retraction of the involved lobe or segment. Cavitation may

be seen inside the parenchymal density. In patients whose disease has been present for a long time before being treated, the lesion may be more extensive, involving more than a lobe of the same lung or the other side (Fig. 4–2). The disease usually spreads by the bronchial route. Occasional dissemination by bloodstream will give rise to miliary tuberculosis. It is characterized on radiographic study by diffuse bilateral small nodular densities.

■ LABORATORY TESTS AND DIAGNOSIS OF PULMONARY TUBERCULOSIS

Tuberculin Test

Tuberculin reaction is an example of delayed hypersensitivity mediated by the lymphocytes. Infection with tubercle bacilli results in sensitization of lymphocytes against tuberculin, which is the biologically active material produced from

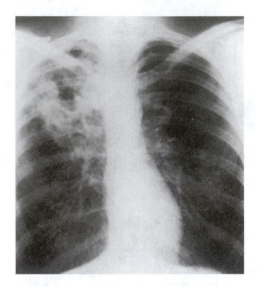

Figure 4–2. Radiograph of far-advanced cavitary pulmonary tuberculosis.

growing *M tuberculosis* in culture media. A purified protein derivative (PPD) of tuberculin is the commonly used substance for skin testing. Tuberculin skin test is the intradermal injection of a small amount of this material, which in sensitized individuals would result in a reaction manifested by an induration mainly from cellular infiltration. This reaction takes place within 48 to 72 hours.

As has been mentioned, a tuberculin test becomes positive 2 to 10 weeks following the start of tuberculous infection and remains so indefinitely, regardless of activity of the infection. Therefore, the result of a tuberculin test simply indicates whether or not an individual has been infected, presently or in the past, with tubercle bacilli. With few exceptions, a negative tuberculin test makes the diagnosis of tuberculosis unlikely.

Conventionally, 0. 1 mL of PPD solution, containing 5 tuberculin units, is injected intradermally with a special tuber-

culin syringe making a small wheal. The injected site is inspected after 48 to 72 hours. The presence of the reaction at the injection site as an area of induration is verified by palpation and its diameter is measured and recorded. Generally, reaction is considered to be positive when the induration measures 10 mm or more in diameter. However, in certain situations, such as HIV-infected persons, or close contacts of infectious cases of tuberculosis, a reaction as small as 5 mm is considered positive. A person without a history of exposure or known risk factor is considered positive only if the skin test results in an induration of 15 mm or more.

Bacteriologic Studies

The most important laboratory study in pulmonary tuberculosis is the examination of sputum for acid-fast bacilli. Although in many instances tuberculosis is strongly suspected from clinical and radiographic data and a positive tuberculin test, its diagnosis is not certain without bacteriologic confirmation. In view of specific staining characteristics of tubercle bacilli, microscopic examination of sputum or other infected material on smear, stained by the acid-fast (Ziehl–Neelsen) technique, is most commonly used. Fluorescent staining (fluorochrome) increases the ease of detection of tubercle bacilli in sputum smear. Concentrated sputum or other suspected specimens increases the diagnostic yield of staining methods. DNA amplification technique (polymerase chain reaction [PCR]) seems to be more sensitive for detecting organisms when their numbers are small. Regardless of the presence or absence of tubercle bacilli by direct examination, the specimen from a suspected case of tuberculosis should be cultured in a special medium. Culture is essential for confirmation of the result of microscopic examination and, if positive, culture allows differentiating *M tuberculosis* from other bacteria with similar staining and morphologic characteristics. It is also necessary for determination of drug susceptibility. Because of emergence of MDR strains, it is now recommended that all isolates of *M tuberculosis* be tested for drug resistance.

The success of bacteriologic identification of tubercle bacilli depends on material submitted for such an examination. Sputum should be expectorated from deep in the lungs, preferably in the morning. Saliva or nasal secretions are not acceptable. (Proper collection of sputum is discussed in Chapter 2.) Sometimes material obtained by gastric washing, laryngeal swab, suctioning, or bronchoscopic material (especially bronchoalveolar lavage [BAL] fluid) is submitted for bacteriologic examination. Pleural fluid, if present, should be likewise examined. In certain circumstances, as in children with hilar lymphadenopathy, bacteriologic proof is not required for a clinical diagnosis. Occasionally, diagnosis of tuberculosis can be made only by pathologic and bacteriologic studies of surgically resected tissue.

Management. Early diagnosis and propertreatment of pulmonary tuberculosis are not only essential for the patient's complete recovery, but are also most important public health measures against tuberculosis. Unfortunately, delay in diagnosis and difficulty with management of many patients with tuberculosis result in the spread of infection to others. Lack of compliance with drug regimens not only results in treatment failure, but also is the major cause of development of drug-resistant strains of *M tuberculosis.* With the significant increase in the number of cases with MDR tuberculosis in recent years, patient management has become complex and therapeutic outcome less successful. Many tuberculous patients are not detected and some are not properly treated; thus, they continue to infect others.

Once a patient with active pulmonary tuberculosis is recognized, he or she may be hospitalized and, during the infective stage of disease, isolated in a negative pressure room. With the institution of appropriate chemotherapy, this stage is often short. Infectivity diminishes rapidly, mainly because of the rapid reduction of the number of organisms in the sputum and decreased cough. Within a few weeks of continuous therapy, patients are considered virtually noninfectious. However, when the patient has, or is likely to have, MDR tuberculosis, duration of infectivity is considered to be much longer. Only repeated negative bacteriologic studies, while the patient is showing clinical and radiographic improvement, would ensure noninfectivity.

Certain measures will reduce the infectivity of the patient with pulmonary tuberculosis. Having the patient wear a mask or at least cover the mouth and nose during coughing and sneezing should be encouraged. Expectorated sputum should be carefully handled and properly disposed. Adequate ventilation of a negative pressure isolation room with 20 or more room-air changes an hour and use of ultraviolet light are very effective in reducing the number of infectious particles in the air. Extreme care should be exercised in using respiratory therapy equipment, with particular attention to decontamination procedures. Health care workers should be safeguarded against *M tuberculosis,* especially MDR strains, by the use of personal respiratory protective devices as indicated by the enforcement policy of Occupational Safety and Health Administration (OSHA) for protection of exposed workers against tuberculosis. Personal items such as clothes, bedding, and dishes are not causes of tuberculosis infection under usual circumstances. It should be emphasized that the most effective way of controlling the infectivity of the patient with active tuberculosis is early proper chemotherapy.

Chemotherapy is the essence of treatment of tuberculosis today. The proper chemotherapeutic regimes for treatment of active tuberculosis should include multiple drugs to which the bacteria are susceptible and should be taken regularly for an adequate length of time. Antituberculosis drugs are included in Appendix I. Isoniazid (INH) remains the most effective drug. It should not be used alone except for prophylaxis. The most effective regimen contains INH and rifampin if the organisms are susceptible. Current recommended initial treatment of active tuberculosis is a four-drug regimen containing INH, rifampin, pyrazinamide, and ethambutol. This regimen is continued until the result of the drug susceptibility study becomes available. With no evidence of drug resistance, ethambutol is discontinued. Two months after the initiation of therapy, pyrazinamide is discontinued and the remaining two drugs (INH and rifampin) are continued for 4 additional months. With evidence of MDR (resistance to at least INH and rifampin), drug regimen is more complex and variable dependent on the susceptibility studies and other factors. As regimens that do not contain INH or rifampin are less effective, include potentially toxic drugs, and require longer duration of treatment, they should be formulated by an expert in tuberculosis. Multidrug resistance not

only adversely affects the therapeutic outcome, but also contributes to prolonged infectious state. Frequent association of MDR tuberculosis with HIV infection, often in noncompliant patients, has created additional problems in its management.

Most of the drug regimens are taken daily with little or no supervision. Many experts now recommend directly observed therapy, which has been shown to reduce the rates of drug resistance and of tuberculosis relapse. Except in MDR cases, directly observed therapy is given twice weekly with proper dose adjustment of the same drugs.

Preventive Measures. The cycle of perpetuation of tuberculosis among the human race can be broken by various preventive and therapeutic measures, as shown in Fig. 4–3. Although the avoidance of contact and preventive therapy soon after contact are measures that would prevent development of infection, they are much less practical because most contacts remain unrecognized. Identification and treatment of infected persons to prevent them from becoming infectious, and the early diagnosis and proper therapy of individuals with infectious tuberculosis to make them noninfectious, are the most effective and practical preventive measures. If both of these objectives are achieved in all cases, the eradication of tuberculosis from the face of the earth would become a reality. Unfortunately, socioeconomic factors in the world make this ultimate goal unrealistic at this time. These measures, however, continue to work in developed and in some developing countries as judged from the steady decline in the incidence of active cases and tuberculin converters in the general population.

Chemoprophylaxis refers to treatment

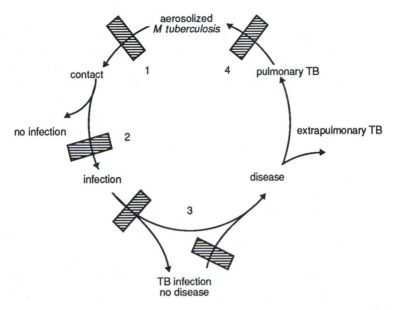

Figure 4–3. Cycle of tuberculosis (TB). Proper intervention at any sites (bars 1 to 4) would break the cycle of perpetuation of TB. Isolating patients during their infectious period, reducing aerosolized tubercle bacilli in the air, and preventing their inhalation by contacts will diminish the rate of new infections (bars 1 and 2). Treatment of infected individuals to prevent them from becoming infectious (bars 3), and treatment of patients with pulmonary TB to make them noninfectious (bar 4), are other effective and practical measures for controlling TB.

of individuals who have no detectable disease, but are at risk of developing it. They include

- Household members and other close associates of recently diagnosed tuberculous patients
- Newly infected persons as manifested by recent tuberculin conversion
- Positive tuberculin reactors in persons infected with HIV
- Others at high risk for developing tuberculosis because of impaired cell-mediated immunity
- Patients with positive tuberculin test and abnormal chest x-ray, suggesting old tuberculous lesion without positive bacteriology and prior TB therapy

- Children with positive tuberculin test

Although every patient with a positive tuberculin test is at higher risk of developing active tuberculosis than nonreactors, the hazard of liver toxicity from INH, the drug of choice for chemoprophylaxis, should be considered in deciding such therapy. Only patients at high enough risk are selected for prophylactic treatment. The usual duration of INH chemoprophylaxis is 9–12 months.

Vaccination with bacille Calmette-Guérin (BCG) derived from an attenuated strain of *M bovis*, confers cellular immunity against tuberculosis with little or no danger of reactivation as seen in naturally infected individuals. Its practical usefulness in countries such as the United

States, where tuberculosis disease occurs mostly in persons who are already infected, is very limited.

Course and Prognosis. Except for patients with severe and overwhelming disease at the time of diagnosis and in patients with MDR tuberculosis, prognosis of pulmonary tuberculosis is generally very good if proper treatment is instituted and continued for an adequate length of time. A majority of patients will be able to return to their usual occupation and live a normal life. The most important cause of therapeutic failure is lack of patient cooperation in taking the prescribed medications. This is more commonly seen among alcoholics and drug addicts, who not only are at higher risk in developing tuberculosis, but also are less compliant in continuing their treatment. It is not uncommon for such patients to have recurrent disease, and some will develop MDR tuberculosis.

With early diagnosis and proper treatment, respiratory functional impairment will be unusual, whereas with advanced and destructive tuberculosis resulting from late diagnosis or improper therapy, significant pulmonary insufficiency will often ensue. Other complications of healed or inactive tuberculosis include hemoptysis from residual bronchiectasis and superinfection with aspergillus in the form of a fungus ball inside a residual cavity.

■ PULMONARY INFECTION SECONDARY TO ATYPICAL MYCOBACTERIA

Certain mycobacteria other than *M tuberculosis* and *M bovis* may occasionally cause pulmonary lesions in humans. These organisms have certain growth and other biologic characteristics that differentiate them from *M tuberculosis*. They are generally known as atypical mycobacteria. Many of them appear to be saprophytic in soil. These bacteria are occasionally isolated from sputum in the absence of demonstrable disease or from the sputum of patients with known pulmonary tuberculosis. Sometimes they are the direct cause of a tuberculosis-like lung disease. Their transmission from person to person has not been proved; therefore, patients infected with these organisms are not considered to be infective and thus need not be isolated.

Pulmonary disease caused by atypical mycobacteria has no characteristic features and is often mistaken for tuberculosis due to typical tubercle bacilli. Diagnosis is established only by repeated demonstration of organisms on culture, as their staining characteristics (acid fastness) are similar to *M tuberculosis.*

Although there are many species of atypical mycobacteria that have been associated with pulmonary infection, the most important ones are *M kansasii, M avium-intracellulare,* and *M scrofulaceum.* The last is an important cause of cervical lymphadenopathy in children. Pulmonary infection with *M kansasii* responds well to the usual antituberculosis drugs. However, most other atypical mycobacteria are often drug resistant, and therefore susceptibility studies are necessary for selection of proper drugs. Occasionally, pulmonary lesions are treated by surgical resection, particularly when the lesions are localized.

As seen in Chapter 6, patients with immunologic deficiency are prone to infection with typical as well as atypical mycobacteria that may result in disseminated and often fatal disease. Patients with acquired immunodeficiency syndrome (AIDS) are especially susceptible to infection with *M avium-intracellulare,* which usually results in systemic disseminated disease, with poor response to therapy.

BIBLIOGRAPHY

ACCP/ATS Consensus Conference. Institutional control measures for tuberculosis in the era of multiple drug resistance. *Chest.* 1995; 108:1690–1710.

American Thoracic Society. Diagnostic standards and classification of tuberculosis. *Am Rev Respir Dis.* 1990; 142:725–735.

American Thoracic Society. Treatment of tuberculosis and tuberculosis infection in adults and children. *Am J Respir Crit Care Med.* 1994; 149:1359–1374.

Bailey WC. Treatment of atypical mycobacterial disease. *Chest.* 1983; 84:625–628.

Barnes PF, Silva C, Otaya M. Testing for human immunodeficiency virus infection in patients with tuberculosis. *Am J Respir Crit Care Med.* 1996; 153:1448–1450.

Blumberg HM, Watkins DL, Berschling JK, et al. Preventing the nosocomial transmission of tuberculosis. *Ann Intern Med.* 1995; 122:658–663.

Centers for Disease Control. Guidelines for preventing the transmission of Mycobacterium tuberculosis in health-care facilities: 1994. *MMWR.* 1994; 43:1–120.

Dannenberg AM Jr. Immunopathogenesis of pulmonary tuberculosis. *Hosp Pract.* 1993; 28:33–40.

Drugs for Tuberculosis. *Med Letter Drugs Ther.* 1995; 37:67–70.

Modilevsky T, Sattler FR, Barnes PF. Mycobacterial disease in patients with human immunodeficiency virus infection. *Arch Intern Med.* 1989; 149:2201–2205.

Reichman LB. Multidrug-resistant tuberculosis: meeting the challenge. *Hosp Pract.* 1994; 29(S):65–74.

Snider DE Jr. The tuberculin skin test. *Am Rev Respir Dis.* 1982; 125(no. 3: part 2):108–118.

Wolinsky E. Nontuberculous mycobacterial and associated diseases. *Am Rev Respir Dis.* 1979; 119:107–159.

5.

Fungal Infection of the Lung

Fungi are widespread throughout the environment. Although the respiratory tract is exposed to the respirable fungal elements, normal host defenses are usually capable of forestalling infection from them, and if infection does occur, host defenses prevent fungal invasion or dissemination. Disease from these organisms develops if the body defenses are weakened or overwhelmed by heavy exposure. Among the fungi causing pulmonary disease in the United States, *Histoplasma capsulatum,* the agent of *histoplasmosis,* and *Coccidioides immitis,* the cause of *coccidioidomycosis,* are the most prevalent (Fig. 5–1). Blastomycosis, although less common, is an important fungal infection caused by *Blastomyces dermatitidis.* These three fungi are dimorphic. In nature, they exist as mold (mycelial form). In the infected host, *H capsulatum* and *B dermatitidis* change to yeast form, where they multiply by budding. *Coccidioides immitis* converts to spherules in the host. These are round, thin-walled cells that produce endospores. With rupture of its wall, the spherule releases endospores, which de-

velop into spherules, and the cycle is repeated. Another fungal disease discussed in this chapter is aspergillosis, commonly caused by *Aspergillus fumigatus.* This fungus is a mold and exists as mycelia (hyphae) in both nature and the infected host.

■ HISTOPLASMOSIS

Epidemiology and Pathogenesis.
Histoplasmosis is one of the most prevalent infections in certain parts of the United States. The causative agent, *H capsulatum,* is a common fungus in soil, particularly when it is enriched by large quantities of droppings from certain birds, such as pigeons, starlings, blackbirds, chickens, and probably many others. The birds themselves do not carry the organisms. Bats, however, whose manure also facilitates the growth of these fungi, may be infected and, thus, may carry the fungi. Chicken coops and starling roosts are some of the common sources of exposure to *H capsulatum.*

The endemic areas in the United

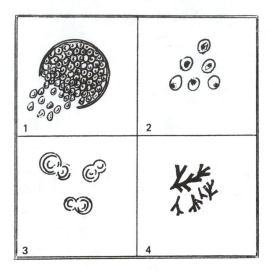

Figure 5–1. Fungi commonly causing respiratory tract infection. (1) *Coccidioides immitis,* (2) *Histoplasma capsulatum,* (3) *Blastomyces dermatitidis,* (4) *Aspergillus fumigatus.*

States are predominantly in the Ohio and Mississippi river valleys, but the infection has also been demonstrated in eastern states along many other river valleys, such as the Potomac, Delaware, Hudson, and St. Lawrence valleys. In certain states, such as Tennessee, Kentucky, Arkansas, and Missouri, histoplasmin skin test, which is a good indicator of prevalence of infection, is positive in as many as 90% of the adult population.

In nature and in culture media at room temperature, *H capsulatum* assumes the mycelial form (mold); in infected tissues and in culture media at 37°C, it is in a yeast form. Human infection is usually the result of inhalation of spores (microconidia) spread in the air from the naturally occurring mycelial form.

As in tuberculosis, implantation of the organisms in the lung results in a primary infection with regional lymph node involvement in a previously uninfected individual. Before the onset of hypersen-sitivity, significant spread of the fungi via the bloodstream takes place. With the development of immunity through a cellular mechanism, the infected tissues react with necrosis and granuloma formation, halting the spread of the disease in both primary and metastatic sites. A positive histoplasmin skin test is an indication of cellular immunity against *H capsulatum.* These foci later become calcified. The primary infection is, therefore, similar to tuberculosis, except for the tendency for multiple pulmonary and extrapulmonary foci, which may undergo extensive calcification.

Postprimary chronic histoplasmosis is most likely due to exogenous reinfection rather than endogenous reactivation, which occurs in tuberculosis. There is evidence that, following primary infection, the organisms do not usually survive very long, and subsequent acute infections from outside sources are common in endemic regions. In comparison with the high prevalence of acute infection, chronic disease is uncommon.

Under certain rare circumstances (especially when there is impaired cellular immunity), histoplasmosis may take a highly invasive form, involving many organs and resulting in death. This form is referred to as *disseminated histoplasmosis.* This occurs especially in the advanced stages of human immunodeficiency virus (HIV) infection.

Clinical Manifestations. The vast majority of adults and older children with acute or primary infection do not have recognizable clinical symptoms; the conversion of skin reactivity to histoplasmin is the only evidence of the infection. Individuals with heavy exposure, however, will develop symptoms of an influenza-like illness, manifested by chills, fever, headache, and generalized aches and pains. Nonproductive cough and substernal chest discomfort may also be present. These symptoms usually subside within a few days without any therapy. In younger children, primary infection is much more serious. Radiographic changes in acute histoplasmosis show patchy parenchymal densities, which may be diffuse and scattered throughout both lung fields. Hilar lymph nodes are frequently enlarged.

Disseminated histoplasmosis is an extremely serious, but fortunately rare, infection. It occurs in young children or in a setting of deficient immunologic state. Pulmonary involvement in disseminated histoplasmosis, which is the rule in children, is usually not significant in adults, in whom clinical manifestations are predominantly extrathoracic. In association with acquired immunodeficiency syndrome (AIDS), histoplasmosis may manifest as a rapidly progressive and severe infection, as discussed in Chapter 6.

Chronic active or *progressive pulmonary histoplasmosis* is mostly a disease of middle-age white males; it is uncommon in females and rare in blacks. There is often evidence of underlying chronic obstructive pulmonary disease. The incident of chronic pulmonary histoplasmosis is very low in comparison with the high infection rate. Symptoms, physical findings, and radiographic changes are similar to pulmonary tuberculosis. Apical and posterior segments of upper lobes are predominantly involved. It is frequently bilateral, and cavitation is common. A less destructive form has been described as *early noncavitary histoplasmosis,* which tends to heal spontaneously. Mediastinal lymphadenopathy may cause compression of adjacent structures. Fibrosing mediastinitis is another complication in which an exaggerated fibrotic reaction to histoplasma antigen results in narrowing or obstruction of blood vessels and/or airways.

Laboratory Studies and Diagnosis. *Histoplasmin* is a filtrate of culture medium in which *H capsulatum* has been growing for several months. Intradermal injection of this material, known as *histoplasmin skin test,* causes a delayed reaction in individuals who have been infected with histoplasma. It becomes positive with primary infection and remains so more or less indefinitely, regardless of disease activity. In certain situations, it may be negative despite the presence of active disease, such as in disseminated histoplasmosis. Histoplasmin skin test, therefore, has limited diagnostic usefulness.

Serologic tests such as *complement fixation* and *immunodiffusion* are more helpful in the diagnosis of histoplasmosis, as they are positive mostly during the active stage of the disease. Detection of antigen in blood or urine, using a sensitive assay, is also considered to be diagnostic.

Demonstration of *H capsulatum* from the sputum or other sources is the only conclusive proof of the diagnosis; however, the result of bacteriologic studies may be unrevealing. Sometimes diagnosis of histoplasmosis is made by biopsy and pathologic examination. Bone marrow examination by smear and culture has a high yield in disseminated histoplasmosis. Blood culture may also be positive. The organisms may also be present on specially stained blood smears in disseminated disease.

Management. The vast majority of patients with acute primary infection will require no therapy. Treatment, however, is indicated in disseminated illness and chronic progressive pulmonary histoplasmosis. As amphotericin B, the agent most effective against histoplasmosis, is potentially toxic, patients are carefully selected for therapy with this drug. Itraconazole is another drug that has proved effective, mostly in mild to moderately severe cases, and it has the advantage of being an oral agent and of being less toxic. Amphotericin B, however, is still the drug of choice for treatment of disseminated disease. Rarely will surgical resection of the involved lung be necessary. Patients with active histoplasmosis need not be isolated, as human-to-human transmission of this infection does not occur under usual circumstances.

Course and Prognosis. The prognosis for acute histoplasmosis in adults and older children is excellent; spontaneous rapid recovery is the rule. With recovery from initial infection, recurrence or reinfection is very uncommon, except in severely immunocompromised patients, as seen with AIDS. The prognosis in infants and patients with disseminated histoplasmosis is usually grave. Chronic progressive pulmonary histoplasmosis with cavitation may result in significant pulmonary functional impairment and eventual respiratory insufficiency.

■ COCCIDIOIDOMYCOSIS

Coccidioidomycosis is a fungal disease, usually self-limited, which primarily involves the lungs but may spread to the lymph nodes, skin, bone, central nervous system, and other organs.

Epidemiology and Pathogenesis. Coccidioidomycosis is endemic in the southwestern United States, particularly the desert areas of California, Arizona, Nevada, New Mexico, Texas, and Utah. In some of these areas the prevalence of positive skin tests is as high as 90%.

The causative agent, *C immitis,* exists in the mycelial form in soil of semiarid regions. Its spores (arthroconidia), after being inhaled and settling in the lung, germinate to form spherules, which make endospores. Initially, the tissue responds to the endospores by nonspecific inflammation; however, once immunity develops, granulomatous reaction takes place and the infection is brought under control. The development of immunity can be demonstrated by positive reaction to the intradermal injection of *coccidioidin* (a filtrate of culture medium growing *C immitis*) or spherulin (a product of the spherule-endospore phase). In occasional patients who do not develop immunity, the infection spreads systemically to involve many organs in the body.

Clinical Manifestations. More than 60% of infected individuals have no symptoms, and the conversion of skin reactivity is the only indication of infection. In the majority of remaining cases, a mild flu-like syndrome develops. This illness, commonly known as "desert fever," manifests by low-grade fever, malaise, headache, body aches and pains, and cough. These symptoms are self-limited and subside in several days. Only a small percentage of these symptomatic patients will have a more prolonged illness from persistent lung involvement lasting for weeks and months. *Disseminated* disease, involving extrathoracic organs, occurs in only a small fraction of the latter group. For some unknown reasons, nonwhite males are much more susceptible to developing the disseminated form, which is very rare in white females. Immunosuppression from various causes is a significant predisposing factor for widespread disease, which is being recognized in increasing numbers in patients with AIDS. Dissemination should be suspected when there is persistent fever, weight loss, or signs of extrapulmonary involvement, such as lymphadenopathy, enlarged liver or spleen, skin or bone lesions, and signs of meningitis. The last is the most serious manifestation of disseminated coccidioidomycosis.

Radiographic Findings. Radiographic changes are variable. Localized parenchymal consolidation with or without hilar or mediastinal lymph node enlargement is the most common x-ray change during acute infection. Sometimes single or multiple nodules may be demonstrated. Cavity formation, with its characteristic thin wall, may occasionally follow these lesions. A thin-walled cavity may be the only radiographic evidence of pulmonary coccidioidomycosis. Diffuse bilateral micronodular pattern is seen in disseminated disease. Pleural effusion may be present in some cases.

Diagnosis. The diagnosis of coccidioidomycosis is often suggested by the clinical presentation and x-ray findings in an appropriate epidemiologic setting. The coccidioidin, or spherulin, skin test becomes positive within 2 to 3 weeks of the onset of infection. It is frequently negative in the disseminated form. Serologic tests commonly performed are immunodiffusion (for precipitating antibody) and complement fixation tests. Precipitin antibodies appear soon after infection; complement fixing antibodies are found later and last longer. Persistence of positive serology beyond 6 months or high complement fixation titer with negative skin test suggests dissemination. With recovery, serologic tests become negative. In certain situations and for conclusive diagnosis, isolation of organisms from the sputum or other infected materials is necessary. The laboratory should be warned if coccidioidomycosis is suspected, as the mold form of *C immitis,* which is the form that grows in culture media, should be handled with utmost care to prevent accidental infection of the personnel. Occasionally, the diagnosis is made by the biopsy method.

Management and Prognosis. As was mentioned earlier, the majority of patients have self-limited and mild disease, which is often unapparent and requires no specific therapy. All patients with pulmonary coccidioidomycosis should be followed closely, especially when there is a cavitary lesion. Lack of spontaneous improvement of lung lesions or their progression and persistence of symptoms may be an indication for specific therapy. Disseminated coccidioidomycosis should always be treated. Although fluconazole and itraconazole seem to be effective in many pulmonary and extrapulmonary lesions, amphotericin B is considered as the therapeutic agent of choice, especially for the treatment of meningitis and disseminated disease. Occasionally, surgical resection may be indicated in persisting localized lesions or when there is recurrent hemoptysis. Disseminated disease, particularly with meningitis, has a poor prognosis.

■ BLASTOMYCOSIS

North American blastomycosis is a chronic fungal infection that originates in the respiratory tract and often spreads to the skin and occasionally to other organs. It is seen mostly in the eastern half of the United States, excluding most of New England and Florida. It affects predominantly middle-age males.

Blastomycosis is a mixed pyogenic and granulomatosus disease. Pulmonary blastomycosis begins as a mild to moderate respiratory infection with cough, expectoration, chest pain, and sometimes hemoptysis. It may heal spontaneously or progress slowly. With progression of the disease, systemic symptoms of fever, night sweats, anorexia, and weight loss become evident. Physical signs are nonspecific and less remarkable. There may be dullness to percussion, decreased breath sounds, or rales over the involved area. The chest x-ray usually shows homogeneous mass lesion or patchy airspace density. Upper lobes are more frequently involved than lower lobes. Cavity formation is uncommon. A more diffuse form may manifest as acute respiratory distress syndrome (ARDS), especially in the advanced stages of HIV infection. Skin lesion is a characteristic feature of blastomycosis, which may be the only manifestation of the disease. It is a chronic, slowly progressive warty and crusting lesion located mostly on the exposed areas of the skin.

Pulmonary blastomycosis is often mistaken for other more common conditions, such as pneumonia, tuberculosis, malignancy, or other fungal infections. Definite diagnosis will depend on demonstration of typical budding yeastlike organisms on smear or culture from the diseased sources, including the sputum. The skin test and the serologic examination have no diagnostic value in blastomycosis.

Although many patients with pulmonary blastomycosis may recover with-

out treatment, because of lack of significant immunity against the infection and the danger of dissemination, blastomycosis is usually treated. Amphoteracin B is the preferred drug, especially in severe and progressive disease. Itraconazole and ketoconazole have been shown to be effective in acute mild to moderate pneumonic form as well as subacute or chronic form of the disease. If untreated, blastomycosis may take a protracted and progressive course, in many cases ending in death. Treated patients generally do well, except AIDS patients who will require chronic suppressive treatment after initial aggressive therapy.

■ ASPERGILLOSIS

Aspergillosis refers to various pathologic conditions resulting from infection with one of many species of *Aspergillus*. This ubiquitous fungus grows as mold on numerous organic materials. It seems, therefore, that exposure to the respirable spores (conidia) of this very common fungus is inevitable. Fortunately, it can cause disease only in a relatively small number of people, and then only under certain circumstances. The fungus may also live as a saprophyte in the respiratory tract, especially in patients with chronic lung disease. Among the species of *Aspergillus* known to cause disease in humans, *A fumigatus* is the most important. In this section, the better-known clinical conditions that result from infection with and/or reaction to this fungus are discussed briefly.

Allergic Bronchopulmonary Aspergillosis. There are two types of hypersensitivity reaction to *Aspergillus* that depend on the immunologic state of the host. In individuals without underlying asthma, heavy or repeated exposure may result in a condition known as *extrinsic allergic alveolitis,* which is discussed in Chapter 13. Malt worker's lung is an example in which exposure to moldy barley from *Aspergillus* results in this type of alveolitis. *Allergic bronchopulmonary aspergillosis,* however, is a disease that occurs in a background of long-standing asthma. It is characterized by episodic asthmatic attacks, expectoration of mucous plugs, transient irregular pulmonary infiltrates, and atelectasis. Peripheral blood eosinophilia, elevated immunoglobulin E (IgE), high specific antibodies against *A fumigatus,* positive skin reactivity to the fungal antigen, and positive sputum culture for the fungus are important for its diagnosis. Recurrent acute episodes may eventually result in chronic changes of pulmonary fibrosis and/ or bronchiectasis. Characteristically, pulmonary fibrosis develops in the upper lobes, and bronchiectasis involves the central bronchi. Allergic bronchopulmonary aspergillosis involves both type I and type III immunologic reactions (see Chapter 13). Systemic corticosteroids are effective in its management, whereas inhaled corticosteroids have no significant role. Although antifungal treatment is generally unnecessary, some patients respond to oral therapy with itraconazole. Proper bronchial toilet, with adequate humidification, use of bronchodilators, and postural drainage, is very important in the management of patients with this disease.

Aspergilloma. Also known as *fungus ball,* aspergilloma is usually the result of colonization of aspergillus in a preformed pulmonary cavity or cyst. Although a variety of cavitary or cystic lung diseases may be the site of aspergilloma, tuberculosis and sarcoidosis are the most common underlying chronic conditions. The cavity in which a fungus ball develops may occasionally result from destructive changes from other types of pulmonary aspergillosis. The ball is formed by tightly matted fungal mycelia with fibrin, mucus, and cellular debris. Most patients with aspergilloma have no symptoms referable to it, although they may be symptomatic from their underlying chronic pulmonary disease. Its most significant complication is hemoptysis, which may be quite severe and life threatening. Characteristic radiographic changes are almost diagnostic (Fig. 5–2). In less obvious cases, standard or computed tomography helps to delineate the intracavitary ball. In some cases, aspergilloma may resolve spontaneously. It rarely causes locally invasive aspergillosis. Unless serious complications develop, treatment of aspergilloma should be conservative.

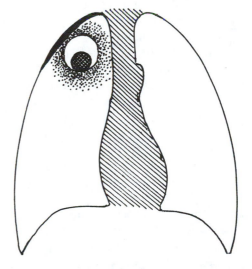

Figure 5–2. A diagram showing a fungus ball (aspergilloma) in a cavity.

Surgical resection is considered if massive or recurrent hemoptysis occurs and if the patient is a reasonable surgical risk. Local antifungal therapy has been used with limited success in some patients. Systemic treatment may be indicated when there is evidence of local invasion.

Chronic Necrotizing Pulmonary Aspergillosis. This is a localized lung infection that has a chronic course and often mimics tuberculosis. Patients with this condition are usually middle-aged and often have underlying chronic conditions such as diabetes, malnutrition, or chronic obstructive lung disease. Radiographic film shows an infiltrative process involving predominantly one of the upper lobes with cavity formation and fibrosis. The cavity is frequently the site of a fungus ball. The disease may be present for a number of months or even years before the diagnosis is made. The clinical course, radiographic finding, repeated isolation of aspergillus from the sputum or bronchoscopically obtained secretions, absence of other pathogenic organisms, and lack of response to antibiotics and antituberculosis drugs should suggest the diagnosis of chronic necrotizing aspergillosis. It is usually confirmed by demonstration of tissue invasion by the fungus on pathologic examination or its response to antifungal drugs. Amphotericin B, with or without the addition of another antifungal drug, flucytosine, is the agent of choice for its treatment. Itraconazole has also been proved to be effective against pulmonary aspergillosis. Surgical resection may be necessary in some cases.

Invasive or Disseminated Aspergillosis. Invasive or disseminated aspergillosis is a most serious and often fatal disease. It is almost exclusively seen in patients with severe debilitating conditions, particularly when they are treated with immunosuppressive drugs and are profoundly granulocytopenic. It is also a serious complication of bone marrow or other organ transplantation. In addition to progressive pulmonary lesion, invasion of other organs is very common. Blood vessels may be invaded, causing their occlusion, which in turn results in tissue infarction and necrosis. Pulmonary manifestations may be overshadowed by severe systemic symptoms and neurologic signs. Diagnosis of invasive aspergillosis is usually made by pathologic examination of resected tissue, although in proper clinical settings it can sometimes be diagnosed by culture of respiratory tract secretions. Generally, treatment is unsuccessful, but some patients respond to antifungal therapy with amphoteracin B or itraconazole, especially after correction of granulocytopenia with recently available human granulocyte colony stimulating factor (Neupogen).

BIBLIOGRAPHY

American Thoracic Society. Fungal infection in HIV-infected persons. *Am J Respir Crit Care Med.* 1995; 152:816–822.

Ampel NM, Dols CL, Galgiani JN. Coccidioidomycosis during immunodeficiency virus infection. *Am J Med.* 1993; 94:235–240.

Davies SF. Fungal pneumonia. *Med Clin North Am.* 1994; 78:1049–1065.

Dismukes WE, Bradsher RW Jr, Cloud GC, et al. Itraconazole therapy for blastomycosis and histoplasmosis. *Am J Med.* 1992; 93: 489–497.

Failla PJ, Cerise FP, Karam GH, Summer WR. Blastomycosis: pulmonary and pleural manifestations. *South J Med.* 1995; 88:405–410.

Horvath JA, Dummer S. The use of respiratory-tract cultures in the diagnosis of invasive pulmonary aspergillosis. *Am J Med.* 1996; 100:171–178.

Kauffman HF, Tomee JFC, van der Werf TS, et al. Review of fungus-induced asthmatic reactions. *Am Rev Respir Crit Care Med.* 1995; 151:2109–2116.

Levitz SM. Aspergillosis. *Infect Dis Clin North Am.* 1989; 3(1):1–18.

Meyer KC, McManus EJ, Maki DG. Over-whelming pulmonary blastomycosis associated with the adult respiratory distress syndrome. *N Engl J Med.* 1993; 329:1231–1236.

Stevens DA. Coccidioidomycosis. *N Engl J Med.* 1995; 332:1077–1082.

Systemic antifungal drugs. *Med Lett Drugs Ther.* 1996; 38:10–12.

Wheat LJ. Histoplasmosis: recognition and treatment. *Clin Infect Dis.* 1994; 19(suppl 1):S19–S27.

6.

Infection with the Human Immunodeficiency Virus: Pulmonary Complications

The term *acquired immunodeficiency syndrome* (AIDS) was coined in 1981 to characterize a newly recognized fatal illness among young homosexual men, manifested by certain unusual opportunistic infections and/or a rare form of cancer. Without a known prior susceptibility to these uncommon diseases, it soon became apparent that these patients had somehow developed a severe immune system deficiency. Intense clinical and laboratory research began to produce a prolific amount of knowledge about this dreadful disease that has continued to afflict and kill an increasing number of young people. Before long, it was realized that AIDS represents only a short terminal stage of a chronic, long-standing infection with a virus that slowly and relentlessly destroys the body's immunologic defense. The virus was named *human immunodeficiency virus* (HIV). Despite extremely rapid scientific advances in the understanding of the molecular structure and biologic behavior of HIV in disabling the body defenses against infections and neoplastic diseases, the AIDS pandemic continues to inflict heavy casualties and immense human suffering throughout the world.

This chapter focuses on the commonly occurring pulmonary complications of HIV infection. For better understanding of these complications, HIV, its pathogenesis and transmission, and the immunologic consequences and clinical spectrum of HIV infection are very briefly discussed. It should be stressed that information on HIV infection and its management will continue to evolve; therefore, the reader should remain up-to-date from current medical publications.

■ HUMAN IMMUNODEFICIENCY VIRUS

HIV is a retrovirus, and as such is about 1/10 of a micron in diameter with a single-stranded RNA genome (Fig. 6–1). Its core, in addition to RNA, contains enzymes, including protease, integrase, and the characteristic *reverse transcriptase.* Surrounding the core is a lipid membrane derived from the infected host cell. The membrane has two layers of glycoproteins (gp). The external layer, known as *gp 120,* has a high affinity to a special receptor (CD4 molecule) on the host cell membrane. The internal layer, known as *gp 41,* is important in fusing the lipid membrane of the virus with that of the target cell, letting the viral core enter the cell. Once inside, the genomic RNA and the enzymes are released into the host cell cytoplasm. Viral reverse transcriptase catalyzes the transcription of viral RNA into a complementary DNA, which is known as *proviral DNA.* This DNA migrates into the nucleus, where it is integrated into the host cells' chromosomes. The viral enzyme integrin mediates this process. Incorporation of proviral DNA into the host cell genome is permanent. The provirus may appear in latent state, but most likely remains active producing new viruses by transcription of viral genomic RNA and formation of viral proteins. The

viral enzyme protease is important for active reproduction of a virus. It hydrolyzes important proteins used to assemble new copies of virus within human cells. Once new viruses are synthesized, they are released to infect other susceptible cells.

■ PATHOGENESIS AND IMMUNOLOGIC CONSEQUENCES OF HIV INFECTION

The cells attacked by HIV are primarily the blood cells with special surface molecules known as CD4, which act as high-affinity receptors for the virus. T lymphocytes with helper and inducer activities have the highest expression of these molecules on their surface and, thus, are primary targets for the viral particles. These cells are known as CD4-positive cells or T4 lymphocytes. Because other cell populations, such as macrophages, blood monocytes, and certain nerve cells, have such viral receptors, they may also be infected. Infection of CD4-positive lymphocytes results in their quantitative and qualitative deficiency. Normally, about 65% of peripheral blood T cells are CD4-positive cells, amounting to more than $1000/mm^3$ of blood. This number reduces to less than $200/mm^3$ in most patients with full-blown AIDS. As only a

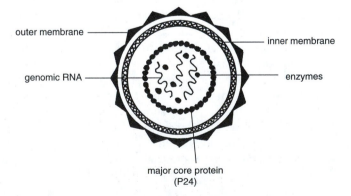

outer membrane

inner membrane

genomic RNA

enzymes

major core protein
(P24)

Figure 6–1. Schematic demonstration of HIV virion and its important components. The actual diameter of the virion is less than 1/400,000 of that shown in this drawing.

small percentage of these cells in peripheral blood becomes infected, marked reduction of CD4-positive T cells cannot be explained by death from their direct viral invasion. It is believed that the ongoing infection of their progenitors in lymph nodes and other lymphatic tissues, even when there is no clinically apparent disease, is the cause of steady decline in the number and dysfunction of these lymphocytes.

Infected macrophages and monocytes are not killed by the virus. They serve as viral reservoirs and as vehicles for transferring HIV to other sites, notably the central nervous system (CNS).

The immunologic effects of HIV infection are mostly related to the reduction of the number and quantitative defect of T helper cells, which have the central role in cell-mediated immunity. Almost all of the immunologic abnormalities in AIDS are explained by the depletion of these cells and their defective helper function, including an inadequate production of lymphokines. Because the cells with CD8 markers, that is, the lymphocytes with suppressor and cytotoxic activities, are not directly affected by the virus, their number is not reduced; in fact, it may even increase. As a result, an imbalance develops between these cells, known as CD8-positive, or T8 lymphocytes, and CD4-positive cells. A so-called T4/T8 ratio, which is normally around 2, therefore may be reduced to less than 1 (reversal of T4/T8 ratio). Infection of macrophages and monocytes by HIV may also alter their function, contributing further to the impairment of cell-mediated immunity.

In addition to the deterioration of cellular immunity, the humoral component of the immune system is also affected by HIV infection. Despite an enhanced polyclonal production of immunoglobulins by B lymphocytes, they are defective in making antibodies against newly acquired infections. Dysfunction of this system may also result in autoimmune disorders, among which thrombocytopenia is the best known. Soon after HIV infection, antibodies against viral antigens are produced. These antibodies, unlike those against most other viruses, are not protective. They are the bases for the serologic diagnosis of HIV infection.

Immunologic impairment resulting from HIV infection is a very slow but steadily progressive process. With a steady decline in immunologic defense, the invasion by pathogenic as well as opportunistic microorganisms becomes inevitable.

■ CLINICAL SPECTRUM OF HIV INFECTION

HIV infection is often silent and remains so for a long period of time before causing any clinically recognizable signs or symptoms. In the past, this was referred to as the *incubation period,* which is a misnomer, as HIV infection is a continuum. During this asymptomatic period, the viral replication continues. *Clinical latency* is a better term to characterize the asymptomatic period. Its duration varies significantly between individuals. Host factors seem to determine the rate of CD4-positive lymphocyte depletion as well as the time of development of pathologic conditions that meet the criteria for definition of AIDS. This terminal stage usually occurs faster in injection drug users (IDUs) than in homosexuals. On average, it takes about 8 years from the time of HIV infection to the development of AIDS. In more than one-half of the cases, prior to the clinical latency, HIV infection results in an acute illness 3 to 6 weeks after the person becomes infected. This self-limited illness has variable severity and is like a viral syndrome. Sometimes it mimics infectious mononucleosis. Common manifestations are fever, headache, sore throat, joint and muscle ache, enlarged lymph nodes, and skin rash. This acute syndrome coincides with increased viremia and transient reduction in CD4-positive lymphocytes (Fig. 6–2). It has been suggested that symptomatic presentation of HIV infection may be predictive of a more accelerated course. With the disappearance of symptoms within one to several weeks, clinical latency begins and viremia abates.

Although HIV-infected patients may remain asymptomatic until the onset of one of the AIDS-defining conditions, many patients develop various manifestations indicative of a chronic illness, such as generalized lymphadenopathy, protracted fever, fatigue, weight loss, diarrhea, oral thrush, anemia, and thrombocytopenia. This type of presentation has been named as *early symptomatic disease.* None of these clinical conditions fulfills the criteria for AIDS-defining illness, but patients with these various syndromes will eventually develop AIDS. The terms *pre-AIDS* and *AIDS-related complex* (ARC) are often applied to these varied clinical states. Generally at this stage of HIV infection, the CD4-positive T cell count is less than $500/mm^3$. Patients with low enough CD4-positive lymphocyte count are considered to have AIDS (see later in this chapter).

Originally, for surveillance purpose, prior to discovery of HIV, *AIDS* was defined by the Centers for Disease Control (CDC) as an immunodeficiency state without a known cause in which certain opportunistic infections developed. Since then, with the identification of HIV, availability of increasing amounts of clinical

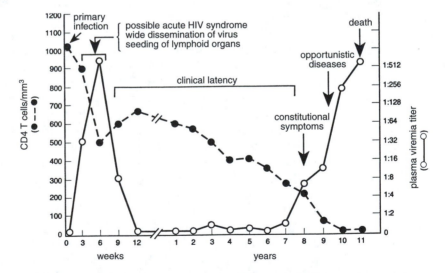

Figure 6–2. Typical course of HIV infection. A sharp increase in viremia after infection is followed by its rapid decline. Low-level viremia continues during the clinical latency, which rapidly rises during the symptomatic period. CD4-positive peripheral blood lymphocyte count, after its initial rapid decline following primary infection, continues to decrease slowly with an accelerated reduction toward the end of the clinical course. (Reprinted by permission of *The New England Journal of Medicine.* Pantleo G, et al. The imunopathogenesis of human immunodeficiency virus infection. *N Engl J Med.* 328:327–335. Copyright 1993, Massachusetts Medical Society.)

data, and careful epidemiologic and statistical analyses, the case definition of AIDS has undergone several revisions. The current definition of AIDS is rather complex and quite lengthy. This strict definition is established only for surveillance purposes. Contrary to general notion, it is not intended for practical patient care. The clinicians caring for HIV-infected patients should pay more attention to the stage of their disease based on clinical and laboratory data, especially their CD4-positive cell count and the presence or absence of complications known to afflict their patients. This type of information is much more useful for proper patient care than the knowledge that the patient does or does not have AIDS.

A CD4-positive cell count of less than $200/mm^3$, or when less than 14% of total lymphocytes are CD4-positive, is one of the most important inclusion criteria in the CDC surveillance case definition for AIDS, as most of the complications included in the case definition occur when the CD4-positive cell count is this low. It should, however, be noted that some of the infectious or neoplastic complications included in the definition can occur with higher counts. Table 6–1 lists the important infections and their resultant clinical conditions in HIV-infected patients, which are included in the CDC case definition of AIDS. For more detailed information, the reader should consult an updated CDC publication on the subject.

TABLE 6–1. CLINICALLY IMPORTANT INFECTIOUS COMPLICATIONS OF HIV INFECTION

Causative Organism	Common Clinical Conditions
Viruses	
Human immunodeficiency virus (HIV)	HIV encephalopathy (AIDS dementia), HIV wasting syndrome
Cytomegalovirus (CMV)	Pneumonia, retinitis, dissemination
Epstein–Barr virus (EBV)	B-cell lymphoma
Herpes simplex virus (HSV)	Recurrent severe and protracted infection, esophagitis, pneumonia
Papovavirus	Progressive multifocal leukoencephalopathy
Protozoa	
Pneumocystis carinii	Pneumonia
Toxoplasma	Encephalitis
Cryptosporidia	Protracted diarrhea
Isospora	Protracted diarrhea
Fungi	
Candida	Mucocutaneous infection, esophagitis, tracheobronchitis, dissemination
Cryptococcus	Meningitis, pneumonia, dissemination
Histoplasma	Disseminated infection
Coccidioides	Disseminated infection
Mycobacteria	
M avium complex	Disseminated infection
M tuberculosis	Pulmonary and extrapulmonary tuberculosis, dissemination
Other Bacteria	
Salmonella	Recurrent sepsis
Encapsulated bacteria, staphylococci	Recurrent pneumonia, septicemia

■ EPIDEMIOLOGY AND TRANSMISSION OF HIV INFECTION

HIV infection is a pandemic in the true sense of the word. AIDS has been reported from almost every country in the world, with sub-Saharan Africa being hit the hardest. By June 1995, more than 1 million AIDS cases had been reported to the World Health Organization (WHO) from various countries around the world. Probably many more cases remain unreported. Reported cases to the WHO were the highest from the United States, where, by the end of 1995, more than half a million cases of AIDS were documented, with more than 300,000 deaths from the disease. After a peak number of cases of AIDS in 1993, the rate showed a downward trend in the United States. However, it is still the number one killer in men 25 to 44 years of age. The number of people infected with HIV can only be estimated. In the United States, 1 million infected persons is the most frequently quoted figure. Minorities represent much higher rates of infection and AIDS. Among the cities, Washington, DC has the highest AIDS rate, followed by Jersey City, San Francisco, New York City, and Miami (each had more than 100 cases per 100,000 residents in 1995).

Transmission of HIV infection occurs by sexual contact (homosexual and heterosexual), through blood, and from an infected mother to her infant. Infection by casual contact, as in households, schools, or workplaces, and transmission by insects are virtually unknown. In developing countries, as in Africa, heterosexual transmission is the most common; while in the United States, homosexual contact remains the predominant way of infection. However, there are an increasing number of cases in which the infection occurs by heterosexual transmission, particularly from HIV-infected IDUs and bisexual men. More than one-third of AIDS cases in the United States are directly or indirectly related to injection drug usage. With heterosexual contact, there is about 20 times greater chance of transmission from an infected man to a woman than from an infected woman to a man.

Transmission by blood mostly occurs among IDUs when a shared needle is contaminated with HIV-infected blood. The risk of occupational transmission in health-care and laboratory workers, although small, has engendered great fear and anxiety. Such a transmission is usually from an accidental skin puncture by a needle or other sharp object contaminated by HIV-infected blood. With strict adherence to *universal precautions,* occupational infection should not occur. By mandatory screening of donated blood for HIV since 1985, transmission of HIV by transfusion of blood or its products has been extremely rare.

Infants born to HIV-infected mothers have about a 30% chance to be infected, which usually occurs during pregnancy or delivery. Occasionally the virus is transmitted postnatally, most likely from breast milk.

Infectivity of individuals with HIV infection is variable, but there is a significant correlation between the severity of HIV-induced immunodeficiency and infectivity. Patients with full-blown AIDS are much more apt to infect others than are asymptomatic individuals with HIV infection. Public health measures for prevention of the spread of this dreadful infection will not succeed without an intense educational campaign. Such measures, together with proper education, seem to have been effective in many homosexual communities. Unfortunately, the spread of infection among IDUs not only remains unabated, but also continues to rise.

DIAGNOSIS AND THERAPEUTIC APPROACH TO PATIENTS WITH HIV INFECTION

As mentioned earlier, during most of its course, HIV infection causes no symptoms. When symptoms occur during the early stages of infection, they are nonspecific. Even at the advanced stage, when one or more of AIDS-defining conditions develops, diagnosis of HIV infection is presumptive. Therefore, the only way of making a definitive diagnosis necessitates demonstration of the virus or its antigenic components. The highly specific and sensitive test for HIV antibody has made it a clinically acceptable means for making or excluding a diagnosis of HIV infection. Except for a period of about 1 to 3 months after infection, the antibody test will become positive. When serum samples are positive by screening with ELISA (enzyme-linked immunosorbent assay) method in two consecutive tests, they are checked with an even more specific Western blot assay for confirmation. With this approach, false-positive test results will be exceedingly rare, especially in the high-risk population. Testing for detection of antibody is advisable in such populations or when HIV infection is suspected on other clinical grounds. HIV testing is done on a patient's request and, if medically recommended, with the patient's consent. The patient is informed of the result, which is kept confidential.

Knowledge of a positive test result will be more useful when the immunologic status of the patient is also determined. Currently, the most useful test for this purpose is measurement of CD4-positive lymphocyte count. In such a patient, the diagnosis of various complicating infectious or malignant disorders should be made expediously. Prophylactic and therapeutic measures will be planned on the basis of these clinical and laboratory data.

Therapeutic measures intended for control of HIV infection are based on the use of antiviral agents, which are inhibitors of viral enzymes important for the life cycle of the retroviruses. The earlier antiretroviral drugs were inhibitors of reverse transcriptase. Zidovudine (ZDV or AZT), which was developed first, has remained the antiviral agent of choice in this class for patients who tolerate it. Other antireverse transcriptases are alternative agents. The beneficial effect of this group of drugs is limited because of the development of resistance by HIV and the significant side effects of the drugs. Recently introduced antiproteases, such as saquinavir, that inhibit a different step in the HIV life cycle, are promising. Combination therapy with different mechanisms of action is additive and may also be synergistic. Development of newer antiviral drugs, results of ongoing clinical trials on various drug regimens, and revision of their indication in different stages of immunosuppression will continue to change the therapeutic recommendations for HIV infection. None of the available drugs so far has been considered to be curative.

Prophylactic and therapeutic regimens aimed at pulmonary complications of HIV infection follow. Discussion of prophylaxis and treatment of other complications is beyond the scope of this book.

■ PULMONARY COMPLICATIONS OF HIV INFECTION

Pulmonary disorders are the major causes of mortality and morbidity in patients with HIV infection. Normally the respiratory tract, in spite of its constant exposure to environmental pathogenic agents, is well protected because of its intricate and highly effective defense system. Alveolar macrophages with their inherent phagocytic activities and their ability to recruit other immunologically competent cells, particularly T lymphocytes, play an essential role in dealing with agents that have eluded the mechanical defenses of the airways. It is, therefore, understandable that deficiency of cellular immunity resulting from HIV infection readily predisposes the lungs to invasion by microorganisms that would normally be held in check. Viruses, mycobacteria, fungi, and protozoa are such organisms that are often considered as opportunistic. Defective B-cell function and quantitative and qualitative abnormalities of phagocytic blood cells resulting from an advanced stage of HIV infection and/or medications facilitate respiratory infection with common bacteria. Easy recognition of respiratory symptoms and signs, ready radiographic detection of lung lesions, and the early effect of lung lesions on pulmonary function and blood gases make pulmonary complications quite apparent. The exact nature of them, however, may not be recognized clinically. A postmortem study of a large number of patients who died of AIDS showed that almost all of them had pathologic evidence of pulmonary disease, many with more

than one pathologic condition, although a significant number of these conditions were not diagnosed correctly before death. Severe and progressive respiratory failure as a consequence of pulmonary complications is considered to be the most common cause of death in patients with AIDS.

Pulmonary complications of HIV infection in the remainder of this chapter are discussed according to their causes, which are either infectious or noninfectious, although the exact cause(s) of some of them is (are) unknown. Infectious complications are by far the most common. Clinical manifestations of these complications almost always include respiratory symptoms of cough and progressive dyspnea. Chest pain is relatively uncommon. Systemic symptoms of fever, malaise, anorexia, and weight loss are frequently present. Radiographic studies may show recognizable patterns; however, they are not by themselves diagnostic. It is the patient's history of either known HIV infection or being in a risk group for such an infection that makes the clinician consider not only the usual but, more often, the unusual causes of respiratory disease.

Pneumocystis carinii Pneumonia

Pneumocystis carinii pneumonia (PCP) was the first opportunistic infection identified in the original cases of AIDS described in 1981. Since then, it proved to be the most common clinically recognizable complication of HIV infection. Although with the introduction of prophylactic measures its incidence has somewhat diminished, it still occurs in the majority of patients at some time during the course of HIV infection. In many patients, it occurs more than once during their shortened lifetime.

Pathogenesis and Pathophysiology. *Pneumocystis carinii* has been recognized as a protozoan, although its exact taxonomy has been questioned and based on molecular biological information, it is now considered to be a fungus by many experts. Identification is by its distinctive morphologic and staining features. It is believed that most healthy persons become infected without developing the disease. In the past, it was thought that PCP developed as a result of reactivation of a dormant infection with the development of a cell-mediated immunodeficiency state. Recent epidemiologic data indicate that most cases develop from reinfection. Lungs are the primary, and often the only, site of active disease. Rarely, other organs have been shown to become infected. The onset of PCP signifies an advanced deficiency of cell-mediated immunity, and there is a strong correlation between its occurrence and the number of CD4-positive lymphocytes. AIDS patients with PCP have a CD4-positive lymphocyte count of less than $200/mm^3$, and at times fewer than $100/mm^3$.

The organisms, unopposed by lung defenses, occupy the surface of alveolar epithelial lining and attach to type I alveolar cells. They go through continual cycles of trophozoite stage and cyst formation and, in the process, multiply rapidly, filling the alveolar spaces. The number of organisms in PCP secondary to AIDS is larger than in PCP due to other immunosuppressed states. Increased alveolar capillary permeability, exudation of fluid, infiltration with inflammatory cells, and loss of surfactant are the pathologic changes that, together with an abundant

number of organisms, result in severe impairment of gas transport.

Clinical Presentation. Clinical manifestations of PCP in AIDS patients usually begin insidiously and progress slowly. Fever, cough, and increasing dyspnea are typical presenting symptoms. Cough is nonproductive, and dyspnea may only be noted with exertion. Chest pain is uncommon, but some patients may complain of peculiar retrosternal discomfort mostly with inspiration. Most patients do not seek medical advice for several weeks from the onset of symptoms. By the time that they consult a physician, most have significant dyspnea.

Physical examination of a patient with PCP usually indicates fever with evidence of associated conditions seen in most AIDS patients, such as oral thrush, wasting, and generalized lymphadenopathy. Signs of respiratory difficulty, such as tachypnea, are often apparent. Examination of the lungs may be normal in spite of significant abnormalities in radiographic film.

Diagnostic Studies. Radiographic study of the chest often suggests the diagnosis in patients with HIV infection or high-risk behavior with the previously mentioned clinical presentation. The study usually shows a diffuse interstitial and sometimes an alveolar pattern of density throughout the lungs (Fig. 6–3). If the study is done earlier, it may show only minimal or no changes. Atypical patterns, such as focal consolidation, perihilar density, or cystic changes, may alsobe seen. Hilar lymphadenopathy and pleural effusions are rarely seen with PCP alone. Their presence should suggest other diagnoses. Radionuclide scanning by gallium-67 or indium-111 is a helpful study when chest

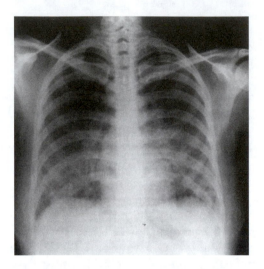

Figure 6–3. A radiograph of a patient with PCP.

radiograph is normal or shows questionable changes. Significant pulmonary uptake of these radioisotopes with normal chest x-ray film is highly suggestive of PCP. Pulmonary function tests indicate restrictive impairment with reduced diffusion capacity. The latter is very sensitive in detecting early disease. A normal diffusing capacity virtually excludes the presence of PCP. It should be noted, however, that reduced diffusion capacity may be secondary to long-standing IV drug use. Blood-gas abnormalities may also be noted early in the course of PCP. Low Po_2, usually with low Pco_2, is common (increased alveolar–arterial O_2 gradient). Besides its diagnostic value, arterial blood gas (ABG) findings help in determining the severity of disease. Serum lactic dehydrogenase (LDH) usually is quite high in PCP.

Although PCP is often suspected on clinical grounds supported by radiographic and other studies, its definitive diagnosis necessitates demonstration of organisms from a specimen of lung secretion or tissue. As patients with PCP usually do not produce sputum spontaneously, it should be induced by hypertonic saline nebulized by an ultrasonic device. Adequate cleansing of the mouth and throat before the sputum induction, and proper collection, processing, and staining of sputum, are essential for a successful result. Diagnostic sensitivity of such a study, if properly done, is close to 70%. With improved staining techniques (such as fluorescent antibody) and introduction of DNA technology (PCR), the yield would be even higher. Bronchoscopy is usually performed when sputum induction is not possible or its result is not diagnostic. Bronchoalveolar lavage is preferred to brushing and transbronchial biopsy, unless other diagnostic possibilities are also seriously considered. Samples obtained bronchoscopically or by sputum induction should always be studied for other organisms, especially for mycobacteria. Figure 6–4 shows an algorithm that is used in diagnostic planning for AIDS or suspected AIDS patients presenting with significant respiratory symptoms.

Treatment and Prophylaxis. Therapeutic management of PCP in AIDS patients consists of treatment with an agent effective against pneumocystis and supportive care. Most patients, being hypoxemic, require oxygen therapy and may even need intubation and mechanical ventilatory support. A commonly used drug regimen at the time of this writing is either a combination of trimethoprim and sulfamethoxazole (TMP–SMX) or pentamidine, which is given for a 2- to 3-week period. Aerosolized pentamidine has proved ineffective for treatment of established PCP. Other regimens considered in patients who are intolerant to TMP–SMX or pentamidine include

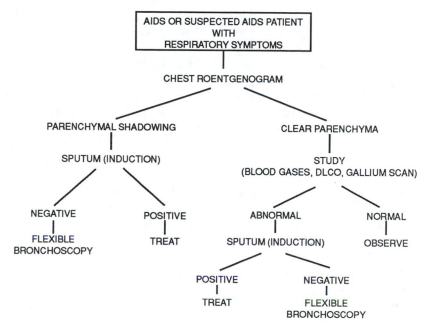

Figure 6–4. An algorithm for clinical approach to HIV-infected patients with respiratory symptoms.

dapsone–trimethoprim or atovaquone. As an adjunctive therapy, corticosteroid administration, along with antipneumocystis drugs, seems to improve survival in patients with AIDS complicated by moderately severe to severe PCP. It may prevent the occurrence of respiratory failure in these patients.

Prophylaxis against PCP is considered to be an essential part in management of HIV-infected persons. It is either primary or secondary. Primary prophylaxis is considered for patients before ever having PCP. It is currently recommended for patients with CD4-positive lymphocyte count below 200 or when less than 20% of blood lymphocytes are CD4-positive. Primary prophylaxis is also advised to HIV-positive patients with oral thrush, and some of the AIDS-defining conditions regardless of CD4-positive cell count. Secondary prophylaxis is given to patients who have recovered from a bout of PCP following adequate treatment. Oral TMP–SMX, given daily or three times weekly, is considered to be the most effective regimen for both primary and secondary prophylaxis. In patients who do not tolerate TMP–SMX, nebulized pantamidine is an acceptable alternative. It is devoid of serious side effects, but is less effective than TMP–SMX. Aerosolized pentamidine is administered every 4 weeks using a Respigard II or equivalent nebulizer with a special filter to remove pentamidine from exhaled air. Cough is a frequent complaint during treatment and wheezing is occasionally noted. These side effects are much more common in smokers and asthmatics. Pretreatment with a bronchodilator is effective in reducing these side effects.

Therapists or other health-care providers administering aerosolized pentamidine should be aware of the possibility of patients having active tuberculosis and should take appropriate measures to prevent exposure. This precaution should also be taken when sputum induction is carried out.

Tuberculosis

For general information on tuberculosis, the reader is referred to Chapter 4. As indicated in that chapter, infection with *Mycobacterium tuberculosis* in most instances remains dormant and suppressed by the body's defense system, and a positive reaction to the tuberculin skin test is the only evidence for such an infection. Reactivation of this latent infection is usually the result of alteration of defense mechanisms, especially weakening of the cell-mediated immunity. The epidemic of HIV infection has caused an extraordinary increase in the population of immunodeficient individuals, predisposing them to active tuberculosis. This disease has emerged as a very important complication of HIV infection, particularly among IV drug users who generally have a high prevalence of preexisting tuberculous infection. Primary infection in individuals with impaired cellular immunity is also known to develop easier than in immunocompetent persons, and it tends to become a progressive disease without going through a dormant stage. Threat of active tuberculosis in HIV-infected patients is therefore from both reactivation of a previous infection and their susceptibility to new infection and its progression. Moreover, once developed, tuberculosis advances more rapidly in such patients. The emergence of multidrug-resistant (MDR) tuberculosis has further compli-

cated the problem. In some cities in the United States, such as New York City, HIV-positive persons are much more likely to have MDR tuberculosis than are HIV-negative persons.

As in every case of active tuberculosis, the importance of its early recognition in HIV-infected patients cannot be overemphasized. Among the numerous infectious diseases complicating AIDS, tuberculosis is the only readily transmittable disease that can infect others, regardless of their immunologic state. Health workers should always be on the alert for tuberculosis whenever they are caring for AIDS patients. Prevalence of MDR tuberculosis in these patients makes such vigilence mandatory.

As in the general population, most common pathogenetic mechanism of tuberculous disease in HIV-infected patients is the reactivation of a latent tuberculous focus. It usually develops before, rather than after, the diagnosis of AIDS. Probably because of higher virulence and pathogenecity of *M tuberculosis* than other truly opportunistic organisms such as *P carinii,* active tuberculosis develops with a lesser degree of immunodeficiency. It has been shown that the number of CD4-positive lymphocytes (an excellent indicator of immunologic state in HIV infection) is only moderately reduced when active tuberculosis is diagnosed. It seems, therefore, that it may be an early clinical manifestation of HIV infection, especially in individuals and populations known to have higher rates of tuberculous infection. The incidence of tuberculosis in patients meeting the criteria for the diagnosis of AIDS may be as high as 10%. When young patients with recently developed tuberculosis are checked for HIV antibody, a significant percentage of them proves positive, indicating that the incidence of HIV-related tuberculosis could be even higher. Therefore, not only is every patient with tuberculosis highly suspected of having coinfection with HIV, every HIV-infected person with symptoms is also suspected of having tuberculosis.

Clinical and radiographic features of tuberculosis occurring in HIV-infected patients vary significantly in relation to the stage of immunologic deficiency. When it develops in the early stage of HIV infection, it tends to have the features of tuberculosis in the general population with an apparently normal immunologic state (see Chapter 4). However, if it occurs when other manifestations of AIDS have developed, the clinical and radiographic characteristics may be quite different. In this setting, extrapulmonary and disseminated forms are much more common. Concurrent presence of other infectious or noninfectious complications in advanced stage of HIV infection makes the clinical picture even less clear. Pulmonary lesions may be atypical in their locations and other radiographic features. Hilar and mediastinal lymphadenopathy, predominant involvement of lower lung fields, the diffuse nature of infiltration, and lack of cavitation result in diagnostic difficulty.

Diagnosis of tuberculosis in HIV-infected patients necessitates a high index of suspicion. Intravenous drug users and other population groups with a history of tuberculosis exposure and/or with positive tuberculin test are primary suspects for active tuberculosis when presenting with respiratory or systemic symptoms. Tuberculin reaction, being a cellular hypersensitivity, may be negative in the late stage of HIV infection despite active tuberculosis. However, in its earlier stages when cellular immunity is still functional, a tuberculin test is useful in detecting tuberculous infection, and its result would be helpful for additional diagnostic and therapeutic planning. With increasing deterioration of immunologic state with HIV infection, reactivity to tuberculin progressively diminishes. To increase the diagnostic sensitivity of the tuberculin test, it has been recommended that a reaction size of >5 mm of induration (instead of >10 mm) at the site of intradermal injection of 5 tuberculin units of PPD be considered as positive when applied to patients with HIV infection. Frequently, negative test results in AIDS patients with active tuberculosis (anergy) indicate that additional diagnostic studies, such as bacteriologic examination of sputum and other available specimens, should be pursued whenever the diagnosis of tuberculosis is suspected, regardless of the result of the tuberculin test. As most patients with HIV infection and respiratory symptoms are studied for PCP, material obtained for this purpose should also be examined for tubercle bacilli. Common occurrence of atypical mycobacterial disease in AIDS makes cultural identification of acid-fast organisms mandatory. Antituberculosis therapy, however, should be initiated whenever acid-fast bacilli are seen in sputum or other specimens while awaiting its definitive identification by culture. The importance of drug susceptibility testing of positive culture for *M tuberculosis* cannot be overemphasized.

As discussed in Chapter 4, because of the likelihood of MDR tuberculosis in HIV-infected patients, an initial four-drug regimen is the currently recommended therapy for HIV-infected patients with active tuberculosis. It contains isoniazid, rifampin, pyrazinamide, and ethambutol. The drug regimen is modified once the result of drug susceptibility becomes available. Prophylaxis with isoniazid seems to be effective in reducing the incidence of tuberculosis in HIV-positive persons with a positive tuberculin test. It is given to such patients for a period of 12 months. In the presence of anergy (lack of reaction to tuberculin and other skin tests) in patients at high risk for tuberculosis, some experts recommend prophylaxis in HIV-positive individuals if active tuberculosis is excluded.

Atypical Mycobacterial Disease

Although other atypical mycobacteria may infect patients with AIDS, *M avium* complex (MAC) is by far the most significant. Infection with this organism in those patients with AIDS usually presents as a widely disseminated disease involving many organs as well as the bloodstream. The portal of entry is thought to be either the gut or the respiratory tract. The lungs may become the primary site of infection, which in normal hosts rarely ever spreads elsewhere. In some patients with an underlying chronic lung disease but normal immunologic state, MAC may cause local lesions. In severe deficiency of cell-mediated immunity, as in full-blown AIDS, it readily disseminates from its primary site. Pulmonary lesions may or may not be radiographically apparent. Disseminated disease with these organisms almost always denotes an advanced stage of HIV infection. This explains the lack of pathologic reaction in the form of granuloma formation, in spite of the presence of extremely large numbers of bacteria in involved organs.

Clinical manifestations of MAC disease in patients with AIDS is often ob-

scured by the concurrent presence of other complications. Systemic signs and symptoms of chills, fever, and weight loss are usually explained by other infectious or noninfectious conditions. Respiratory manifestations, if present, are nonspecific. Chest radiograph may be normal despite demonstration of acid-fast organisms in sputum. In many instances, the diagnosis is made on postmortem examination. In suspected patients, bone marrow biopsy may reveal the organisms. It can also be cultured from blood, bone marrow, or stools.

MAC is universally resistant to first-line antituberculosis drugs. The efficacy of most other drugs in various combinations has been disappointing. Regimens containing one of the new macrolides, especially clarithromycin, seem to show some efficacy against MAC disease. As the differentiation from *M tuberculosis* is not possible on morphologic or staining characteristics of the organisms, most patients with positive smear of sputum or other pathologic material are treated with antituberculosis drugs until proper identification of causative bacteria is made by culture.

Viral Pneumonia

Three prevalent herpesviruses, namely cytomegalovirus (CMV), herpes simplex virus (HSV), and varicella-zoster virus (VZV), may infect the lungs in AIDS patients. After infection earlier in life, under normal conditions these viruses live in a dormant state, contained by the body's cell-mediated immunity. Reactivation of this latent infection occurs when this important defense system weakens. Cytomegalovirus infection is by far the most common, and pulmonary involvement is a frequent occurrence in AIDS. It also infects other organs such as the eye, liver, and gastrointestinal tract. Although CMV is often isolated from respiratory-tract secretions or lung tissue from AIDS patients with pneumonic infiltration, its role is usually uncertain. Its association with PCP is very common. However, as most such patients improve after treatment for PCP, it appears that CMV has no clinically significant part in this situation. Uncommonly, CMV may be the sole agent responsible for pneumonia. Dyspnea and nonproductive cough are the usual symptoms in patients with CMV pneumonia. Isolation of the virus from pulmonary secretions is not diagnostic of CMV pneumonia. Its definitive diagnosis requires histologic and/or cytologic evidence of infection with this virus. There is no satisfactory treatment for CMV pneumonia.

Both HSV and VZV behave as opportunistic infections in AIDS patients; in addition to causing recurrent skin lesions, they may disseminate and involve other organs. Pulmonary involvement, although uncommon, may be the cause of severe hypoxemic respiratory failure. In view of the treatable nature of these infections, their early diagnosis is important. Acyclovir is effective against infection by both of these viruses.

Among other viruses implicated in causing pulmonary complications in AIDS patients, Epstein–Barr virus (EBV) is noteworthy. B-cell lymphoma in these patients is considered to be related to infection with EBV. Its role in causing interstitial pneumonia has also been suggested. Herpesvirus-like DNA sequence detected in Kaposi's sarcoma is supportive of the earlier view that this neoplastic lesion is caused by a virus.

Pulmonary Mycoses

Infection with *Candida albicans,* the most common fungal infection in AIDS, is the cause of oral thrush and may result in painful esophagitis. It uncommonly affects the tracheobronchial tree and rarely results in pneumonia. Clinically more significant mycotic diseases involving the lungs are histoplasmosis, coccidioidomycosis, and cryptococcosis, which may occur in patients with AIDS. As was mentioned in Chapter 5, both histoplasmosis and coccidioidomycosis may manifest as widespread disease in immunocompromised patients.

Cases of disseminated histoplasmosis in AIDS patients are being reported mostly from the endemic areas, although some have occurred in patients from nonendemic regions, most likely as a result of activation of an earlier infection. Its clinical manifestations are nonspecific and difficult to differentiate from those of other conditions occurring in AIDS. Pulmonary involvement may mimic PCP or tuberculosis and may progress to respiratory failure. Diagnosis of disseminated histoplasmosis can only be made by demonstration and identification of its causative fungus, *Histoplasma capsulatum,* from involved tissues or blood. The clinical course of histoplasmosis is more severe and its response to amphotericin B and other antifungal agents is less satisfactory in AIDS than in other immunosuppressed states.

Disseminated coccidioidomycosis in AIDS patients has been reported only from endemic areas. Whether it is the result of reactivation of a dormant infection or progression of a recent infection is not known. It seems that either mechanism may cause dissemination in severely immunocompromised persons. The lungs are almost always involved and pleural effusion is common. Both systemic and pulmonary manifestations are nonspecific. Central nervous system (CNS) signs and skin lesions are not uncommon. The diagnosis is made by identification of the fungus *Coccidioides immitis* from sputum, bronchoscopically obtained material, pleural effusion, or other tissues. Serologic tests are less useful for the diagnosis of coccidioidomycosis in AIDS. Treatment, although less effective, is the administration of amphotericin B.

Cryptococcal disease in AIDS patients is predominantly a CNS disorder in the form of meningitis or cerebral infection. The primary infection, however, occurs in the lungs in a more or less silent manner, from which it disseminates to other organs, especially the CNS. Clinically apparent pulmonary disease from *Cryptococcus neoformans* often coexists with CNS infection. It may cause pneumonic consolidation, interstitial infiltration, or pleural effusion. Diagnosis is usually made by the examination of bronchoscopically obtained material. In patients suspected to have cryptococcal infection, cerebrospinal fluid should always be examined. Fluconazole or itraconazole are effective against pulmonary cryptococcal infection. In some patients, treatment with amphotericin B with flucytosine will be necessary.

Because of frequent relapses after initial response, lifelong suppressive treatment with one of the oral antifungal agents is often recommended for fungal pneumonias in HIV-infected patients.

Bacterial Pneumonia

Although earlier the most frequent infections in HIV-positive patients were from opportunistic organisms, in recent years the common pathogenic bacteria have become the predominant causes of pneumonia in this patient population. In view of its high morbidity and mortality in untreated or improperly treated patients, bacterial pneumonia should always be considered in the differential diagnosis of pulmonary disease in HIV-infected patients. Response to adequate antibacterial treatment in these patients is generally good. *Streptococcus pneumoniae* and *Haemophilus influenzae* are the organisms most commonly involved. Infection with these bacteria is much more prevalent in HIV-infected individuals than in an age-matched control group. Sinusitis from these organisms is very prevalent in all stages of HIV infection. As mentioned earlier in this chapter, a higher incidence of infection with bacteria, especially encapsulated organisms, is related mainly to the abnormality of humoral immunity that occurs in patients with HIV infection. Deficiency of antibody production in response to new infections is compounded by impaired phagocytic activity of macrophages and, perhaps, granulocytes. Bacterial pneumonia occurs more frequently in IV drug users than other risk groups with HIV infection. Other bacteria that are known to cause pneumonia in this population include *Moraxella catarrhalis*, *Klebsiella pneumoniae,* and *Staphylococcus aureus.* In advanced stage of HIV infection in patients with granulocytopenia (usually drug induced), pulmonary infection from *Pseudomonas aeruginosa* is being encountered in an increasing number of patients.

Clinical manifestations of bacterial pneumonia in HIV-infected or AIDS patients are not much different from those seen in immunocompetent hosts. The onset of symptoms of chills, fever, and cough is abrupt and more acute than those due to PCP. Other distinguishing features are sputum production and pleuritic chest pain, which are usually lacking in PCP. Chest x-ray film may show lobar, segmental, or diffuse infiltrations. Bacterial pneumonia may coexist with an opportunistic pulmonary infection, such as PCP. Both the rate of recurrence and frequency of bacteremia are higher when the pneumonia occurs in HIV-infected patients than in the general population.

Diagnosis of bacterial pneumonia is based on clinical presentation and the result of sputum examination. Blood cultures should always be obtained. Its treatment is similar to the treatment of community-acquired pneumonia in the general population as discussed in Chapter 3. Active immunization with pneumococcal vaccine is recommended for HIV-infected individuals. Its effectiveness, however, is generally inadequate. In patients with recurrent bacterial pneumonia, antibacterial prophylaxis has been advocated. TMP–SMX for PCP prophylaxis seems to reduce the incidence and recurrence rate of bacterial pneumonia.

Malignant Disease Involving the Lungs

Although immunologic deficiency as a contributing factor in the pathogenesis of the malignant process has been known for a long time, AIDS has added a new dimension to this intriguing oncologic phenomenon. Among neoplastic diseases, Kaposi's sarcoma (KS) stands alone as a highly prevalent malignancy in AIDS. There is also a relatively increased incidence of non-Hodgkin's lymphomas.

Although recognized for more than a century before the AIDS epidemic, KS in the Western world occurred only rarely as a slow-growing malignancy in older individuals. In association with HIV infection, this neoplasm behaves as a highly aggressive multicentric cancer whose onset often signifies an advanced stage of immunodeficiency. For no apparent reason, it is more prevalent among homosexuals than IV drug users or hemophiliacs. This marked difference in its incidence and other epidemiologic data suggest that KS is related to infection with a virus that is transmitted mainly through homosexual activity along with or in proximity to HIV infection. This virus has recently been identified to have herpesvirus-like DNA sequences (Kaposi's sarcoma–associated herpesvirus, or KSHV). KS may occur relatively early with HIV infection with only mild reduction in CD4-positive cell count. In recent years its incidence has been declining, but its prognosis is becoming worse. Earlier in AIDS epidemics, almost 60% of homosexuals with AIDS developed KS in the course of their illness; recently, it occurs in about 20%. Skin and mucous membranes are the most common sites of Kaposi's lesions, which appear as purplish to bluish nodules or plaques of various sizes. The gastrointestinal tract and lungs are often involved, usually following, but occasionally without, skin lesions. From autopsy studies, about 60% of patients with KS show evidence of pulmonary involvement, which may not have been clinically recognized. Tumors may develop in the lung parenchyma, bronchi, lymph nodes, and pleura. Although uncommon, bronchoscopically demonstrable changes appear as discrete, bright red mucosal lesions at the branching points of the bronchi, which are highly characteristic of pulmonary KS.

Clinically, pulmonary KS has no characteristic manifestations. Diagnosis is usually suspected when unexplained radiographic changes are seen in patients with cutaneous or mucosal KS. This cancer is responsible for about one-third of the episodes of pulmonary lesions in patients with known KS elsewhere in the body. Radiographic changes are more suggestive of KS when focal parenchymal or perihilar densities are seen with pleural effusion and intrathoracic lymph node enlargement. Pathologic diagnosis from bronchoscopically obtained material is not usually successful, even when apparent endobronchial lesions are biopsied. As thoracotomy is rarely performed for the evaluation of lung lesions in AIDS, the diagnosis of pulmonary KS remains uncertain in most incidences. Although pulmonary KS denotes a poor prognosis, most patients succumb to other, mostly infectious, complications of AIDS. Various treatment modalities are under investigation. Alpha interferon, although effective in cutaneous KS, has not been proved to benefit intrathoracic disease.

The AIDS-associated lymphomas constitute the second most common malignant complication. They are mostly B-cell tumors, probably caused by EBV infection. They behave differently from histologically similar tumors in immunocompetent patients. Extranodal lesions, which occur in the CNS, gastrointestinal tract, and intrathoracic organs, are common. These lymphomas are high-grade malignancies, progress rapidly, and often terminate fatally. Intrathoracic lesions may appear as pulmonary nodules, masses, interstitial infiltrates, pleural effusion, and/or mediastinal lymphadenopathy. The response of these lymphomas to chemotherapy is poor. With improvement in management of infectious complications of AIDS, patients are now living longer with advanced stage of immunodeficiency. As a result, the incidence of malignancy, particularly lymphoma, is increasing.

Other Noninfectious Pulmonary Complications

Diffuse interstitial pattern is a common radiographic change due to pulmonary complications of AIDS. The vast majority of cases are infectious in nature and occasionally are due to a malignancy. In association with HIV infection, however, other interstitial lung diseases develop whose etiology and pathogenesis are poorly understood. Two forms of interstitial lung disease of unknown cause have been described: nonspecific interstitial pneumonitis (NIP) and lymphocytic interstitial pneumonitis (LIP). NIP has been reported in up to one-third of HIV-infected patients with interstitial lung disease. Histologically, it is characterized by alveolar cell hyperplasia and interstitial inflammatory infiltrates by lymphocytes, macrophages, and plasma cells. Clinical manifestations include fever, nonproductive cough, and mild dyspnea. Diagnosis is usually reached by exclusion of often suspected PCP and other specific causes of interstitial pneumonia. Definitive diagnosis requires lung biopsy. Clinical course of NIP is usually benign and spontaneous improvement is common.

LIP occurs rather frequently in children with HIV infection and meets the criteria for the diagnosis of AIDS if the patient is younger than 13 years of age. LIP has been reported in adults only sporadically, and occurs more commonly in blacks than in whites. Diffuse infiltration of the lungs by lymphocytes is the main pathologic finding. These cells have CD8 markers. Frequent association with peripheral blood lymphocytosis with an increased number of CD8-positive T cells suggests that these cells have a pathogenetic role in this disease. Clinical manifestations of cough and dyspnea have an insidious onset. Chest radiograph shows bilateral reticulonodular densities predominantly involving the lower lung fields, often mimicking PCP. Although transbronchial biopsy may suggest the diagnosis, it can only be proved by open lung biopsy. As spontaneous improvement may take place, a period of observation is recommended before deciding for treatment with corticosteroids.

Other intrathoracic complications of HIV infection that should be mentioned are pleural effusions, pneumothorax, bullous lung disease, primary pulmonary hypertension, and cardiac pulmonary edema.

BIBLIOGRAPHY

Agostini C, Trentin L, Zambello R, Semenzato G. HIV-1 and the lung: infectivity, pathogenic mechanism, and cellular immune responses taking place in the lower respiratory tract. *Am Rev Respir Dis.* 1993; 147:1038–1049.

American Thoracic Society. Fungal infection in HIV-infected persons. *Am J Respir Crit Care Med.* 1995; 152:816–822.

Ampel NM, Dols CL, Galgiani JN. Coccidioidomycosis during immunodeficiency virus infection: result of a prospective study in a coccidioidal endemic area. *Am J Med.* 1993; 93:235–240.

Barnes PF, Silva C, Otaya M. Testing for human immunodeficiency virus infection in patients with tuberculosis. *Am J Respir Crit Care Med.* 1996; 153:1448–1450.

Beck JM, Shellito J. Effects of human immunodeficiency virus on pulmonary host defenses. *Semin Respir Infect.* 1989; 4:75–84.

Bozzette SA, Finkelstein DM, Spector SA, et al. A randomized trial of three antipneumocystis agents in patients with advanced HIV infection. *N Engl J Med.* 1995; 332:693–699.

Cadranel J, Mayaud C. Intrathoracic Kaposi's sarcoma in patients with AIDS. *Thorax.* 1995; 50:407–414.

Centers for Disease Control. AIDS associated with injecting-drug use—United States. *MMWR.* 1996; 45:392–398.

Centers for Disease Control. Guidelines for prophylaxis against *Pneumocystis carinii* pneumonia in persons infected with human immunodeficiency virus. *MMWR.* 1992; 41(RR-4):1–11.

Centers for Disease Control. HSPHS/IDSA guidelines for prevention of opportunistic infections in persons infected with human immunodeficiency virus: a summary. *MMWR.* 1995; RR-8:1–34.

Centers for Disease Control and Prevention. 1993 revised classification system for HIV infection and expanded surveillance definition of AIDS among adolescents and adults. *MMWR.* 1992; 41(RR-17):1–19.

Chaisson RE. Bacterial pneumonia in patients with human immunodeficiency virus infection. *Semin Respir Infect.* 1989; 4:133–138.

Davey RT Jr, Lane HC. Laboratory methods in the diagnosis and prognostic staging of infection with human immunodeficiency virus type 1. *Rev Infect Dis.* 1990; 12:912–930.

DeLorenzo LJ, Huang CT, Maguire GP, Stone DJ. Roentgenographic patterns of *Pneumocystis carinii* pneumonia in 104 patients with AIDS. *Chest.* 1987; 91:323–327.

Fauci AS. Multifactorial nature of human immunodeficiency virus disease: implications for therapy. *Science.* 1993; 262:1011–1018.

Fish DG, Ampel NM, Galgiani JN, et al. Coccidioidomycosis during human immunodeficiency virus infection. *Medicine.* 1990; 69:384–391.

Gagnon S, Boota AM, Fischl MA, et al. Corticosteroids as adjunctive therapy for severe *Pneumocystis carinii* pneumonia in the acquired immunodeficiency syndrome. *N Engl J Med.* 1990; 323:1444–1450.

Gallant JE, Moore RD, Chaisson RE. Prophylaxis for opportunistic infections in patients with HIV infection. *Ann Intern Med.* 1994; 120:932–944.

Godwin CR, Brown DT, Masur H, et al. Sputum induction: a quick and sensitive technique for diagnosing *Pneumocystis carinii* pneumonia in immunosuppressed patients. *Respir Care.* 1991; 36:33–39.

Graham NMH, Chaisson RE. Tuberculosis and HIV infection: epidemiology, pathogenesis, and clinical aspects. *Ann Allergy.* 1993; 71:421–428.

Graybill JR. Histoplasmosis and AIDS. *J Infect Dis.* 1988; 158:623–626.

Horsburgh CR Jr. *Mycobacterium avium* complex infection in the acquired immunodeficiency syndrome. *N Engl J Med.* 1991; 324:1332–1338.

Ioannidis JPA, Cappelleri JC, Skolnik PP, et al. A meta-analysis of the relative efficiency and toxicity of *Pneumocystis carinii* prophylaxis regimens. *Arch Intern Med.* 1996; 156:177–188.

Janoff EN, O'Brien J, Thompson P, et al. *Streptococcus pneumoniae* colonization, bacteremia, and immune response among persons with human immunodeficiency virus infection. *J Infect Dis.* 1993; 167:49–56.

Kramer EL, Sanger JH, Garay SM, et al. Diagnostic implications of Ga-67 chest scan patterns in human immunodeficiency virus–seropositive patients. *Radiology.* 1989; 170:671–676.

Lane HC, Laughton BE, Falloon J, et al. Recent advances in the management of AIDS-related opportunistic infections. *Ann Intern Med.* 1994; 120:945–955.

Leoung GS, Feigal DW, Montgomery AB, et al. Aerosolized pentamidine for prophylaxis against *Pneumocystis carinii* pneumonia. *N Engl J Med.* 1990; 323:769–775.

Levy JA. The transmission of HIV and factors influencing progression to AIDS. *Am J Med.* 1993; 95:86–100.

Masur H. Prevention and treatment of pneumocystis pneumonia. *N Engl J Med.* 1992; 327:1835–1860.

Masur H, Ognibene FP, Yarchoan R, et al. CD4 counts as predictors of opportunistic pneu-monias in human immunodeficiency virus (HIV) infection. *Ann Intern Med.* 1989; 111:223–231.

Medin DL, Ognibene FP. Pulmonary disease in AIDS: implications for respiratory care practitioners. *Respir Care.* 1995; 40:832–854.

Meduri GU, Stein DS. Pulmonary manifestations of acquired immunodeficiency syndrome. *Clin Infect Dis.* 1992; 14:98–113.

Miller RF, Mitchell DM. *Pneumocystis carinii* pneumonia. *Thorax.* 1995; 50:191–200.

Mitchell DM, Miller RF. New development in the pulmonary diseases affecting HIV infected individuals. *Thorax.* 1995; 50:294–302.

Murphy RL, Lavelle JP, Allan JD, et al. Aerosol pentamidine prophylaxis following *Pneumocystis carinii* pneumonia in AIDS patients. *Am J Med.* 1991; 90:418–426.

New drugs for HIV infection. *Med Lett Drugs Ther.* 1996; 38:35–37.

O'Brien WA, Hartigan PM, Martin D, et al. Changes in plasma HIV-1 RNA and CD4+ lymphocyte counts and the risk of progression to AIDS. *N Engl J Med.* 1996; 334:426–431.

O'Riordan TG, Smaldone GC. Exposure of health care workers to aerosolized pentamidine. *Chest.* 1992; 101:1494–1499.

Pantaleo G, Graziosi C, Fauci AS. The immunopathogenesis of human immunodeficiency virus infection. *N Engl J Med.* 1993; 328:327–335.

Polish LB, Cohn DL, Ryder JW, et al. Pulmonary non-Hodgkin's lymphoma in AIDS. *Chest.* 1989; 96:1321–1326.

Pulmonary complications of HIV infection. *Semin Respir Crit Care Med.* 1995; 16:161–260.

Rosen MJ. Pneumonia in patients with HIV infection. *Med Clin North Am.* 1994; 78: 1067–1079.

Safrin S, Finkelstein OM, Feinberg J, et al. Comparison of these regimens for treatment of mild to moderate *Pneumocystis carinii* pneumonia in patients with AIDS. *Ann Intern Med.* 1996; 124:792–802.

Schooley RT. Cytomegalovirus in the setting of infection with human immunodeficiency virus. *Rev Infect Dis.* 1990; 12(suppl 7):S811–S819.

Shelhamer JH, Gill VJ, Quinn TC, et al. The laboratory evaluation of opportunistic pulmonary infections. *Ann Intern Med.* 1996; 124:585–599.

Smith GH. Treatment of infections in the patient with acquired immunodeficiency syndrome. *Arch Intern Med.* 1994; 154:949–973.

Taylor IK, Coker RJ, Clarke J, et al. Pulmonary complications of HIV disease. *Thorax.* 1995; 50:1240–1245.

Tindall B, Cooper DA. Primary HIV infection: host responses and intervention strategies. *AIDS.* 1991; 5:1–14.

Wachter RM, Russi MB, Bloch DA, et al. *Pneumocystis carinii* pneumonia and respiratory failure in AIDS: improved outcomes and increased use of intensive care units. *Am Rev Respir Dis.* 1991; 143:251–256.

Walworth CM, Tavel JA, Kovacs JA. Treatment and prevention of opportunistic infections in patients with human immunodeficiency virus infection. *Adv Intern Med.* 1996; 41:31–84.

Wasser L, Talavera W. Pulmonary cryptococcosis in AIDS. *Chest.* 1987; 92:692–695.

Weiss JR, Pietra GG, Scharf SM. Primary pulmonary hypertension and the human immunodeficiency virus. *Arch Intern Med.* 1995; 155:2350–2354.

Wheat LJ, Connolly-Stringfield PA, Baker RL, et al. Disseminated histoplasmosis in the acquired immunodeficiency: clinical findings, diagnosis, and treatment, and review of the literature. *Medicine.* 1990; 69: 361–374.

White DA, Matthay RA. Noninfectious pulmonary complications of infection with the human immunodeficiency virus. *Am Rev Respir Dis.* 1989; 140:1763–1787.

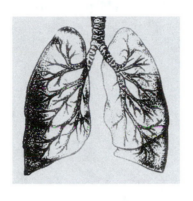

OBSTRUCTIVE
AIRWAYS DISEASES

7.

Diseases of the Upper Respiratory Tract: Upper Airway Obstruction

The upper respiratory tract includes the nose, paranasal sinuses, pharnyx, larynx, and trachea. The pharynx is divided into three continuous components: nasopharynx, the section above the soft palate; oropharynx, the part that can be seen when the mouth is wide open and the tongue is depressed; and hypopharynx or laryngopharynx, the part below the level of the epiglottis to the level of the cricoid cartilage. The last two parts make a common pathway for both food and air. The nasopharynx above and the larynx below are protected by the proper function of the soft palate and the epiglottis, which close them respectively with the act of deglutition and/or vomiting. The larynx is also divided into three regions: supra-glottic, glottic, and subglottic (Fig. 7–1). The trachea is divided into extrathoracic and intrathoracic portions.

In the course of their physiologic functions of warming, humidifying, and cleansing inspired air, the upper airways are exposed to a variety of irritants, allergens, and infectious agents. Upper respiratory infections, which include the common cold, are the most prevalent disorders of the respiratory tract. There are several noninfectious pathologic conditions that may also involve the upper respiratory tract. As some of these disorders may result in clinically significant respiratory complications by impeding airflow, they are discussed briefly in this chapter.

129

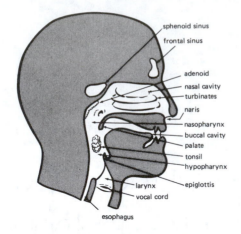

Figure 7–1. Upper respiratory tract.

■ NASAL AND NASOPHARYNGEAL OBSTRUCTION

Because of the presence of dual pathways to the pharynx through the nose and the mouth, obstruction of the nose and the nasopharynx usually does not result in ventilatory impairment. The long-held belief that newborn infants are obligate nasal breathers has recently been refuted. It has been demonstrated that infants become able to mouth-breathe after a short but variable interval following nasal obstruction. Chronic obstructive lesions in these locations, as seen in individuals with chronically enlarged adenoids, have been implicated in sleep-related breathing disorders (see Chapter 25). Obstruction in these areas may be the cause of some difficulties encountered during oxygen administration by the nasal route, nasopharyngeal or nasotracheal intubation, and suctioning. Moreover, with mouth breathing, inspired air may not be properly warmed or humidified, resulting in dryness and irritation of the upper air passages.

■ OROPHARYNGEAL AND HYPOPHARYNGEAL OBSTRUCTION

As a common pathway for both food and respired air, this part of the pharynx is endowed with several deglutitory muscles, not the least of which is the tongue. It has been demonstrated that the respiratory control system also regulates the tone of muscles in this area, preventing their relaxation and their tendency to collapse during inspiration. As the weight of the tongue tends to displace it backward in the supine position, the importance of adequate muscle tone in this position is obvious. A common problem in unconscious patients is the obstruction of the airway as a result of total relaxation of the jaw muscles, the tongue, and the pharyngeal wall (Fig. 7–2).

In the obstructive form of sleep apnea, as discussed in Chapter 25, the obstruction to airflow during inspiration most commonly occurs in the oropharynx. It results from periodic loss of muscle tone of the tongue and the pharynx during certain stages of sleep. During apnea, the tongue is displaced backward, touching the soft palate and the uvula;

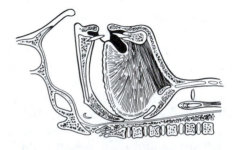

Figure 7–2. Hypopharyngeal obstruction in comatose patient in supine position. Obstruction results from relaxation of the muscles of the jaw, tongue, and pharyngeal wall, causing backward displacement of the base of the tongue.

the relaxed pharyngeal wall at this level is sucked toward the base of the tongue with inspiratory effort, thus completing the obstruction. Snoring, which is an invariable feature of this type of obstructive sleep apnea, is from vibration or flutter of the soft palate and uvula between the base of the tongue and the posterior pharyngeal wall when the air passage is incompletely obstructed.

Sudden upper airway obstruction may develop from the impaction of a large piece of food in the hypopharynx (Fig. 7–3). This may occur as a result of poor eating habits, particularly when the victim attempts to swallow an improperly chewed and excessively large bite of meat. This catastrophic event, known since antiquity, has been highly publicized, and its on-site emergency treatment effectively popularized in recent years, thanks to H. J. Heimlich's innovative effort.

Other causes of pharyngeal obstruction include neoplastic lesions, traumatic injury, and marked inflammatory swelling of the pharyngeal wall. Retropharyngeal abscess is an important cause of upper airway obstruction at the pharyngeal level, especially in children younger than 6 years of age.

■ LARYNGEAL OBSTRUCTION

Because of peculiarities of structure and anatomic position of the larynx, this organ is a frequent site for upper airway obstruction from a variety of causes. The small size of the larynx in young children especially predisposes them to laryngeal obstruction. The most common cause in this age group is inflammation of laryngeal structures due to infection. Epiglottitis and croup, two major infectious causes of laryngeal obstruction, are discussed in more detail.

Obstruction at the level of the larynx has several other causes, which include foreign body aspiration, allergic or traumatic edema of the larynx, neoplastic lesions, congenital defects, and vocal cord dysfunction. Foreign body aspiration is fairly common in young children, mostly in toddlers. Although most small objects will pass through the larynx and lodge inside a bronchus, larger objects may cause laryngeal obstruction, which may be partial or complete. With complete obstruction, only a witness (usually a family member or babysitter) capable of performing maneuvers that can dislodge the obstructing object will be able to save the child's life. Edema of the larynx may be from an allergic reaction (angioedema) or a traumatic injury. Edema following removal of an endotracheal tube is well known. Laryngeal obstruction may result from lack of function of abductor muscles of vocal cords as in bilateral vocal cord paralysis. Increased activity of its adductor muscles will also cause closure of the glottis. Normally, the *glottic* opening widens during inspiration and narrows

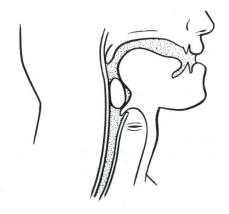

Figure 7–3. Hypopharyngeal obstruction by a bolus of food.

during expiration. A paradoxical vocal cord adduction during inspiration may occur with no obvious organic cause resulting in partial laryngeal obstruction. In the past, laryngeal diphtheria was one of the common causes of upper airway obstruction in the United States. With regular immunization, it is rarely seen in this country, but is still common in most developing countries. Recent resurgence of diphtheria in many eastern European countries, especially in the former Soviet Union, underscores the importance of a diligent vaccination program in preventing the outbreak of this potentially fatal disease.

Epiglottitis

Supraglottic obstruction is commonly due to *epiglottitis,* which is one of the most serious infectious diseases in young children. It is usually caused by *Haemophilus influenzae* type b. Since the widespread immunization of infants and children with vaccine against this organism, the incidence of epiglottitis in children has significantly declined. It should be noted that epiglottitis occurs in adults with increasing frequency. In adults, its cause is not always obvious. Besides *H influenzae,* other organisms such as *Staphylococcus aureus, Streptococcus pneumoniae,* beta-hemolytic streptococcus, and *Moraxella catarrhalis* may be involved. Although epiglottitis in adults can also result in upper airway obstruction, it does so much less often than in young children. It can occur at any time of year, but occurs more commonly during the winter and early spring. Infection and resulting inflammation in epiglottitis, despite its name, are rarely limited to the epiglottis, but involve other supraglottic structures, including

aryepiglottic folds and adjacent loose connective tissues. Pharynx, uvula, the base of the tongue, and false vocal cords may also be involved, especially in adults. *Supraglottitis* may be a more appropriate term. A swollen and enlarged epiglottis, however, seems to be the main cause of airway obstruction in this disease.

The onset of epiglottitis is quite sudden, especially in children. Sore throat, fever, odynophagia (painful swallowing), and muffled voice develop rapidly within several hours, followed by progressive respiratory distress and exhaustion. The afflicted child will be seen sitting up, leaning forward, drooling, and breathing rapidly. There is inspiratory retraction of intercostal and supraclavicular spaces. *Stridor* is, however, less common. In adults, the onset of epiglottitis is slower and presentation is less dramatic, but it may progress to respiratory difficulty from airway obstruction. The diagnosis of supraglottitis in adults is often delayed. However, in children, because of its striking and rapidly progressive symptomatology, epiglottitis is more readily recognized, or at least suspected, once they are brought to an emergency department. An attempt at direct visualization of the epiglottis should not be made without the presence of an anesthesiologist or otolaryngologist, as a marginal opening at supraglottic level may become compromised further. A lateral radiographic examination of the neck is usually diagnostic by showing an enlarged and swollen epiglottis ("thumb sign"), but should be done only if the diagnosis is in doubt and if there is no immediate danger of airway obstruction. This study is not indicated in severely ill patients with respiratory difficulty when epiglottitis is suspected. Because of a need for proper airway management, they should be under immediate care of an otolaryngologist or qualified anesthesiologist. A definitive diagnosis can be established when an adequate airway is established. Although in the past tracheostomy was preferred, endotracheal intubation now is considered to be the method of choice.

Diagnosis of supraglottitis in adults usually is made by direct examination of the supraglottic area by fiberoptic (flexible) pharyngolaryngoscopy. If findings confirm the diagnosis, patients' respiratory status should be closely monitored. Most adult patients will improve with conservative management. Only about 15% may need intubation. Antimicrobials for treatment of epiglottitis in both children and adults should be effective against *H influenzae* and other bacterial pathogens known to cause epiglottitis. A third-generation cephalosporin is the most commonly used antibiotic. A blood culture result may identify the offending pathogen, allowing for revision of antibiotic coverage. Although corticosteroids are used by some, there is no definite proof that they alter the clinical course of epiglottitis.

Croup

Croup is the most common cause of *subglottic* obstruction in children 6 months to 6 years of age. It is the result of a viral infection of the subglottic area of the larynx, trachea, and bronchi and is also known as laryngotracheobronchitis. By far the most common infectious agent is parainfluenza virus. Croup occurs most frequently in the late fall and early winter. Croup is characterized by a distinctive harsh barking or "croupy" cough, which may or may not be associated with hoarseness. Fever, if present, is of low grade. For

some unknown reason, male children are affected more often than female children. Croup has a rather fluctuating course, usually with nocturnal worsening, lasting for several days before full recovery. Stridor is usually appreciated during the inspiratory phase of cough; sometimes it is present with regular breathing. Occasionally croup may present as a life-threatening upper airway obstruction.

The diagnosis of croup, in most cases, is made by history and clinical presentation alone. It should be differentiated from epiglottitis. A radiographic study of the neck in posteroanterior (PA) and lateral views may be necessary in some cases, and may show characteristic narrowing of the subglottic larynx in croup. Most children with croup are treated on an outpatient basis, with proper instruction to parents regarding adequate humidification of the child's room. They may be given inhalational treatment with racemic epinephrine (or L-epinephrine) if symptoms warrant. If the child shows any indication of impaired airway or if supraglottitis cannot be excluded, he or she should be hospitalized for close observation and necessary treatment. Humidification with oxygen supplementation is the usual treatment. Aerosolized epinephrine (racemic or L-epinephrine) is administered with any indication of airway compromise. In recent years, corticosteroid therapy in the form of injectable dexamethasone has been used increasingly for treatment of croup. There are some studies indicating that corticosteroid-treated children show more rapid resolution of their stridor and the need for tracheal inhalation is lessened. Although endotracheal intubation is relatively infrequent in croup, patients with evidence of increasing airway obstruction, progressive hypoxemia, and respiratory failure should have establishment of an adequate airway as the essential part of their medical care.

Spasmodic croup is referred to as a recurrent and transient condition in children. It has the characteristics of viral croup except that spasmodic croup occurs suddenly, without evidence of an infection. The symptoms usually develop suddenly at night, often improve without any treatment, and recur with no obvious cause. An allergic mechanism has been proposed. In severe cases, its treatment is the same as that for viral croup.

■ TRACHEAL OBSTRUCTION

Tracheal lesions are uncommon causes of upper airway obstruction. Well-recognized conditions resulting in tracheal obstruction are tracheal stenosis (following tracheostomy, prolonged tracheal intubation, or trauma) and tumors. The latter may be an intralumenal growth such as tracheal carcinoma or an extralumenal mass lesion compressing the trachea, particularly its intrathoracic portion. Another cause of airway obstruction at this area in children 3 years of age and younger is bacterial tracheitis, which is a superinfection of a viral respiratory illness. The most common organism causing bacterial tracheitis is *S aureus,* but other organisms such as *S pneumoniae, M catarrhalis,* and *H influenzae* may be involved. This condition, because of sloughing of the epithelial lining of the trachea and its clinical similarity to croup, is also called *pseudomembranous croup.* Findings on endoscopic examination are diagnostic. The majority of children with this condition will require endotracheal intubation

while being treated with an appropriate antibiotic.

■ DIAGNOSIS OF UPPER AIRWAY OBSTRUCTION

Prompt and accurate diagnosis of upper airway obstruction, its location, and its cause is the key for its proper management. Complete obstruction with no airflow should be diagnosed and treated on the scene immediately. In confronting an unconscious patient who may or may not be breathing, the possibility of airway obstruction should always be considered, and the establishment and maintenance of an adequate airway should be given the highest priority. In a situation in which there is no airflow, obstructed airway will be recognized in the process of resuscitation when the lungs cannot be inflated by artificial means or by mouth-to-mouth respiration. The diagnosis of

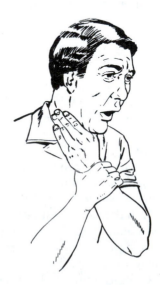

Figure 7–4. Universal distress signal for choking.

complete airway obstruction from food lodged in the hypopharynx is often made by individuals witnessing the incident. The victim, while eating, suddenly stops breathing and is unable to make any sound or cough, becoming pale and agitated. If the "universal distress sign for choking" is known, the person choking may grab his or her neck over the larynx with the thumb and index finger (Fig. 7–4).

Partial upper airway obstruction usually is suspected and diagnosed from a history and a physical examination. History of aspiration of a foreign object; traumatic injury or infection in or around the upper airways; alteration of voice; and respiratory symptoms, such as dyspnea, cough, wheezing, and stridor, should alert one to the possibility of partial obstruction. Physical findings of hoarseness or aphonia, inspira-

tory stridor, inspiratory and expiratory wheezes originating from the upper airway, inspiratory retraction of intercostal spaces and supraclavicular regions, and mass lesions in the pharynx are helpful diagnostic clues. Diagnosis of epiglottitis, croup, and bacterial tracheitis is discussed on pages 132–134.

The diagnosis of less acute or chronic airway obstruction from other causes, suspected from a history or a physical examination, is made by direct visualization or by endoscopy of the suspected area and appropriate radiologic studies, including computed tomography (CT) scanning. These studies also help in estimating the severity of the obstruction and selecting as well as timing the necessary therapeutic measures.

Partial upper airway obstruction is sometimes mistaken for disease of the

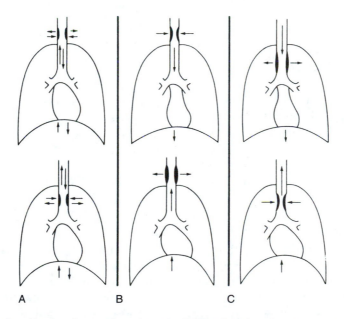

Figure 7–5. Extrathoracic and intrathoracic upper airway obstruction. (A) With a fixed obstruction, either extrathoracic (*top*) or intrathoracic (*bottom*), the obstruction size does not change with forced inspiration or expiration. (B) With variable extrathoracic obstruction, the obstruction is increased during forced inspiration (*top*) and is decreased during forced expiration (*bottom*). (C) With variable intrathoracic obstruction, the obstruction is diminished with forced inspiration (*top*) and increased with forced expiration (*bottom*).

lower respiratory tract, particularly asthma. Vocal cord dysfunction without an organic cause may sometimes result in significant respiratory difficulty, which is often erroneously diagnosed as asthma. Longstanding upper airway obstruction may also mimic chronic obstructive lung disease by its respiratory symptoms and complications, including hypoxemia, hypercapnia, and cor pulmonale. It also may manifest itself as sleep apnea syndrome (see Chapter 25).

Routine spirometry of a forced expiratory vital capacity may suggest the presence of partial upper airway obstruction. The maximum expiratory–inspiratory flow-volume loop, however, is most informative. Airways are subjected to changes in their lumen during a respiratory cycle according to the location of the airway inside or outside of the thorax. Intrathoracic airways will tend to widen during inspiration and narrow during expiration. The reverse is true with extrathoracic airways. This is because of changes in transmural pressure (the difference between the intraluminal and external pressure) during the respiratory cycle. If an obstructing lesion is pliable and thus influenced by the transmural pressure, it is called *variable;* if stiff and unyielding to pressure changes, it is termed *fixed* (Fig. 7–5). Therefore, in upper airway obstruction, a fixed lesion, regardless of its intrathoracic or extrathoracic location, will limit the airflow during both expiration and inspiration. A flow-volume loop obtained in a patient with this type of obstruction will show flattening of both the inspiratory and expiratory curves (Fig. 7–6B).

With an extrathoracic variable obstruction, the inspiratory half of the loop is mostly affected and thus flattened (Fig.

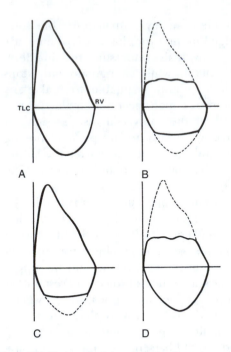

Figure 7–6. Maximum expiratory–inspiratory flow-volume loop. (A) Normal, (B) fixed (extrathoracic or intrathoracic) obstruction, (C) variable extrathoracic obstruction, and (D) variable intrathoracic obstruction. TLC, Total lung capacity; RV, residual volume.

7–6C); whereas with intrathoracic variable obstruction, the expiratory curve is flat (Fig. 7–6D).

■ MANAGEMENT OF UPPER AIRWAY OBSTRUCTION

The therapeutic strategy in upper airway obstruction will depend on several factors, which include the degree of obstruction; its progression, nature, and location; and associated conditions. However, the immediate therapeutic goal is the same; that is, establishing and maintaining adequate airflow.

In the management of unconscious patients with an obstruction resulting from backward displacement of the jaw and tongue, extending the neck and moving the mandible forward by chin lift will usually correct the pharyngeal obstruction. Extending the neck separates the posterior wall of the pharynx from the base of the tongue, while displacing the mandible forward by chin lift widens the pharynx further (Figs. 7–7 and 7–8). It should be emphasized, however, that whenever a traumatic cause for unconsciousness is suspected, the possibility of concomitant injury to the cervical spine should be considered and necessary precautions undertaken. Any foreign material or secretion should be removed by suctioning or other means. Insertion of an oropharyngeal or nasopharyngeal airway will help to maintain airway patency in unconscious patients.

The principle of management of complete airway obstruction occurring as

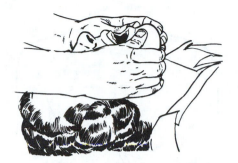

Figure 7–8. Maneuver for backward tilting of the head, forward displacement of the mandible, and opening of the mouth.

the result of impaction of food in the hypopharynx is the dislodgement of the obstructing material. As this should be done immediately and at the scene by a layperson, the maneuvers used are indirect and are based on exerting sudden pressure over the chest or below the diaphragm. An increase in intrathoracic pressure by its transmission to the upper airway jolts the occluding material loose, and it is subsequently ejected. These maneuvers include the well-known *Heimlich maneuver* (abdominal thrust, as in Fig. 7–9), chest thrust, and back blows. As they are abundantly popularized in lay publications and graphically displayed in restaurants, they are not discussed in this book. Readers interested in further information should consult the publications on the subject, some of which appear in the references at the end of this chapter. Management of epiglottitis, croup, and bacterial tracheitis is discussed on pages 132–134. Allergic swelling of the upper airway (angioedema of the larynx) is treated with systemic epinephrine, antihistamines, and corticosteroids. Rarely, mechanical airway restoration will be needed.

Most causes of less acute or chronic

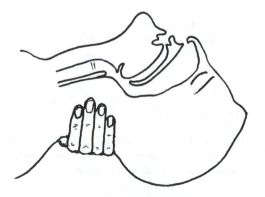

Figure 7–7. Extension of the neck results in opening of the obstructed airway from loss of consciousness.

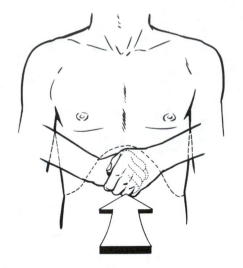

Figure 7–9. Position of hands and direction of pressure in the Heimlich maneuver.

upper airway obstruction are due to lesions treatable only by surgical intervention. Tracheostomy for lesions located in the larnyx or proximal to it will often be necessary. For unresectable tracheal cancer, laser therapy has shown excellent short-term success.

A temporizing measure useful in some instances of upper airway obstruction is the administration of a low-density gas mixture, which reduces the resistance due to obstruction in the large airways. One such mixture is helium–oxygen (heliox), which is given in a ratio of 80/20, unless a higher oxygen concentration is desired. Although restoration of an adequate airway is the primary objective of treatment in upper airway obstruction, sometimes because of technical difficulty or patient refusal, administration of a low-density gas mixture may provide rapid relief. If the obstruction is nonprogressive and reversible, it may obviate the necessity for surgery. This method can

also improve a marginal airflow to one that would allow adequate time for changing an emergency bedside procedure to one that can be done in an operating room.

BIBLIOGRAPHY

Aboussouan LS, Stoller JK. Diagnosis and management of upper airway obstruction. *Clin Chest Med.* 1994; 15(1):35–53.

Acres JC, Kryger MH. Clinical significance of pulmonary function tests: upper airway obstruction. *Chest.* 1981; 80:207–211.

American Heart Association. Guidelines for cardiopulmonary resuscitation and emergency cardiac care. *JAMA.* 1992; 268: 2171–2302.

Bank DE, Krug SE. New approaches to upper airway disease. *Emerg Med Clin North Am.* 1995; 13:473–487.

Frantz TD, Rasgon BM, Quesenberry CP Jr. Acute epiglottitis in adults. Analysis of 129 cases. *JAMA.* 1994; 272:1358–1360.

Heimlich HJ, Uhley MH. The Heimlich maneuver. *Clin Symp.* 1979; 31(3):3–32.

Hoffman JR. Treatment of foreign body obstruction of the upper airway. *West J Med.* 1982; 136:11–22.

Hoffstein V. Snoring. *Chest.* 1996; 109: 201–222.

Levin DL, Muster AJ, Pachman LM, et al. Cor pulmonale secondary to upper airway obstruction. *Chest.* 1975; 68:166–171.

Mayo-Smith MF, Spinale JW, Donskey CJ, et al. Acute epiglottitis. *Chest.* 1995; 108:1640–1647.

O'Hollaren MT, Everts EC. Evaluating the patient with stridor. *Ann Allerg.* 1991; 67: 301–305.

Olsen KD, Kern EB, Westbrook PR. Sleep and breathing disturbance secondary to nasal obstruction. *Otolaryngol Head Neck Surg.* 1981; 89:804–810.

Rodenstein DO, Stanescu DC. The soft palate

and breathing. *Am Rev Respir Dis.* 1986; 134: 311–325.

Schroeder LL, Kapp JF. Recognition and emergency management of infectious causes of upper airway obstruction in children. *Semin Respir Inf.* 1995; 10:21–30.

Sheikh KH, Mostow SR. Epiglottitis—an increasing problem for adults. *West J Med.* 1989; 151:520–524.

Skrinskas GJ, Hyland RH, Hutcheon MA. Using helium–oxygen mixtures in the management of acute upper airway obstruction. *Can Med Assoc J.* 1983; 128:555–558.

Stretton M, Newth CJL. Croup and epiglottitis: key to successful therapy. *J Respir Dis.* 1991; 12:86–94.

Chronic Obstructive Pulmonary Disease

Chronic obstructive pulmonary disease (COPD) is a clinical term used to include groups of conditions associated with chronic obstruction to airflow within the lungs. Although in the past asthma and sometimes bronchiectesis and cystic fibrosis were included, the term *COPD* is now applied only to chronic bronchitis and emphysema. Also known as *chronic airflow obstruction (CAO)*, COPD is by far the most common chronic pulmonary disorder. It has been estimated that more than 14 million Americans have the disease. Disability from COPD is second only to that from heart disease.

Chronic bronchitis and emphysema have many common features and frequently they coexist in the same patient. In this chapter, for descriptive purposes, they are discussed separately by delineating their distinctive pathologic, pathogenetic, physiologic, and clinical features before addressing their common diagnostic and therapeutic management. It

should be underscored that in most patients, a definitive differentiation between chronic bronchitis and emphysema cannot be made. This is because the manifestations of these two conditions often overlap and patients frequently have both conditions at the same time. The term COPD, therefore, can be more appropriately applied to such patients.

■ CHRONIC BRONCHITIS

Chronic bronchitis is defined in clinical terms as chronic excessive production of mucus from the bronchi not due to known specific disease such as tuberculosis or bronchiectasis. It manifests clinically by cough and increased sputum for at least 3 consecutive months each year for 2 successive years. The anatomic correlate is an increase in size and number of the mucus-producing elements in the bronchi. Chronic bronchitis is named appropriately, as the condition is chronic and airway inflammation is its essential pathologic feature.

Etiology. The major factors associated with chronic bronchitis are the smoking of tobacco products and age. There is also a significant difference in its incidence among males and females; middle-age males are most commonly afflicted. By far, the most important etiologic factor is *cigarette smoking*. A direct relationship exists between the amount and the duration of cigarette smoking and the severity of bronchitis, although significant individual variation occurs in the effect of smoking on the respiratory tract. The etiologic role of other factors, without the effect of smoking, appears to be much smaller.

Severe and recurrent respiratory infection in childhood has been implicated as a cause of increased susceptibility to the harmful effects of smoking later in life and, therefore, may have an ancillary role. A direct role for infection, however, has not been definitely established in the etiology of chronic bronchitis. The role of infection is more significant in exacerbation of symptoms and progressive deterioration of the clinical course. Earlier in the course of chronic bronchitis, the sputum consists only of mucus, indicating lack of infection. A change, however, in the sputum to a more purulent state in the course of the disease is indicative of intercurrent bacterial infection. Thus, the role of bacterial infection in chronic bronchitis is mainly a secondary one. Infection with respiratory viruses is probably a common precipitating cause of acute exacerbations, but there is no evidence to implicate viruses as a primary factor in the etiology of chronic bronchitis. Recurrent acute bronchitis in non-smokers with otherwise normal lungs does not seem to proceed to chronic bronchitis.

The role of airway reactivity in chronic bronchitis is less clear. It is known that with airway hyperreactivity associated with chronic bronchitis, the rate of decline in pulmonary function is accelerated. Airway inflammation, on the other hand, increases its nonspecific reactivity. The cause and effect between chronic bronchitis and airway hyperreactivity therefore seems to be mutual.

Compared with cigarette smoking, the significance of air pollution as an etiologic factor in chronic bronchitis is much less. Chronic bronchitis is a rare disease among the nonsmoking population. Heavy atmospheric pollution with sulfur dioxide (SO_2) and particulate matter is an important factor in exacerbation of this condition. Considering all possible etiologic factors in chronic bronchitis, the effect of smoking far outweighs the effect of all other factors put together.

Pathology and Pathogenesis. There has been no general agreement on morphologic criteria for pathologic diagnosis of chronic bronchitis. The increased mucus production is due to enlargement of bronchial *mucous glands* and an increase in the number of *goblet cells.* They are the most consistent pathologic changes. Other pathologic changes include infiltration of mucosa and submucosa by variable numbers of chronic and acute inflammable cells, loss of cilia, and squamous metaplasia. In membranous bronchioles, there is mucus plugging and peribronchiolar inflammation and fibrosis with distortion of small airways.

The pathogenic mechanism of chronic bronchitis is not entirely clear. There is ample evidence, however, that chronic and protracted irritation of bronchial mucosa is the major factor in causing hypertrophy and hyperplasia of mucus-producing glands and cells, as well as in perpetuating the mucosal inflammation. Different mediators of inflammation (cytokines) released from the lower respiratory tract cells, including epithelial cells and macrophages, maintain inflammation and also stimulate fibroblastic proliferation and activity. As a result, more or less permanent changes in airway architecture develop. Decrease in ciliary function and alteration in physicochemical characteristics of bronchial secretions impair their clearance, predisposing the patient to recurrent respiratory infection. Damaged and inflamed mucosa enhances the sensitivity of the irritant receptors, which, in turn, causes bronchial hyperreactivity.

Pathophysiology. Physiologic changes in chronic bronchitis are related to narrowing of the airways. Most patients with chronic bronchitis, however, have normal airway resistance. In this so-called *simple bronchitis,* maximal expiratory flow rates are normal, although more sensitive tests for determining obstruction of small airways are frequently abnormal. With continuation of the inflammatory process and development of peribronchiolar fibrosis, increased airway resistance becomes easily recognizable by simple spirometry (obstructive bronchitis). Increased secretions in airways, with or without infection, contribute to airflow limitation. Bronchoconstriction and airway hyperreactivity may also be present. For unknown reasons, airway reactivity in association with chronic bronchitis is more common in women than in men. In addition to the alteration of lung mechanics due to airflow obstruction,

maldistribution of ventilation is almost always present. Mismatching of ventilation with perfusion of blood causes abnormality of gas exchange as reflected in the alteration of blood gases. With advancing disease and increasing airway obstruction, progressive hypoxemia and hypercapnia (respiratory failure) develop. Increased pulmonary vascular resistance, right-side heart failure, and sometimes polycythemia are other late complications.

Clinical Manifestations. The majority of patients with chronic bronchitis are so accustomed to the symptoms of cough and expectoration that they will not be disturbed by them and, therefore, will not seek medical care. Many will deny any symptoms, and only on careful and repeated questioning will they admit having cough and sputum production. The patients whose symptoms consist of only cough and expectoration of mucus for many years are considered to have *simple uncomplicated chronic bronchitis.* Other patients will give a history of frequent "chest colds" with exacerbation of symptoms: cough becoming more severe and sputum more abundant and often purulent. It may also be bloody. Chronic bronchitis is probably the most common cause of hemoptysis. The onset of dyspnea, which indicates the development of significant airway obstruction, is usually insidious, but may show abrupt exacerbations with bouts of respiratory infection. These patients are considered to have *obstructive* chronic bronchitis. Dyspnea is at first mild and brought about only by exertion. Some patients will adjust their way of life and activities to avoid this symptom. With the progression of disease, the patients will become more and more dyspneic with less and less effort, eventually remaining dyspneic all the time. At this stage, other symptoms of respiratory failure will be evident.

The physical examination usually reveals no significant abnormal findings in patients with the *simple* form of chronic bronchitis. In the *obstructive* form, there may be evidence of prolonged expiration and wheezing. Rales, which usually clear with coughing, are due to presence of secretions in the airways. In the more advanced stage of chronic bronchitis, patients are dyspneic at rest and signs of right-side heart failure may be present. By this time, characteristic features of a "blue bloater" may also develop. Signs of respiratory failure are discussed elsewhere (see Chapter 26).

Management. As therapeutic measures in chronic bronchitis are also applicable to pulmonary emphysema, to avoid repetition, they are discussed under the heading, "Management of Chronic Obstructive

Pulmonary Disease," at the end of this chapter.

■ PULMONARY EMPHYSEMA

Pulmonary emphysema is defined in anatomic terms as permanent abnormal enlargement of airspaces distal to terminal bronchioles associated with destructive changes of alveolar walls.

Pathology and Classification. The terminal bronchiole is a purely conducting structure, but the generations of airways distal to it have increasingly more alveoli in their walls (Fig. 8–1). The portion of the lung distal to the terminal bronchiole is called *acinus*, which is considered by some to be the anatomic unit of the lung. There are some 25,000 such units, which make up about 300 million total alveoli of the lungs. Simple overdistension of the airspaces without destructive

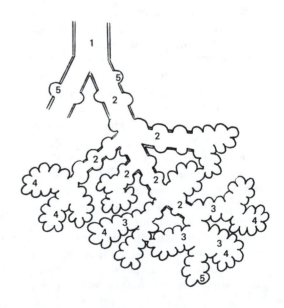

Figure 8–1. Schematic drawing of normal distal airways and airspaces (acinus). (1) Terminal bronchiole, (2) respiratory bronchiole, (3) alveolar duct, (4) alveolar sac, (5) alveoli.

lesions, seen in an asthmatic attack, old age, or compensatory overdistension of remaining lung after pneumonectomy, should not be considered as emphysema (Fig. 8–2).

Depending on the site of involvement in the acinus, emphysema has been divided into several forms. The most common ones are centrilobular and panlobular. In *centrilobular* or *centriacinar emphysema,* the lesion is in the center of the lobules, which corresponds to enlargement and destructive changes in the respiratory bronchioles (Fig. 8–3). This form of emphysema often involves the upper lung fields and is almost always associated with chronic bronchitis. It rarely occurs in nonsmokers.

In *panlobular* or *panacinar emphysema* (Fig. 8-4), which is less common than the centrilobular variety, the entire acinus is more or less involved. The normal architecture of the alveoli and other airspaces is lost. They are enlarged and their septa

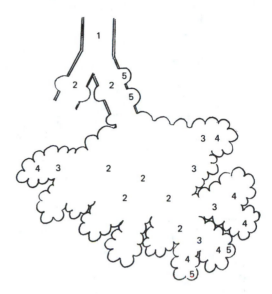

Figure 8–3. Centrilobular emphysema. Numbers represent various parts of an acinus as in Fig. 8–1.

are destroyed, resulting in significant loss of pulmonary parenchyma. Many bullae of various sizes are often present. Panlobular emphysema occurs throughout the lung, but lower and anterior lung fields are more predominantly involved. Its correlation with cigarette smoking is less than in centrilobular emphysema. Emphysema in association with familial alpha$_1$-antiprotease deficiency (see later) is usually panlobular.

Bullous emphysema or bullous disease of the lung usually refers to a pulmonary condition in which there are isolated emphysematous changes with development of bullae, in the apparent absence of underlying generalized emphysema. A *bulla* is defined as an airspace that measures more than 1 cm in diameter in its distended state. Superficial subpleural collection of air is referred to as a *bleb*. The sizes of bullous lesions vary considerably;

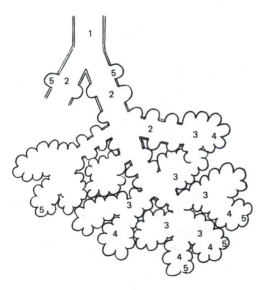

Figure 8–2. Simple hyperinflation. Numbers represent various parts of an acinus as in Fig. 8–1.

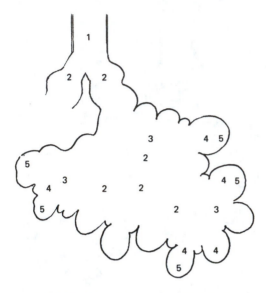

Figure 8–4. Panlobular emphysema. Numbers represent various parts of an acinus as in Fig. 8–1.

sometimes a single or several bullae may occupy a large portion of the hemithorax (giant bulla), compressing the adjacent lung tissue. Bullous changes are not uncommonly seen with generalized emphysema.

Etiology and Pathogenesis. Because of a definite relationship between cigarette smoking and chronic bronchitis, which is frequently associated with emphysema, it is inevitable to conclude that smoking is the major known etiologic factor in pulmonary emphysema. Emphysema, however, is known to occur in individuals who have never smoked, and many patients with long-standing chronic bronchitis do not develop clinically significant emphysema. Therefore, it seems that other factors, some genetic and familial, are involved in the pathogenesis of emphysema, especially when it develops in early age.

The only known and well-studied genetic abnormality that leads to emphysema is alpha$_1$-antitrypsin defciency. Only a small minority (less than 1%) of patients with COPD are known to have deficiency of this serum compound, which is also known as alpha$_1$-antiprotease. Normally, it inhibits the effect of proteases (enzymes that digest proteins) on elastin and collagen, the major protein compounds of lung architecture. Its deficiency is transmitted as a Mendelian recessive trait. Only homozygotes have severe enough deficiency of alpha$_1$-antiprotease to cause COPD, especially panacinar emphysema. It seems that the destructive changes of emphysema are the result of an unprotected effect of proteases, including elastase produced by the inflammatory cells. The effect of smoking in patients with deficiency of inhibitors of these enzymes accelerates development and progression of emphysema. Based on this information and experimental studies of papain-induced emphysema in animals, the "protease–antiprotease" hypothesis of pathogenesis of emphysema has developed. According to this theory, the major factor resulting in alveolar disruption in emphysema is the elastin-attacking enzyme (elastase) released from the phagocytic cells, unopposed by its inhibitor. Protease/antiprotease imbalance may result from factors such as infection, respiratory irritants, and inactivation of inhibitors. In cigarette smokers, increased neutrophilic white blood cells produce an increased amount of elastase in the lungs. Although alpha$_1$-antiprotease is increased in smokers, much of it is inactivated (oxidized) by cigarette smoke.

Pathophysiology. Although commonly associated chronic bronchitis contributes to airway obstruction in emphysema, *airflow limitation* in pure emphysema has a different mechanism. The fragmentation and disruption of pulmonary elastic tissue, which also supports noncartilagenous distal airways, cause reduced *elastic recoil* of the lung. Increased intrathoracic pressure during expiration results in the collapse and the premature closure of the airways that lack the support of radial traction by the elastic parenchyma. As this is the major mechanism of increased flow resistance in pure emphysema, flow rates are affected only during expiration; unless there is associated obstructive bronchitis, inspiratory flow rates are normal. *Large residual volume,* another characteristic feature of emphysema, is due to early closure of airways (air trapping) as well as overdistended airspaces. Lung capacities that include residual volume (functional residual capacity [FRC], total lung capacity [TLC]) are also increased. The area of gas-exchanging surface of the alveolar-capillary membrane is reduced as a result of disruption and destruction of alveolar walls. This pathologic change is responsible for the *reduction of diffusing capacity* in emphysema. Static compliance of lungs is increased; however, both compliance and airway resistance in different regions of the lung in emphysema are quite variable due to nonuniformity of pathologic changes. This is the cause of *uneven ventilation* and *mismatching of ventilation with blood flow,* which, in turn, explain the *increased physiologic dead space* and *abnormal blood gases* demonstrated in emphysema.

Clinical Manifestations. The symptoms of pulmonary emphysema are variable and by no means specific. Patients with localized emphysema usually have no symptoms. Frequently, the symptoms of chronic bronchitis with cough and expectoration predominate the clinical picture, at least in the early stage. Dyspnea, which initially occurs only with exertion, gradually increases in its intensity. It is almost impossible to be certain in patients with chronic bronchitis if or when emphysema has occurred. Patients without preceding or complicating bronchitis may develop exertional dyspnea as the only symptom, cough and expectoration being absent. The rate of progression of dyspnea is variable. Some patients will have a very slow and imperceptible increase in their shortness of breath; others will have a more rapid progression of dyspnea and onset of disability. Most patients will adjust their physical activities to avoid or minimize their symptoms. Nevertheless, dyspnea will occur with less and less effort until the patient remains short of breath even at rest.

Severity of dyspnea does not always correlate with the degree of pathologic or physiologic abnormalities. Although some patients with chronic airway obstruction will increase their ventilation to maintain relatively normal blood gases, others with the same amount of disease will show less, if any, change in their ventilatory effort. Patients in the first group have more dyspnea than patients in the latter group and often are referred to as "pink puffers." This difference in response is probably due to a difference in sensitivity of the respiratory centers or their chemoreceptors.

As in chronic bronchitis, the course of pulmonary emphysema is frequently interspersed by periods of exacerbation of symptoms, usually related to intercurrent infections or other complications. The onset of respiratory failure is also usually precipitated by such events.

Physical findings may be normal in

mild or localized emphysema. In more advanced cases, there is evidence of an enlarged thoracic volume with an increase in the anteroposterior diameter of the chest. Dorsal kyphosis, prominent anterior chest, elevated ribs, flaring of costal margin, and widening of costal angle give the chest the appearance of a barrel (Fig. 8–5). The patient may appear dyspneic, using his or her accessory respiratory muscles. To facilitate their use, some patients assume a sitting position, bend over, and rest the elbows on their thighs. The expiratory phase of respiration is prolonged, and the patient may be breathing against pursed lips. Overdistension of the lungs manifests by increased resonance to percussion, which may include areas that are normally dull (eg, over the heart or liver). Breath

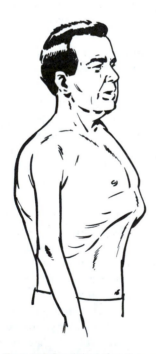

Figure 8–5. Barrel chest of emphysema.

sounds are reduced in intensity and may be difficult to hear. Sometimes expiratory wheezes may be heard. Heart sounds appear distant. Other physical findings, such as cyanosis and other signs of respiratory failure, may be present in the advanced stage of emphysema (see Chapter 26).

■ DIAGNOSTIC STUDIES IN CHRONIC OBSTRUCTIVE PULMONARY DISEASE

As chronic bronchitis is defined in clinical terms, its diagnosis is usually established by the patient's medical history. In its advanced stage, pulmonary emphysema can be diagnosed by physical examination. However, in most cases clinical information is inadequate or questionable and additional investigation will be necessary. Two of the most commonly performed studies are radiographic examination of the chest and pulmonary function tests.

Radiographic Examination. Radiographic examination in patients who present with chronic cough and expectoration indicative of chronic bronchitis most often shows no significant abnormalities. It is more useful to exclude conditions that may mimic chronic bronchitis, such as tuberculosis and bronchiectasis, or for identification of certain complications. Coexistent emphysema may also be suggested by a chest radiograph. Being defined in anatomic terms, pulmonary emphysema is often diagnosed by radiographic study. Changes in chest x-ray film from emphysema are variable and depend on type, extent, and severity of the disease. Typical changes include depression and flattening of the diaphragm, hyperlucency, reduced vascular markings, widened space between the sternum and the heart, and increased anteroposterior diameter of the chest (Figs. 8–6 and 8–7). Most of these changes are indicative of overinflation. Demonstration of bullous lesions, however, is an unequivocal x-ray sign of emphysema. Sometimes chest radiograph may show increased markings without x-ray evidence of hyperinflation. Computed tomography (CT), especially high-resolution computed tomography (HRCT), has been shown to be much more sensitive and specific than standard radiographic study for diagnosis of emphysema and identification of its various anatomic types. HRCT is therefore more useful when patients with emphysema are being considered for resection of bullae or lung-volume reduction surgery.

Pulmonary Function Tests. Pulmonary function tests (PFTs) are important for diagnosis, determination of severity, and evaluation of progression of COPD. Chronic bronchitis in its early stage will show no significant abnormality in routine spirometry. More sensitive tests that identify obstruction of small airways such as measurement of closing volume may be abnormal. In more advanced stages of chronic bronchitis, with further airway obstruction and superimposition of emphysematous changes, forced expiratory flow rates are diminished. Total lung capacity (TLC) in chronic bronchitis without emphysema is usually normal, but residual volume (RV) is increased, resulting in a high RV/TLC ratio.

In emphysema, in addition to reduced forced expiratory flow rates, TLC is increased, which is mainly the result of large RV (Fig. 8–8). The latter may be as high as several times the normal in advanced cases. RV/TLC ratio, therefore, is also increased. Reduced expiratory flow rates alone cannot differentiate between airway obstruction from chronic bronchi-

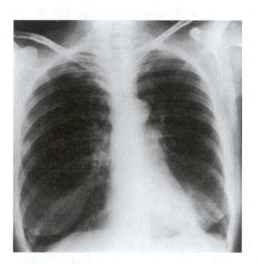
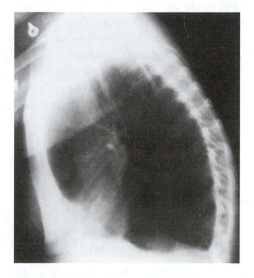

Figures 8–6 and 8–7. Posteroanterior and lateral radiographs of the chest in a patient with severe emphysema.

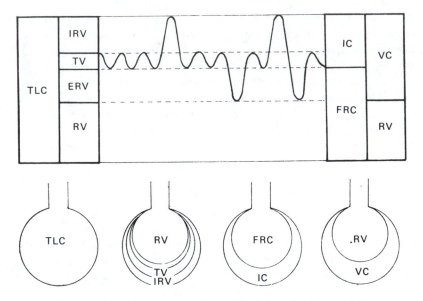

Figure 8–8. Lung volumes and capacities in COPD. Note significant increase in RV.

tis and that caused by emphysema. A large TLC, however, is more consistent with emphysema than with chronic bronchitis. Normal maximum inspiratory flow rate with significantly reduced forced expiratory flow rates, as determined by flow-volume loop, is indicative of emphysema. This is because in emphysema airway obstruction occurs as a result of dynamic compression of collapsible airways during expiration, whereas during inspiration they remain open. One test of pulmonary function that more accurately determines the presence of emphysema is low diffus-

ing capacity, which is usually normal in chronic bronchitis without emphysema.

It should be emphasized that the main practical purpose of PFTs in COPD is the determination of the disease's severity, progression, and response to therapeutic interventions. A simple spirometry with measurement of various flow rates (especially FEV_1) usually suffices (Fig. 8–9). For determination of the presence and magnitude of reversibility of airway obstruction, the study is repeated after inhalation of a beta-agonist bronchodilator.

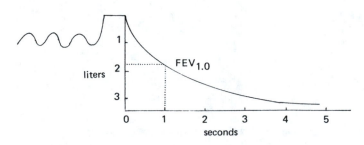

Figure 8–9. Forced spirogram in COPD. FEV_1 is less than 50% of vital capacity, which is also reduced.

Arterial blood studies may show normal findings in mild, or even moderate, COPD, but they are abnormal in more advanced cases. Reduced arterial P_{O_2} is the most common abnormality, particularly during exacerbations. Although often normal, arterial P_{CO_2} may be chronically elevated and/or may show an acute rise during an intercurrent infection or other complications.

■ MANAGEMENT OF CHRONIC OBSTRUCTIVE PULMONARY DISEASE

In view of the well-established role of smoking tobacco products in the pathogenesis of chronic bronchitis, complete cessation of smoking is the most effective preventive measure against this disease and the only certain means of favorably affecting its course (see Chapter 16). Early changes of chronic bronchitis, when the obstruction is limited to the small airways, are more or less reversible when the inciting factors are eliminated. With the prevailing uncertainty about the pathogenesis of emphysema, it is almost impossible to predict (except in individuals with alpha$_1$-antiprotease deficiency) who will develop the disease under the influence of environmental factors such as cigarette smoking. It is, therefore, important to avoid factors that are known or suspected to play a major role in the pathogenesis of emphysema. Unfortunately, the structural changes in well-established disease, particularly with emphysema, are irreversible; thus, prevention, or slowing of the progression of disease by avoiding further insults, should be one of the main objectives of its management.

Preliminary results of treatment of patients with alpha$_1$-antiprotease deficiency with the recently marketed drug Prolastin are promising in slowing the progression of emphysema. The drug, also known as alpha$_1$-proteinase inhibitor, should be administered intravenously throughout the patient's life. Its long-term effectiveness remains to be determined.

The most important phase of treatment of established COPD is *outpatient management,* which should include measures to control the progression of the disease, to prevent complications and the need for frequent hospitalizations, to control or at least alleviate the symptoms, and to teach the patient how to cope with his or her illness and disability. Although the individual patient's needs are variable, these general measures are applicable to almost all patients with COPD.

In addition to cigarette smoke, other respiratory irritants should be avoided as much as possible. Patients should be instructed about proper bronchial hygiene by adequate hydration, humidification of inspired air, postural drainage, and other respiratory physiotherapeutic maneuvers. These simple and inexpensive measures would be adequate for treatment of the majority of patients with uncomplicated chronic bronchitis, and should also be considered as an important part of the therapeutic regimen in more advanced disease.

Bronchodilators are the most commonly used drugs in outpatient treatment of COPD. Unfortunately, not every patient benefits from their use. It has been estimated that, in only about one-third of patients, the spirometric study shows any significant improvement (increase in FEV_1). However, some patients may have symptomatic benefit with no spirometric improvement. Inhaled beta$_2$-

agonists are fast acting and, in addition to their bronchodilatory effect, they improve mucous clearance. Anticholinergic bronchodilators, such as ipatropium bromide, may be more effective than beta$_2$-agonists in COPD, but they have slower onset of action that lasts longer. Therefore, they are more suitable for regular maintenance use than for acute relief of dyspnea. Inhaled anticholinergics have no significant side effects and can also be used with other bronchodilators. Oral theophylline is used in many patients who have more troublesome symptoms. Slow-release preparations are particularly convenient for patients who have difficulty in using inhaled medications. Although theophylline is a mild bronchodilator, it has additional therapeutic effects including improvement in mucociliary transport, stimulation of respiratory center, reduction of pulmonary vascular resistance, improvement of cardiac function, and increase in respiratory muscle strength. Its potential toxicity and a need for blood level determination are the major disadvantages of theophylline. Oral corticosteroids may improve a small percentage of patients with COPD. It is usually given to patients who do not improve with more conservative therapy. If no objective benefit can be demonstrated after a few weeks of trial, the corticosteroids should be stopped. If systemic steroids prove to be beneficial, an inhaled preparation may be substituted to avoid side effects of long-term use of systemic steroids. Expectorants and mucolytic agents probably have no significant therapeutic benefit in COPD.

Infection, bacterial as well as viral, plays a major role in the exacerbation of COPD and contributes significantly to the disability from this condition. In fact, it seems to be partly responsible for progressive deterioration of respiratory function in these patients. Preventive measures, such as immunization against pneumococcal infection and influenza, should be undertaken. In patients with frequent *bacterial* respiratory infections, antibiotic prophylaxis sometimes is considered. Most clinicians, however, prefer prompt use of antibiotics when there is evidence of bacterial infection, often judged by change in cough and characteristics of sputum to a more purulent form and sometimes supported by bacteriologic studies. The choice of antibiotic is based on the frequent isolation of pneumococci, *Haemophilus influenzae,* and *Moraxella catarrhalis* from the sputum of such patients. Routine sputum culture before antibiotic treatment usually does not provide useful additional information. In choosing from a variety of antimicrobials for outpatient treatment of suspected infection in COPD, the cost of drugs should be taken into consideration.

One of the most important aspects of outpatient management of COPD is the proper education of the patients, and/or their families, about their disease and adequate explanation of the therapeutic regimen. Success in their cooperation and compliance with treatment often depends on their understanding of the illness and the measures directed toward it. Proper reconditioning exercise programs, breathing retraining, adequate nutrition, psychosocial support, and vocational counseling are essential for comprehensive care and rehabilitation of these patients.

When indicated, bronchodilators and sometimes corticosteroids are preferably administered in aerosolized form by hand nebulizers or metered dose inhalers. There is no significant advantage of intermittent positive pressure breathing (IPPB) therapy over simpler inhalation therapy in COPD patients, as was concluded in a recent multicenter trial. The use of IPPB for home management is not recommended.

Exercise programs are intended to help more efficient use of the respiratory muscles and to improve endurance. Although not resulting in any significant improvement in pulmonary function as determined by the usual tests, these programs are known to increase exercise tolerance and enhance the sense of well-being in patients.

Patients with advanced disease remain in a state of chronic respiratory failure manifested by severe hypoxemia with or without hypercapnia. Such patients should be considered for continuous oxygen therapy if their arterial Po_2 is chronically lower than 55 torr or if there is evidence of cor pulmonale or secondary polycythemia with a Pao_2 of less than 60 torr. It should be documented that hypoxemia persists despite optimal medical management. Some patients with COPD develop severe hypoxemia, sometimes to an alarmingly low level, during sleep, while they have only mild to moderate hypoxemia during wakefulness. These patients are candidates for nocturnal oxygen therapy. Newer methods of oxygen delivery, such as the use of oxygen-conserving devices (reservoir cannulas and demand pulsing oxygen delivery system) and transtracheal oxygen (TTO) seem to be more effective in refractory hypoxemia in COPD.

Hospitalized patients with COPD usually have serious complications, including pneumonia and respiratory failure, or they are hospitalized for unrelated conditions. The management of patients with respiratory failure due to COPD is discussed in Chapters 26 and 28. Patients with COPD undergoing major thoracic or abdominal surgery are at much higher risk for developing respiratory complications (see Chapter 19). Surgery for pulmonary emphysema is being done for resection of giant bullae, and, more recently, patients with other subsets of emphysema are subjected to a procedure called *lung-volume reduction surgery*. There is still no well-established patient selection criteria for this procedure. Advanced COPD has become the most common indication for lung transplantation. There are many who are awaiting their turn to receive an appropriate donor lung. Unfortunately, only a small percentage of them succeed and many die from the disease while waiting.

Course and Prognosis of COPD. The course of chronic bronchitis is quite variable. Most patients with chronic cough and expectoration for many years will have no impairment of lung function. However, some patients will progress rapidly to a more symptomatic stage with increasing dyspnea and disability. Some will have frequent respiratory tract infections and ensuing exacerbations. Pulmonary emphysema may supervene and accelerate the deterioration of pulmonary function. Cessation of smoking, especially in the early stages of chronic bronchitis, may stop or at least slow down the disease progression. The natural history of pulmonary emphysema is also variable. Some patients have early-onset emphysema with rapid progression, while others develop emphysema in older age with a slower rate of change in lung function. In most patients, however, the rate of decline in pulmonary function is predictable as judged from yearly deterioration of expiratory flow rates. It has been estimated that the average time from the onset of the disease to the stage of severe respiratory impairment is about 25 to 30 years. There is a good correlation between the severity of airway obstruction, as judged by FEV_1, and mortality from COPD. With an FEV_1 below 750 mL, very few patients will survive 5 years. The onset of respiratory failure indicates even a worse prognosis.

BIBLIOGRAPHY

Alpha$_1$-proteinase inhibitor for alpha$_1$-antitrypsin deficiency. *Med Lett Drugs Ther.* 1988; 30:29–30.

ATS Statement. Standards for diagnosis and care of patients with chronic obstructive pulmonary disease. *Am J Respir Crit Care Med.* 1995; 152(suppl):S78–S121.

Ball P. Epidemiology and treatment of chronic bronchitis and its exacerbation. *Chest.* 1995; 108(suppl):43S–52S.

Bégin P, Grassino A. Inspiratory muscle dysfunction and chronic hypercapnia in chronic obstructive pulmonary disease. *Am Rev Respir Dis.* 1991; 143:905–912.

Brenner M, Yusen R, McKenna R Jr., et al. Lung volume reduction surgery for emphysema. *Chest.* 1996; 110:205–218.

Burrows B. Airways obstructive diseases: pathogenetic mechanisms and natural histories of the disorders. *Med Clin North Am.* 1990; 74:547–559.

Celli BR. Pulmonary rehabilitation in patients with COPD. *Am J Respir Crit Care Med.* 1995; 333:710–714.

Crofton J, Masironi R. Chronic airways disease: the smoking component. *Chest.* 1989; 96(suppl):349S–355S.

Crystal RG. α_1-Antitrypsin deficiency: pathogenesis and treatment. *Hosp Pract.* 1991; 26(2):73–86.

Ferguson GT, Cherniack RM. Management of chronic obstructive pulmonary disease. *N Engl J Med.* 1993; 328:1017–1022.

Goldstein RS, Ramcharan V, Bowes G, et al. Effect of supplemental nocturnal oxygen on gas exchange in patients with severe obstructive lung disease. *N Engl J Med.* 1984; 310:425–429.

Griffith DE, Garcia JGN. Tobacco cigarettes, smoking, smoking cessation, and chronic obstructive pulmonary disease. *Semin Respir Med.* 1989; 10:356–371.

Gross NJ. The use of anticholinergic agents in the treatment of airways disease. *Clin Chest Med.* 1988; 9:591–598.

Hodgkin JE. Prognosis in chronic obstructive pulmonary disease. *Clin Chest Med.* 1990; 11:555–569.

Idell S, Garcia JGN. Mechanisms of smoking-induced lung injury. *Semin Respir Med.* 1989; 10:345–355.

Jansen HM, Sachs APE, van Alphen L. Predisposing conditions to bacterial infections in chronic obstructive pulmonary disease. *Am J Respir Crit Care Med.* 1995; 151:2073–2080.

Murphy TF, Sethi S. Bacterial infection in chronic obstructive pulmonary disease. *Am Rev Respir Dis.* 1992; 146:1067–1083.

O'Connor GT, Sparrow D, Weiss ST. The role of allergy and nonspecific airway hyperresponsiveness in the pathogenesis of chronic pulmonary disease. *Am Rev Respir Dis.* 1989; 140:225–252.

O'Donohue WJ Jr. Home oxygen therapy. *Med Clin North Am.* 1996; 80 (3):611–622.

Petty TL. Home oxygen—a revolution in the care of advanced COPD. *Med Clin North Am.* 1990; 74:715–729.

Proteases and antiproteases. *Am J Respir Crit Care Med.* 1994; 150(6 suppl):S109–S189.

Renston JP, DiMarco AF, Supinski GS. Respiratory muscle rest using nasal BiPAP ventilation in patients with stable severe COPD. *Chest.* 1994; 105:1053–1060.

Rosen RL, Bone RC. Treatment of acute exacerbations in chronic obstructive pulmonary disease. *Med Clin North Am.* 1990; 74:691–700.

Samet JM, Tager IB, Speizer FE. The relationship between respiratory illness in childhood and chronic air-flow obstruction in adulthood. *Am Rev Respir Dis.* 1983; 127:508–523.

Snider GL. Chronic obstructive pulmonary disease: risk factors, pathophysiology, and pathogenesis. *Am Rev Med.* 1989; 40:411–429.

Stubbing DG, Mathur PN, Roberts RS, Campbell EJM. Some physical signs in patients with chronic airflow obstruction. *Am Rev Respir Dis.* 1982; 125:549–552.

Sweer L, Zwillich CW. Dyspnea in the patient with chronic obstructive pulmonary disease. *Clin Chest Med.* 1990; 11:417–445.

Swinburn CR, Mould H, Stone TN, et al. Symptomatic benefit of supplemental oxygen in hypoxemic patients with chronic lung disease. *Am Rev Respir Dis.* 1991; 143: 913–915.

Tarry SP, Celli BR. Long-term oxygen therapy. *N Engl J Med.* 1995; 333:710–714.

Ziment I. Pharmacologic therapy of obstructive airway disease. *Clin Chest Med.* 1990; 11:461–486.

9.

Asthma

Asthma is a respiratory disease characterized by an increased reactivity of the airways to various stimuli and manifested clinically by periodic wheezing, dyspnea, and cough. Clinical manifestations, which are the result of widespread narrowing of bronchi and bronchioles caused by mucosal inflammation, increased secretions, and smooth muscle contraction, improve either spontaneously or with therapy.

■ ETIOLOGY AND PATHOGENESIS

Asthma is a common respiratory disease that may begin at any age. In about half of the cases, however, the onset is before age 10. In more than one-third of patients, there is a history of asthma in members of the immediate family. It is estimated that about 5% to 7% of the population in the United States and Europe has asthma.

Hyperreactivity of the airways, the central feature of asthma, is a condition in which the trachea and bronchi show an exaggerated sensitivity to the bronchoconstrictive effect of a variety of physical, pharmacologic, and biologic agents. Although the exact mechanism of airway hyperresponsiveness is unknown, several factors, including genetic predisposition, autonomous nervous imbalance, and the alteration of adrenergic receptors have been implicated in its development. An essential component of asthma is airway inflammation, which together with epithelial damage, resulting from various causes, plays a major role in causing, augmenting, and sustaining bronchial hyperreactivity.

Depending on whether or not a *specific* external cause for asthma can be demonstrated, asthma is classified into extrinsic and intrinsic categories. As *nonspecific* stimuli may result in asthmatic reaction in both of these categories, they have no discriminating role in this classification. Because extrinsic asthma is most frequently the result of an allergy, the terms *allergic asthma* and *extrinsic asthma* are often used interchangeably. However, there are other causes of extrinsic asthma besides allergies, in which case it is known as *extrinsic nonallergic asthma*. Most cases of occupational asthma are considered to be nonallergic but related to exposure to specific agents. In *intrinsic asthma,* no specific cause can be identified, there is no personal or family history of allergy, and it is most common in individuals whose asthma begins later in life. Despite this apparent distinction, a significant overlap exists between extrinsic and intrinsic asthma. Different factors in various combinations may be responsible in many cases, and thus, it may be impossible to categorize them.

Regardless of the underlying causes of asthma, many factors trigger an asthma attack as nonspecific stimuli. Specific stimuli may also act as triggers, but only in sensitized asthmatics. In addition, airway reactivity is enhanced by some of the nonspecific, and almost all of the specific, factors when they cause airway inflammation and/or mucosal epithelial damage. It seems, therefore, that interaction of various stimuli with hyperresponsive airways not only causes an acute asthmatic episode, but also, by causing inflammation of airways, increases their reactivity.

Important factors that may precipitate or exacerbate an asthma attack are listed in Table 9–1. It should be noted, however, that in many instances the provoking cause of the asthma attack remains undetermined. Bronchial narrowing during an attack is from a varying combination of several changes. They include contraction of smooth muscles, increased secretions by mucous glands and goblet cells, edema of the bronchial wall, cellular infiltration, and the dilation of small blood vessels. The mechanism of production of these changes under di-

TABLE 9–1. PRECIPITATING OR EXACERBATING FACTORS IN ASTHMA

Allergens*
Viral infection of respiratory tract
Irritating dusts, fumes, or gases
Tobacco smoke
Exercise—cold air
Occupational exposure to certain substances*
Aspirin and related anti-inflammatory drugs
Certain food additives and preservatives
Emotions
Esophageal reflux
Sleep

*Denotes specific factors; others are nonspecific.

verse provoking factors may differ. The role of these factors and some of the well-recognized categories of asthma are discussed briefly. Understanding their various pathogenetic mechanisms is very important in making rational therapeutic decisions. Some of these factors are well recognized and studied, while others remain speculative. It should be stressed that in many cases of asthma, there is more than one stimulus that can trigger it and initiate inflammatory response. Therefore, any classification based on mechanisms of airway narrowing must be arbitrary. The following discussion is intended to address some of the important factors known to have a role in asthma.

Allergy

Allergy in asthma is an *immediate* or *type 1* hypersensitivity reaction that requires the presence of specific immunoglobulin E (IgE) class of antibodies. This type of reaction occurs in individuals who have *atopy*, which is a hypersensitivity state with a genetic predisposition characterized by the production of an excessive amount of IgE antibodies against a variety of antigens. About 10% to 20% of the general population are atopic and have the tendency to develop hay fever, asthma, eczema, and other IgE-mediated allergic reactions. These types of hypersensitivity reactions result from the interaction of antigens (allergens) with their specific IgE antibodies, which tend to attach to the mast cells, basophilic granulocytes, and perhaps other cells. Mast cells have the highest concentration of IgE molecules on their surface. The cross-linking of two IgE antibody molecules by specific antigen signals the initiation of a series of intracellular biochemical events, resulting in the release of several mediators. Some of these mediators are preformed and stored as specially stainable granules, and many others, before being released, are rapidly synthesized as a result of the signal from the antigen–antibody interaction.

Among the many chemical mediators identified thus far, important ones are *histamine, eosinophil chemotactic factor of anaphylaxis (ECF-A), neutrophil chemotactic factor (NCF), leukotrienes* (formerly known as *slow-reacting substance of anaphylaxis,* or *SRS-A*), *prostaglandins,* and *platelet-activating factor.* The first three substances are preformed, while the last three are freshly synthesized from arachidonic acid, which is a phospholipid constituent. The respiratory tract is one of the few sites in which there is a large number of mast cells. In addition to mast cells, other cells, including macrophages, neutrophils, eosinophils, and endothelial cells, are known to produce many of these mediators as well as many cytokines. Both T lymphocytes and B lymphocytes are also active participants and interact with other cells in causing and maintaining airway inflammation and their heightened reactivity. Plasma cells, made

from B-lymphocytes, are responsible for production of IgE antibody.

Some of the mediators released from the mast cells and other inflammatory cells are potent constrictors of the airways by causing contraction of smooth muscles in their wall. In addition, they result in microvascular congestion, increased tracheobronchial secretions, and mucosal edema. As mentioned earlier, these changes, together with infiltration of mucosa by inflammatory cells, constitute the mechanism of airway obstruction in asthma. Among the inflammatory cells, eosinophils and their products have been recognized to cause injury and desquamation of respiratory tract epithelial cells, thus enhancing airway hyperresponsiveness. The common allergenic substances often incriminated in allergic asthma include pollens of trees, grass, and weeds; antigens of molds; house dust mites; and animal feathers or dander. Allergens are not only important as triggers in asthma, they also seem to play a role in the pathogenesis of the disease itself. It appears that repeated exposure to allergens sustains airway hyperresponsiveness in genetically susceptible individuals. House dust mites are probably the most potent allergen in this regard. Recent studies have also shown the importance of cockroaches in children's asthma.

There are certain patterns of asthmatic response to allergenic exposure. *Early response* occurs within several minutes of exposure to an inhaled antigen and resolves within about an hour. *Late asthmatic response* begins several hours after exposure and lasts much longer. A late asthmatic reaction may or may not follow an early response; it may also occur without an early reaction. When an immediate response is followed by a late one, it is called a *dual asthmatic response.* As a result of a late asthmatic reaction, airways become even more susceptible to the bronchoconstrictive effect of both specific and nonspecific stimuli. This increased hyperresponsiveness, which may persist long after antigenic exposure has stopped, has been considered to be one of the reasons of the self-perpetuating state that is seen in some of the cases of untreated asthma.

The increased production and release of various substances by mast cells are not limited to IgE-mediated allergic response. Many nonallergic causes of asthma may also operate through these mediators and share the same mechanism of airway obstruction, with the exception of the involvement of IgE antibodies (Fig. 9–1). In many clinical situations, the distinction between allergic and nonallergic asthma is almost impossible.

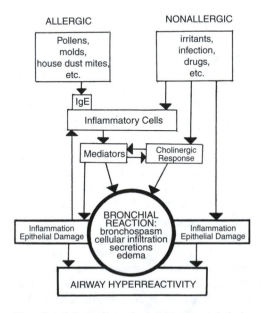

Figure 9–1. Pathogenetic mechanisms of asthma in both allergic and nonallergic forms. Note their close interrelationship.

Cholinergic Response

The vagus nerve plays a significant role in bronchospasm and increased mucosal secretions in asthma. *Cholinergic response* is a mechanism of bronchospasm in which the vagus nerve is involved. The airways are richly innervated by both the sensory and motor fibers of this nerve. Irritant receptors on the tracheobronchial mucosa are the sensory nerve endings, and the smooth muscles of the airways are innervated by its motor fibers. Stimulation of the vagus, either directly or indirectly, causes bronchospasm and increases mucosal secretions. It seems that mediators released from the mast cells and other inflammatory cells interact with the action of the vagus nerve. Histamine, in addition to its direct effect on smooth muscles, may cause reflex bronchoconstriction by stimulating the sensory nerve endings of the vagus. Some of the mediators may sensitize the smooth muscles, making them more susceptible to the bronchoconstrictive effect of vagal stimulation; and stimulation of the vagus nerve facilitates mediator release by the mast cells. This interaction may create another positive feedback loop that sustains inflammation and bronchial narrowing (see Fig. 9–1).

Occupational and Environmental Factors

Common atmospheric pollutants, including sulfur dioxide, nitrous oxide, ozone, and a variey of other noxious gases and aerosolized particulate matters are known to provoke or exacerbate bronchospasm in asthmatics, which can occur in various environments, including workplaces. When asthma develops as a result of prolonged exposure to specific inhaled substances in the work environment, it is referred to as *occupational asthma.* It should be differentiated from aggravation of symptoms in a known asthmatic exposed to nonspecific triggers in the workplace. In occupational asthma, a period of exposure from a few weeks to several years is necessary for the disease to develop (*latency period*). Although an allergy may be the underlying mechanism in some workers, most patients with occupational asthma are not atopic and there is no evidence of an IgE-mediated hypersensitivity reaction. Chemical effects of some of the causative agents, other types of immunologic processes, and resultant inflammation have been considered in its pathogenesis. The percentage of workers who develop occupational asthma depends on the agent involved. For example, among workers exposed to toluene diisocyanate, an important cause of occupational asthma, about 10% develop asthma. As in allergic asthma, exposure to the specific inhaled substances in the workplace not only results in asthma attacks, but also increases airway responsiveness to the same agents and to nonspecific asthma-provoking factors.

More than 200 agents have been recognized to cause occupational asthma. The more common and important causes are isocyanates in workers involved with polyurethane, plastics, and varnish and car spray painters; trimellitic anhydride among workers with epoxy resins; organic dusts from various woods, plants, and grain flours in sawmill operators, tea workers, and bakers; animal products in laboratory workers or other animal handlers; enzymes among detergent and pharmaceutical manufacturers; and a variety of other chemicals in different workplaces. There is enough evidence to consider *byssinosis,* a chronic lung disease due to cotton dust exposure, as a form of occupational asthma.

Infection

Respiratory tract infection is often suspected in acute asthmatic attacks. Although bacterial infection may occasionally be a complicating condition of asthma, viral upper respiratory tract infection is a much more frequent preceding event. Because of a lack of an obvious precipitating cause of nonallergic asthma, infection is considered to play a more important role. It seems, however, that common viral respiratory tract infection also acts as a nonspecific factor in provoking bronchospasm in allergic asthma. Asthmatic episodes in children, whose asthma is most often allergy-related, are frequently precipitated by a viral respiratory tract infection. It has been demonstrated that infection with certain viruses, such as respiratory syncytial virus, rhinovirus, and influenza virus, can cause transient airway hyperreactivity in normal subjects. In asthmatics, infection with such viruses may not only precipitate an asthma attack, but they may also increase airway responsiveness to other nonspecific provoking factors and, if sensitized, to certain specific agents. Inflammatory changes and epithelial injury are suggested to be the cause of increased airway responsiveness, as in allergic asthma. The relationship of *Aspergillus* infection and asthma is discussed in Chapter 5.

Exercise

It is well known that many asthmatic subjects, especially children and young adults, develop bronchoconstriction following exercise. Commonly known as *exercise-induced asthma,* it may be the first manifestation of asthma. Exercise usually has to be vigorous (eg, running fast for several minutes) to have a clinically significant effect on the airways, as it is the high minute ventilation that is essential for provoking an attack. It occurs *after* rather than during exercise. The maximal bronchoconstriction occurs 5 to 10 minutes after the completion of exercise. Both the cooling and drying of the airway mucosa occur with the increased ventilation of exercise. The inspired air, before reaching the alveoli, is conditioned to be saturated with water vapor and to have a temperature of 37°C. This is accomplished by heat exchange with, and evaporation of water from, the airway mucosa. Although both heat exchange with inspired air and evaporation cause mucosal cooling, the latter is more important, as it also causes water loss. With a high minute ventilation, the cooling and drying effect is increased. Exercise in cold dry air, such as cross-country skiing, is more likely to provoke a bronchoconstrictor response than exercise in a warm and humid environment, such as swimming in a heated pool. As it has been shown that hypertonicity of the periciliary fluid in the bronchi can by itself cause bronchospasm, it seems that the water loss from the airways during vigorous exercise, especially in cold dry air, has a role in causing bronchoconstriction. Microvascular congestion of airways, which develops with rewarming of the mucosa after being cooled during exercise, is probably a major contributing factor. Both cholinergic reaction as a result of the stimulation of irritant receptors of the airways and mediator release from the mast cells are most likely involved in bronchial narrowing. Figure 9–2 shows changes in FEV_1 that occurs during and after exercise in a typical case.

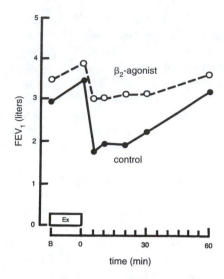

Figure 9–2. Typical change of forced expiratory flow rate in exercise-induced asthma with and without prior therapy with a beta-2 agonist. Note that the rapid decline in FEV_1 in untreated patient occurs after exercise. (Reprinted by permission of *The New England Journal of Medicine.* McFadden ER Jr, Gilbert IA. Exercise-induced asthma. *N Engl J Med.* 330:1362–1367. Copyright 1994, Massachusetts Medical Society.)

Pharmacologic Factors

Aspirin and other nonsteroidal anti-inflammatory drugs (NSAIDs) are known to precipitate or exacerbate asthma. About 10% to 20% of asthmatics have an associated sensitivity to aspirin or related drugs. Nasal polyps are often present in these patients, who are usually adults and have a more chronic and unremitting asthma. It is postulated that the mechanism of action of these drugs is through their effect on arachidonic acid metabolism, which results in the formation of an additional amount of leukotrienes. Sensitivity to aspirin and other NSAIDs has no definable immunologic basis and is considered to be an idiosyncratic reaction. There is a significant cross-reactivity between these agents.

Beta-adrenergic blocking agents, commonly used for the treatment of hypertension and some cardiac and noncardiac diseases, are known to cause or enhance an asthmatic attack. Most of these agents are nonselective—that is, they block both beta-1 (predominantly cardiac) and beta-2 (predominantly bronchial) adrenergic receptors. Even beta-1–selective drugs may have some bronchospastic effect.

Among the food additives, tartrazine, a yellow food-coloring agent, is known to provoke an asthma attack. Patients sensitive to aspirin usually react to this agent. Bisulfites and metabisulfites are used in the food-processing industry as preservatives and antioxidants. Restaurant food, especially from salad bars, contains significant amounts of these agents. They are also used in certain wines, beers, dried fruits, and many other preserved food items. Asthmatic reactions occur in about 5% of patients with asthma following the intake of food or drink containing sulfites. The mechanism of sulfite sensitivity is not clearly understood.

Nocturnal Exacerbation

Many asthmatic patients are known to have more difficulty with their asthma in the late night and early morning hours. The worsening of asthma may be associated with sleep at any time of the day, as the factors considered in its pathogenesis are mostly sleep related. The contributing factors include gastroesophageal reflux; retained airway secretions from a suppressed cough reflex during sleep; late asthmatic reactions from daytime exposure to irritants or allergens in the bedroom; sleep-related changes in the function of the autonomic nervous system; and circadian variation in circulating factors such as epinephrine, cortisol, and histamine. It seems that patients who have more severe asthma and a higher degree of bronchial hyperreactivity are also more prone to nocturnal exacerbation of their bronchospasm. The prolonged dosing interval of medications in patients who are on certain antiasthmatic drugs may be another important cause of the nocturnal exacerbation of asthma.

Clinical studies strongly suggest that in subjects with hyperreactive airways, gastroesophageal reflux, which occurs more commonly in the supine position, may result in nocturnal asthma independent of other factors. It seems that the incidence of reflux is higher in asthmatics than in the general population. Bronchodilators, such as theophylline preparations and beta-adrenergic agonists, are known to reduce the lower esophageal sphincter tone, further increasing the likelihood of regurgitation of gastric juice. Bronchospasm resulting from gastroesophageal reflux is mostly a cholinergic reflex mediated by the vagus nerve. Rarely, aspiration of regurgitated material may occur and incite an asthmatic response.

Emotional Factors

Stress and other psychological factors are known to affect asthma. Symptoms of asthma have been shown to worsen or improve with suggestion in many asthmatics. The mechanism of effect of emotional factors on asthma is the result of complex interactions between the central nervous system (CNS), neuroendocrine pathway, and immune system. It appears that efferent activity of the vagus nerve by its effect on airway smooth muscles and mediator release plays a significant role.

Psychological factors probably influence the efficacy of therapeutic interventions in asthma.

Pathologic Changes. Pathologic examination of the lungs of patients dying from asthma, which represents the most severe form of the disease, shows evidence of a widespread obstruction of the airways from mucous plugs and inflammation of the airway walls. Lungs are hyperinflated from trapped air. The infiltration of the bronchial walls with various inflammatory cells (especially eosinophils and neutrophils), thickening of airway walls, prominent bronchial smooth muscles, hypertrophy of mucous glands, increased number of goblet cells, and epithelial desquamation are usually seen. Some of these changes, to a lesser extent, can be seen in less severe asthma attacks. A limited number of bronchoalveolar lavage studies in asthma following exposure to inhaled antigens shows a predominance of eosinophils and neutrophils, indicating that inflammation is part of the asthmatic reaction in many patients.

Pathophysiology. The pathophysiologic changes during an asthma attack are based on narrowing of the airways caused by contraction of smooth muscles, mucosal and submucosal edema, infiltration with inflammatory cells, microvascular congestion, and increased secretions. Increased airway resistance results in decreased forced expiratory flows and hyperinflation. Increased respiratory workload is related to both airflow resistance and hyperinflation. In addition to mechanical disadvantage during an asthma attack, abnormal distribution of both ventilation and blood flow with their mismatching results in the alteration of arterial blood gases (ABGs), particularly hypoxemia. More severe and prolonged asthma attacks may culminate in hypercapnia from worsening of ventilation–perfusion mismatching and respiratory muscle fatigue.

Clinical Manifestations. The history is often the key to the diagnosis of bronchial asthma. A history of episodic attacks of wheezing and shortness of breath with symptom-free intervals is characteristic. Many patients give a history of frequent emergency room visits and hospital admissions for their asthma attacks. Some patients have a less clear-cut history and may be seen during their first attack. Many asthmatics, mostly adults, have a more chronic form of the disease without entirely symptom-free intervals. One remarkable feature of asthma is the tremendous variation in the severity and the duration of attacks. Even in the same patient, each attack may be quite different from the others. Asthma attacks are commonly more frequent and more severe late at night or the early morning hours.

The onset of an asthmatic attack is usually insidious; mild initial wheezing and cough progress to increasingly severe dyspnea. In a fully developed attack, the patient has a sense of pressure or tightness in the chest and sometimes a feeling of suffocation, and will sit upright or lean forward to obtain maximum use of the accessory respiratory muscles. Cough, which frequently accompanies the dyspnea, is at first nonproductive, but becomes more and more productive of stringy and mucoid sputum near the end of the attack. Duration of an untreated asthma attack varies considerably, but usually is more than 1 hour, often several hours, and sometimes even several days.

The history of the precipitating event, such as an upper respiratory infection or exposure to allergens or respiratory irritants, may be elicited. Frequently, however, such a history is lacking. Occupational asthma is suggested by a history of prolonged exposure to a specific agent in the workplace and typical temporal relationship of symptoms to re-exposure following a weekend off work.

Physical examination will show evidence of varying degrees of respiratory difficulty, from no apparent distress to a most severe respiratory struggle. Wheezing may be audible at a distance. The chest is usually held in an expanded position, indicating hyperinflation of the lungs. Intercostal and supraclavicular retraction with inspiration may be evident, particularly in children. The patient often uses the accessory respiratory muscles. Perspiration is common, and cyanosis is sometimes observed. On auscultation of the chest, rhonchi with variable pitch and tone are heard throughout the lung fields. They are mostly expiratory, but may be inspiratory as well in more severe attacks. Sometimes, with severe airway obstruction, breath sounds may be markedly diminished or absent in certain lung regions. A valuable physical finding during an asthma attack is variation of systolic blood pressure with phases of respiration. A positive sign, known as *paradoxical pulse,* is present when the systolic blood pressure during expiration is 10 mm Hg or more higher than during inspiration. A paradoxical pulse of more than 20 mm Hg is often associated with a severe asthma attack. Marked tachycardia (pulse rate of more than 120/min), a respiratory rate of more than 30/min, and use of accessory muscles of respiration are other clinical indicators of severity.

Although symptoms of a typical asthma attack consist of the triad of dyspnea, cough, and wheezing, in some patients cough may be the only manifestation. Asthma, therefore, should be considered in the differential diagnosis of unexplained chronic or recurrent cough.

Radiographic Study. Roentgenographic examination of the chest during an asthmatic attack usually shows evidence of hyperinflation, manifested by increased lung volumes with hyperlucency of the lung fields. Less commonly, chest x-ray may reveal areas of atelectasis, peribronchial infiltration, or other densities due to bronchial obstruction with mucous plug or concomitant infection. Radiographic study should be done sparingly and only when there is question of complications, such as pneumothorax, or if the diagnosis of asthma is uncertain.

Pulmonary Function Tests. The abnormalities of pulmonary function tests (PFTs) in asthma vary appreciably from patient to patient and in the same patient, depending on activity of the disease at the time of study and severity of the attack. The most consistent changes detected by pulmonary function testing in asthmatics are indicative of increased airway resistance, which is demonstrated by expiratory flow studies. These studies will help to evaluate the severity of airway obstruction, progression of disease, and response to therapy.

Some patients, between their attacks, may be in complete remission, having entirely normal pulmonary function. Most asthmatic patients, however, will show evidence of small airway obstruction during their symptom-free intervals. This abnormality can be detected by more sensitive tests, such as closing volume determination. Some asthmatics will continue to show significant airway resistance identifiable by usual spirographic study, even after they are over their acute attacks. When physical examination and routine spirometric studies are inconclusive, a bronchial provocation test (see Chapter 2) may be performed. Such a test is often considered in patients whose asthma may manifest as chronic or recurrent cough.

During the asthmatic attack, there is marked reduction in flow rates. The forced vital capacity and its derivatives are severely reduced. A simple and practical method for evaluating the severity of asthma and assessing its response to therapy is the use of a peak expiratory flowmeter. A characteristic spirographic tracing can be seen in Fig. 9–3. The flow abnormalities will be corrected, at least partially, by administration of a bronchodilator (eg, inhalation of a beta-2 agonist).

Lung volumes and capacities are significantly affected by the asthmatic attack. Hyperinflation, a characteristic finding, is indicative of increased residual volume (RV) and functional residual capacity (FRC) at the expense of vital capacity (VC) and inspiratory reserve volume (IRV), which are reduced (Fig. 9–4). Variation in airway obstruction in different lung regions results in nonuniformity of distribution of ventilation and abnormality of ventilation–perfusion ratio.

The result of these various PFTs seems to be similar to their result in pulmonary emphysema, except for the reversibility of the abnormalities in asthma. Furthermore, diffusion capacity is often normal and may even be increased in asthma, whereas it is significantly reduced in emphysema.

Arterial blood gas analysis has had a tremendous impact on understanding the problem of gas transport abnormalities in asthmatics and on proper management of patients with severe and intractable asthma. This test helps to identify the patients who will require hospitalization and more intensive and aggressive treatment. It is essential for monitoring the progress of patients and their response to the therapeutic measures, particularly when they are supported by mechanical ventilation.

Abnormal ABGs during an asthma attack are almost the rule. The most common finding is mild to moderate hypoxemia, usually with some degree of hypocapnia. Hyperventilation may be partly due to increased hypoxemic stimulation, but frequently it is the result of neurogenic reflexes from irritant and stretch receptors and the patient's anxiety and apprehension. With more severe attacks, hypoxemia may be more pronounced. Low arterial Po_2 is due to ventilation–perfusion mismatching, which

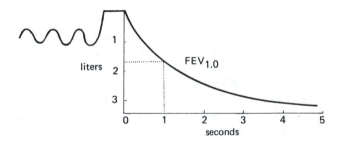

Figure 9–3. Forced spirogram during an asthma attack.

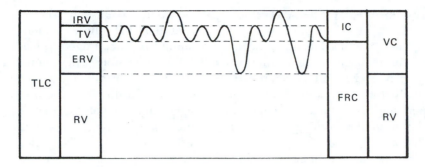

Figure 9–4. Lung volumes and capacities during an asthma attack. Note marked increase in RV and FRC.

is a most common physiologic disturbance in asthma. With further clinical deterioration, arterial P_{CO_2} rises, reaching hypercapnic levels. This is a potentially life-threatening situation and should be considered a medical emergency. Rapidity of the onset of ventilatory failure (CO_2 retention) is not only related to the severity of airway obstruction, but may also be due to other factors, such as oversedation with drugs, uncontrolled oxygen administration, and patient exhaustion. There is also individual variation of responsiveness of the respiratory center and/or chemoreceptors, which may explain earlier CO_2 retention in some patients.

Differential Diagnosis. Because there are many other causes of dyspnea and wheezing, and asthma may manifest in atypical ways, several conditions are considered in its differential diagnosis. Chronic obstructive lung disease with its exacerbations and remissions, especially chronic obstructive bronchitis, is sometimes difficult to differentiate from asthma. Congestive heart failure and pulmonary embolism among cardiovascular

diseases may mimic asthma. Respiratory symptoms in the early stage of bronchiolitis in young children are often suggestive of asthma.

Disorders most likely to be mistaken for asthma and treated as such long before their exact nature is recognized are some of the conditions that result in obstruction of upper airways, including the trachea (see Chapter 7). The symptoms from these disorders may be chronic, unremitting, and unresponsive to bronchodilators, or they may be intermittent and even responsive to antiasthmatic medications. Vocal cord dysfunction without an identifiable organic cause is another condition that simulates asthmatic attacks. A high index of suspicion together with information from adequate history taking, proper physical examination, and radiographic study will help to reach an accurate diagnosis in most cases. When upper airway obstruction is suspected, a study of inspiratory and expiratory flow-volume loop is most helpful. Computed tomography (CT) scan of the upper airways and endoscopic studies may also be needed for a proper diagnosis.

■ MANAGEMENT OF ASTHMA

Proper management of asthma begins with its accurate diagnosis, determination of its severity and its effect on the patient's daily function, identification of the underlying pathogenetic mechanism, and recognition of provoking and exacerbating factors.

As in any chronic disease, patients with asthma should have a thorough understanding of their disease and therapeutic measures. The importance of the role of health professionals in this regard cannot be overemphasized. The treatment plan, its objectives, and implementation should be properly explained to patients and/or their families for assuring their cooperation and compliance with the therapeutic decisions. Because asthma is a heterogeneous disease, its management should be tailored to meet individual therapeutic needs of each patient. As self-administration of metered-dose inhalers (MDIs) has become the mainstay of asthma therapy in outpatient settings, and their efficacy depends on their proper use; thorough instruction of patients about their correct application is the responsibility of physicians, therapists, and nurses. They should be able to demonstrate and verify the optimal method of MDI use. Spacer devices and special reservoir systems may be necessary to help self-administration of MDIs, especially when the patients have difficulty with hand–breath coordination.

Adjunctive measures such as proper hydration by adequate fluid intake and humidification of rooms during the cold months should be emphasized. Some patients may have underlying emotional problems that may be at least partly responsible for their asthma attacks. Proper psychiatric counseling should be recommended for these patients. Patients should be encouraged to lead as normal a life as possible. They should not be restrained from physical activities. On the contrary, asthmatics should be encouraged to participate in regular graded exercises. Children, in particular, should not be discouraged from sports activities. With proper medical management, the majority of asthmatic children will be able to partake in physical education programs at school. There are good indications that exercise-induced bronchospasm diminishes with more training; furthermore, it can be prevented by proper medications.

Prevention of Asthma Attacks

Preventive measures play an essential part in management of patients with asthma. As asthma attacks are usually the result of interaction between a predisposed individual and provoking factors that are predominantly environmental, the elimination or avoidance of these factors and alteration of the patient's reactivity constitute the basic principle in asthma prevention. Exposure to allergenic substances, particularly the ones known to be associated with the patient's asthma; to agents causing occupational asthma; to respiratory irritants such as dust, chemicals, fumes, cigarette smoke, and cold air; and to infectious agents should be avoided as much as possible. As discussed earlier in this chapter, basic pathogenetic abnormality, namely hyperreactivity of airways, can also be altered by reducing exposure to allergens, asthma-producing agents in the workplace, and other factors known to cause airway inflammation.

Skin testing with various allergens is

being extensively used in evaluation of patients with asthma. The majority of these patients show positive skin reaction to the commonly used test materials. Although skin testing is helpful in identifying the causative allergens and for planning of a preventive and therapeutic regimen in some asthmatics, it may be misleading. Skin tests do not provide an accurate measurement of sensitivity and hyperreactivity of the bronchi in most patients. Many asthmatics with a positive reaction to a known allergen may have no difficulty on repeated or continuous exposure to that agent. Basing the patient management decision solely on the results of these tests may cause an unnecessary burden and suffering to the patients and their families without a significant benefit. Bronchial inhalation challenge tests with antigen extracts, which are not yet readily available, seem to be more specific in demonstrating the causative roles of airborne allergens in asthma. Changing the allergenic reactivity in patients with allergic asthma by immunotherapy (hyposensitization) may be beneficial in selected subjects. Although not as effective as in allergic rhinitis, hyposensitization consists of regular injections of minute but gradually increasing amounts of the extracts of antigens recognized as specifically responsible for asthma attacks.

With the knowledge that airway inflammation is a major factor in maintaining bronchial hyperresponsiveness, anti-inflammatory drugs (eg, corticosteroids, cromolyn, nedocromil) play an important role in preventing asthma attacks. Long-acting beta-2 agonist bronchodilators, such as salmeterol, are also mainly used for their preventive action (see later in this chapter).

Antiasthmatic Drugs. The five major categories of drugs used in the management of asthma are

1. Sympathomimetics
2. Theophylline and its salts
3. Anticholinergics
4. Corticosteroids
5. Cromolyn and nedocromil

Drugs in the first three categories are primarily known for their bronchodilatory effect by relaxing bronchial smooth muscles. Corticosteroids, cromolyn, and nedocromil, which have more complex modes of action, are used mainly for their anti-inflammatory effects in prophylactic and chronic treatment of asthma. Another agent, recently introduced for the latter purpose, is the leukotriene receptor antagonist (LTRA). Various preparations of antiasthmatic drugs are included in Appendix I.

The most commonly used sympathomimetics are selective beta-2 agonists administered in aerosolized form. Inhaled drugs can be given with a jet or ultrasonic nebulizer or they can be more conveniently used from an MDI, either as a propellant-generated aerosol or breath-activated devices for dry-powder preparations. Except for beta agonists with slower onset and long duration of action (eg, salmeterol), these drugs are primarily used on an "as needed" basis for relief of an acute asthma attack. Frequent requirement for these drugs indicates the necessity for anti-inflammatory therapy (see later in this chapter). Salmeterol, the only long-acting inhaled beta-2 agonist approved in the United States at the time of this writing, is more suitable for its preventive effect against exacerbations that occur at night ("nocturnal asthma"), following exercise, or other ircumstances known to trigger an asthma attack. It is not recommended for children younger than 12 years of age. Its duration of action is about 12 hours, versus 3 to 4 hours for other commonly used beta-2 agonists (albuterol or terbutaline). Salmeterol is not a substitute for an anti-inflammatory drug and it should not be used on an "as needed" basis for acute symptoms of asthma. Proper instruction on the use of self-administered MDIs cannot be overemphasized. Some of the beta-2 agonists are also available for oral and parenteral use (see Appendix I).

Theophylline and its salts are among the commonly used agents for the prevention and treatment of asthma attacks. Aminophylline is the only preparation in this category that is available for IV use. Theophylline is better known for its potent smooth-muscle relaxing property, although the exact mechanism of its action is not fully understood. It has other pharmacologic effects besides its bronchodilatory action. Because of the narrow margin between the therapeutic and toxic levels of theophylline, the determination of its plasma concentration is frequently needed. Slow-release oral preparations have facilitated its clinical use. Some asthmatics with frequent attacks may benefit from chronic theophylline therapy for preventive purpose. With the development of safe and effective topical bronchodilators, the use of theophylline in treatment of acute asthma is waning.

Ipratropium bromide, available in MDI form, is the most commonly used anticholinergic agent. It may be used in asthma for its additive bronchodilator effect in conjunction with other antiasthmatic agents. Because of its negligible cardiac stimulatory effect, it may be used in place of adrenergic drugs in patients with certain heart conditions. Although its bronchodilatory effect is less than that of beta-2 agonists in asthma, it is somewhat more effective in chronic obstructive bronchitis.

Corticosteroid preparations are playing an increasingly important role in the management of asthma. The exact mechanism of their action in asthma is not known, but several of their interrelated effects have been ascertained. The most important effect is the reduction and prevention of inflammation through the inhibition of various mediators of inflammation. With the increasing knowledge on the importance of inflammation in pathogenesis of asthma and with the recognition of its role in late asthmatic response and airway hyperreactivity, the anti-inflammatory effect of corticosteroids has proved to be the key to their effectiveness. These agents also enhance and potentiate the effects of beta-adrenergic drugs and also reduce mucous secretion. As their prolonged systemic administration is known to cause many significant side effects, a decision for such therapy should be made with a great deal of circumspection. Fortunately, topical preparations for inhalational use result in fewer and much less serious undesired effects. The most commonly reported problem of oral *Candida* infection can be prevented, at least partly, by rinsing the mouth and throat after each treatment. Rarely, inhaled steroids affect the laryngeal muscles, resulting in dysphonia. The aerosol preparations are excellent substitutes for more hazardous oral corticosteroids in the long-term management of steroid-dependent asthmatics. These inhalational drugs are assuming an increasingly more prominent role in outpatient management of asthma, especially when there is a heightened airway hyperreactivity. Different types of corticosteroid preparations for use in asthma are described in Appendix I.

Cromolyn sodium (Intal) and related compound nedocromil sodium (Tilade) are anti-inflammatory agents used for the preventive management of asthma. They have no role in treatment of an acute attack. By inhibiting pulmonary mast-cell degranulation, they prevent bronchospasm induced by antigens, exercise, or some agents responsible for occupational asthma. These drugs block both early and late asthmatic responses and therefore are effective in preventing an attack when used 15 to 20 minutes before exposure to such triggers. Both cromolyn and nedocromil are available in MDI form. The former is also used in powder form with a special device (Spinhaler).

Zafirlukast (Accolate), an oral agent that opposes the bronchoconstrictive and inflammatory effects of leukotrienes, was recently approved for prophylactic and chronic treatment of asthma in adults and children 12 years of age and older.

Treatment of an Asthma Attack

The therapeutic approach to the patient with asthma attacks depends on severity of the episode. Mild attacks without complicating factors, such as a bacterial infection, usually can be successfully treated with a bronchodilating agent taken from a MDI. Most patients are familiar with these episodes and are or should be properly instructed in their management. They should be alerted against abuse of their medications, particularly nebulizers. Patients requiring frequent use of inhaled bronchodilators are usually candidates for a preventive regimen with inhaled corticosteroids or cromolyn.

More severe attacks and lack of response to initial self-treatment are an indication for seeking further medical help and institution of more vigorous therapy; otherwise, the asthmatic attack may become self-perpetuating and reach the intractable stage (status asthmaticus). The attacks of patients who are seen in emergency rooms usually have begun a few hours earlier, if not longer. A thorough and objective evaluation, including the determination of arterial blood gases and the measurement of peak expiratory flow, will help in the management plan and the decision for hospitalization. Most such patients, at least for the first few hours, are treated in the emergency room. As dehydration is common at this stage, intravenous fluid therapy should be started. Oxygen therapy by the nasal route is often indicated. An adrenergic bronchodilator, by inhalation or sometimes by injection, is given as the first drug. Some recommend intravenous aminophylline together with adrenergic drugs as indicated. A short course of an oral corticosteroid preparation with rapidly tapering dose is sometimes recommended. The efficacy of treatment should be closely monitored clinically and by repeat measurements of peak expiratory flow rate. Most patients will improve and may be discharged after a few hours of close observation. They should be instructed on the proper use of their maintenance medications and about their outpatient follow up.

Some patients will be refractory to this treatment and continue to have significant airway obstruction and increasing respiratory difficulty. By definition, this is an *intractable asthma,* which is also known as *status asthmaticus.*

Status Asthmaticus and Its Treatment

Status asthmaticus has been defined as a severe asthmatic attack that does not respond to treatment with an adequate amount of commonly used bronchodilators—that is, beta-adrenergic stimulant and aminophylline—within a few hours. This condition should not be confused with *chronic asthma,* which may also respond poorly to bronchodilators. Chronic asthma is fairly stable and tolerated by the patient despite significant functional impairment, whereas status asthmaticus is an acute progressive and life-threatening event that will rapidly lead to acute respiratory failure if not treated properly. The intractability of asthma usually is related to inflammation and mucous plugging of the airways. Mucosal damage and inflammation increase the airway hyperreactivity and contribute to perpetuation of bronchospasm. Hypoxemia, acidosis, and probably other factors may result in refractoriness to the bronchodilators. Progression to this critical stage and fatal outcome may sometimes be alarmingly rapid from the outset of an asthma attack, which is appropriately termed *sudden asphyxic asthma.* More commonly, however, status asthmaticus is the result of increasing respiratory difficulty taking place within a few days of its onset prior to emergency room visit.

Patients in status asthmaticus are in acute and severe respiratory distress. They appear apprehensive and anxious, perspiring and unable to lie down. Respirations are rapid and shallow, and heart rate is fast with evidence of pulsus paradoxus. They use accessory respiratory muscles and are often unable to speak. Although wheezing is common, patients with very severe airway obstruction may have a more or less silent chest, which may indicate impending respiratory arrest. The clinical presentation and response to bronchodilator therapy are often sufficient to evaluate the severity of airflow obstruction. Bedside measurements of peak expiratory flow rates will be most helpful for determination of an objective response to initial therapeutic measures. ABGs are usually measured in severe asthma for assessment of the degree of hypoxemia, adequacy of alveolar ventilation, and acid–base status. Generally, hypercapnia indicates severe airway obstruction and respiratory muscle fatigue in severe asthma. However, it is not by itself an indication for mechanical ventilatory support. Contrarily, normocapnia does not exclude severe disease and impending respiratory arrest. Patients' deteriorating condition, altered sensorium, and physical exhaustion despite optimal therapeutic measures are better indicators for tracheal intubation and mechanical ventilation. Radiographic examination of the chest is mostly indicated for detection of barotrauma and other pleuropulmonary complications.

Therapeutic interventions for status asthmaticus are determined by the patients' condition at presentation in the emergency department. In some instances, immediate intubation will be the highest priority measure. In most other cases, however, emergency intubation is not required and patients can be properly assessed and started on antiasthmatic medications, which include oxygen, beta-agonist bronchodilators, and corticosteroids. Sometimes intravenous aminophylline is also administrered. Beta agonists are commonly given in inhalational form, usually in larger and more frequent doses. Some experts recommend continuous administration of beta agonists for patients with severe airflow obstruction. MDIs with a proper spacing device may be as effective as nebulizers if properly administered. When a patient cannot properly use one form of bronchodilator delivery system, another form should be tried to ensure adequacy of treatment. Parenteral preparations (terbutaline or epinephrine) have no advantage over properly administered inhalational bronchodilators. They are used for patients who are unable to cooperate with aerosol treatment because of impaired sensorium or severity of dyspnea. A systemic corticosteroid, given intravenously, is essential for the management of intractable asthma.

Although not yet considered part of therapeutic measures of status asthmaticus, *heliox* (a blend of helium and oxygen) seems to reduce the work of breathing in some asthmatics by decreasing resistance in airways with turbulent flow. Whether it would reduce the need for intubation and mechanical ventilation remains to be studied.

Patients who, on arrival to the emergency department or shortly thereafter, are desperately ill from severe asthma, who fail to respond to adequate therapy, who show evidence of exhaustion and decreased alertness, and who seem on the verge of respiratory arrest should be intubated for mechanical ventilatory support. General principles of mechanical ventilation, discussed in Chapter 28, are applicable to such patients. There are, however, certain specific considerations in asthmatic patients who are being treated with a respirator. Complications of mechanical ventilation, including barotrauma, hypotension, and respiratory acidosis, are usually the result of *air trapping* (dynamic

hyperinflation). Therefore, ventilator settings should minimize dynamic hyperinflation by increasing expiration time, which usually is accomplished by reducing minute ventilation and increasing inspiratory flow rates. Minute ventilation, being the product of respiratory rate and tidal volume, can be diminished by reducing either or both. Reducing respiratory rates in severe asthmatics who are tachypneic requires heavy sedation and even administration of neuromuscular blocking agents. Because of high airway resistance, which is also present during inspiratory phase, increasing flow rates will result in very high peak inspiratory pressures. As long as inspiratory plateau pressure remains below 35 mm H_2O, high peak inspiratory pressures resulting from increased airway resistance are not considered to be a significant cause of barotrauma or increased intrapleural pressure. Controlled (*permissive*) hypoventilation with or without bicarbonate infusion (to keep arterial blood pH higher than 7.2) is an acceptable strategy in the treatment of status asthmaticus in patients who develop prohibitive degree of dynamic hyperinflation with normocapnic ventilation. While on a ventilator, patients should continue receiving their inhaled bronchodilator therapy. There are still controversies regarding optimal delivery of inhaled beta-2 agonists to intubated, mechanically ventilated patients. Both nebulizers and MDIs (usually with spacer devices) are being used. Regardless of the method used, only a small percentage of nebulized drug reaches the lungs; therefore, proper adjustment of dosing should be made.

As patients with severe and intractable asthma may have similar episodes in the future, they should be on an appropriate regimen of antiasthmatic medications after their discharge from the hospital. Such patients would benefit from chronic corticosteroid therapy, preferably in topical form if possible.

Course and Prognosis of Asthma.
Asthma is a chronic disease with periodic recurrences over many years, if not for the patient's life. There is no actual curative treatment for it, although spontaneous recovery is not uncommon, mostly in childhood asthma. Approximately one-third of cases beginning in early childhood will recover by their adult age. Beyond that age, tendency to spontaneous recovery is much less. Appropriate therapeutic measures, however, have a significant impact on the course and prognosis of asthma. Inadequately treated patients will continue to be vexed by it throughout their lives. The attacks may become progressively worse and more frequent, and remissions less complete. Nonspecific provoking factors such as respiratory infections will assume more importance. Some patients may have more chronic and continuous airways obstruction interspersed by acute exacerbations, which may be mistaken for chronic bronchitis. Actually, there are reasons to believe that chronic bronchitis and even changes of emphysema may take place in many of these patients later in the course of their disease. Although pure allergic asthma does not predispose to emphysema, many intrinsic asthmatics may show the pathologic changes of emphysema.

The fatality rate from asthmatic attacks is relatively small, but patients with severe status asthmaticus and respiratory failure have considerable mortality, which has increased in recent years.

BIBLIOGRAPHY

Abramson MJ, Puy RM, Weiner JM. Is allergen immunotherapy effective in asthma? A meta-analysis of randomized controlled trials. *Am J Respir Crit Care Med.* 1995; 151:969–974.

American Thoracic Society. Progress at the interface of inflammation and asthma. *Am J Respir Crit Care Med.* 1995; 152:385–424.

Ariyananda PL, Agnew JE, Clarke SW. Aerosol delivery systems for bronchial asthma. *Postgrad Med J.* 1996; 72:151–156.

Barnes PJ, Pedersen S. Efficacy and safety of inhaled corticosteroids in asthma. *Am Rev Respir Dis.* 1993; 148:S1–S26.

Bone RC. Goals of asthma management: a step-care approach. *Chest.* 1996; 109:1056–1065.

Busse WW. Long- and short-acting β_2-adrenergic agonists: effects on airway function in patients with asthma. *Arch Intern Med.* 1996; 156:1514–1520.

Busse WW, Kiecolt-Glaser JK, Coe C, et al. Stress and asthma. *Am J Respir Crit Care Med.* 1995; 151:249–252.

Chan-Yeung M, Malo JL. Occupational asthma. *N Engl J Med.* 1995; 333:107–112.

Chapman KR, Verbeek PR, White JG, Rebuck AS. Effect of a short course of prednisone in the prevention of early relapse after the emergency room treatment of acute asthma. *N Engl J Med.* 1991; 324:788–794.

Christopher KL, Wood RP, Eckert RC, et al. Vocal cord dysfunction presenting as asthma. *N Engl J Med.* 1983; 308:1566–1570.

Cockcroft DW. Occupational asthma. *Ann Allergy.* 1990; 65:169–175.

Corbridge TC, Hall JB. The assessment and management of adults with status asthmaticus. *Am J Respir Crit Care Med.* 1995; 151:1296–1316.

Creticos PS, Reed CE, Norman PS, et al. Ragweed immunotherapy in adult asthma. *N Engl J Med.* 1996; 334:501–506.

Durham SR. Late asthmatic responses. *Respir Med.* 1990; 84:263–268.

George RB, Owens MW. Bronchial asthma. *Dis Mon.* 1991; 37: 142–196.

Hanania NA, Chapman KR, Kesten S. Adverse effects of inhaled corticosteroids. *Am J Med.* 1995; 98:196–208.

Harding SM, Richter JE, Guzzo MR, et al. Asthma and gastroesophageal reflux. *Am J Med.* 1996; 100:395–405.

Hopp RJ, Townley RG, Biven RE, et al. The presence of airway reactivity before the development of asthma. *Am Rev Respir Dis.* 1990; 141:2–8.

Horwitz RJ, Busse WW. Inflammation and asthma. *Clin Chest Med.* 1995; 16:583–602.

Kamada AK, Szefler SJ, Martin RJ, et al. Issues in the use of inhaled glucocorticoids. *Am J Respir Crit Care Med.* 1996; 153:1739–1748.

Kauffman HF, Tomee JFC, van der Werf JG, et al. Review of fungus-induced asthmatic reactions. *Am J Respir Crit Care Med.* 1995; 155:2109–2116.

Lawrence ID, Patterson R. Topical respiratory therapy. *Adv Intern Med.* 1990; 35:27–43.

Leatherman J. Life-threatening asthma. *Clin Chest Med.* 1994; 15:453–479.

Leff AR. Endogenous regulation of bronchomotor tone. *Am Rev Respir Dis.* 1988; 137:1198–1216.

Manthous CA. Management of severe exacerbation of asthma. *Am J Med.* 1995; 99: 298–308.

Martin RJ. Nocturnal asthma. *Ann Allergy.* 1994; 72:5–10.

McFadden ER Jr, Gilbert IA. Exercise-induced asthma. *N Engl J Med.* 1994; 330:1362–1367.

Meeker DP, Wiedemann HP. Drug-induced bronchospasm. *Clin Chest Med.* 1990; 11: 163–175.

Moss RB. Alternative pharmacotherapies for steroid-dependent asthma. *Chest.* 1995; 107: 817–825.

Nelson HS. β-adrenergic bronchodilators. *N Engl J Med.* 1995; 333:499–506.

Newman LS. Occupational asthma: diagnosis, management and prevention. *Clin Chest Med.* 1995; 16:621–636.

NIH Conference. Asthma. *Ann Intern Med.* 1994; 121:698–708.

O'Connell EJ, Rojas AR, Sachs MI. Cough-type asthma: a review. *Ann Allergy.* 1991; 66:278–285.

O'Neil CE. Mechanics of occupational airways diseases induced by exposure to organic and inorganic chemicals. *Am J Med Sci.* 1990; 299:265–275.

Parker SR, Mellins RB, Sogn DD. Asthma education: a national strategy. *Am Rev Respir Dis.* 1989; 140:848–853.

Sandford A, Weir T, Pare P. The genetics of asthma. *Am J Respir Crit Care Med.* 1996; 153:1749–1765.

Weersink EJM, Postma DS. Nocturnal asthma: not a separate disease entity. *Respir Med.* 1994; 88:483–491.

Weinberger M, Hendeles L. Theophylline in asthma. *N Engl J Med.* 1996; 334:1380–1388.

10.

Bronchiectasis

Bronchiectasis is a chronic disease of bronchi and bronchioles characterized by irreversible dilatation of their lumen and associated with inflammation and destruction of their walls. Because of the impairment of bronchial clearance, increased bronchial secretion becomes stagnant and secondarily infected. This in turn causes further destruction of bronchial structure and dilatation and, therefore, results in a self-sustaining, sometimes progressively advancing, pathologic process.

Etiology and Pathogenesis. Although bronchiectasis is seen in all ages, its onset in many patients is in childhood. The exact basic abnormality that sets the stage for the pathologic changes of bronchiectasis is not always known. Per-sistent or intermittent bacterial colonization and infection and the resultant inflammation seem to be the mechanism of perpetuating damage and dilatation of bronchi. Among the various conditions predisposing to bronchiectasis, congenital or familial factors are most common (Table 10–1). Nearly half the cases are associated with cystic fibrosis, which is discussed in Chapter 11. Abnormalities of systemic as well as local defenses, important causes of recurrent respiratory tract infection, are therefore expected to play a crucial role in damaging and dilating the bronchi. As bronchiectasis by itself is a known cause of repeated lung infection, a vicious circle seems to be an essential part of this disease process. Both congenital and acquired immunodeficiency states may be its underlying cause. Congenital agammaglobulinemia is a well-recognized condition in which bronchiectasis occurs frequently. In addition to cystic fibrosis, local factors predisposing to bronchiectasis include abnormality of mucociliary function and partial or complete obstruction from foreign body aspiration, deformation of scarring, and mucous impaction. All of these result in stasis of bronchial secretions and recurrent infection. A congenital disorder of motility of the cilia, known as *primary ciliary dyskinesia* or *immotile cilia syndrome,* has added significantly to our understanding of the pathogenesis of recurrent airway infec-

TABLE 10–1. SOME OF THE KNOWN OR SUSPECTED CAUSES OF BRONCHIECTASIS

1. Cystic fibrosis
2. Ciliary dyskinesia, including Kartagener's syndrome
3. Congenital and acquired immunodeficiency states (agammaglobulinemia, AIDS)
4. Bronchial obstruction
5. Foreign body
6. Aspiration and inhalation injury
7. Allergic bronchopulmonary aspergillosis
8. Childhood pulmonary infection (complication of pertussis or measles)
9. Healed tuberculosis and other necrotizing lung infection
10. Smoke inhalation
11. Rheumatoid lung
12. Transplant rejection

tion and bronchiectasis. This condition not only affects the cilia of the respiratory epithelial cells, but also the other ciliated cells, as well as sperm tails. Several different ultrastructural changes in cilia have been demonstrated to be the cause of their abnormal motility. The impairment of mucociliary transport leads to recurrent infections of the respiratory tract, including the nasal sinuses. Abnormal motility of sperm tails causes sterility in male patients. Well defined and best recognized among congenital ciliary dyskinesias is Kartagener's syndrome, which is characterized by bronchiectasis, chronic sinusitis, and situs inversus (transposition of the internal organs from one side to the other).

Acquired changes in the structure of the lung and the bronchi as seen following tuberculosis or other necrotizing infections are known to result in bronchiectasis. Obstruction of a bronchus, as it may occur following the impaction of a foreign body, in addition to causing inflammatory damage to its wall also results in distal atelectasis. Dilatation of weakened bronchial wall is therefore further aggravated by the negative pressure exerted by

atelectasis around it. Allergic bronchopulmonary aspergillosis (see Chapter 5), by causing repeated mucous plugging, is also a recognized cause of bronchiectasis.

In many patients, bronchiectasis develops with known cause and in others, it is difficult to explain the sequence of events. A history of pulmonary infection developing as a complication of measles, whooping cough (pertussis), or other childhood diseases is frequently obtained. With routine immunization against measles and pertussis, the incidence of pneumonia as their complication has markedly diminished. The role of most of these conditions in the pathogenesis of bronchiectasis remains conjectural. With an increasing use of computed tomography (CT) imaging technology for investigation of lung disease, bronchiectasis has been recognized to be a complication of other conditions such as rheumatoid lung disease, acquired immunodeficiency syndrome (AIDS), smoke inhalation (a late sequela), and transplant rejection.

Pathology. Bronchiectasis usually affects the segmental and subsegmental bronchi and may involve one or more segments of a lobe or several lobes. It is frequently bilateral, with a predilection for basilar segments of the lower lobes, mostly the posterior ones. Right middle lobe and lingular segments are next as common sites for bronchiectasis. Upper lobe bronchiectasis is likely to be secondary to destructive tuberculosis, histoplasmosis, and other chronic infections involving this lobe.

Dilatation of bronchi may have a different configuration, which is the basis for the classification of bronchiectasis into various morphologic types: cystic or saccular, varicose or fusiform, and cylindrical (Fig. 10–1).

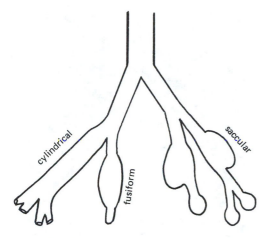

Figure 10–1. A diagram showing various morphologic types of bronchiectasis.

Pathologic examination shows that the normal structure of bronchial wall is destroyed, the mucosa is atrophied, the ciliated columnar epithelium is lost or replaced by flattened squamous epithelium, the dilated lumen is often filled with purulent material, and the bronchi and bronchioles distal to ectatic areas are obstructed by secretions, inflammation, and fibrosis.

Clinical Manifestations. The most common symptoms of bronchiectasis are *cough* and *expectoration* of an unusually large amount of sputum. The latter symptom, when chronic, is characteristic of bronchiectasis. Other common manifestations are hemoptysis and recurrent localized pneumonia. The amount of expectoration is variable. Some patients have copious amounts of sputum exceeding several hundred milliliters daily; others have much less or, occasionally, no expectoration at all. Bronchiectasis without increased sputum production is referred to as *dry* bronchiectasis. Generally, the amount of expectoration is largest in

bronchiectasis involving the dependent bronchi; upper lobe disease is more often "dry."

Sputum is usually mucopurulent. The purulent component will vary with and depends on the associated infection, which may be intermittent or continuous. In some cases, the presence of anaerobic infection gives the sputum a foul odor.

Hemoptysis is a common occurrence with bronchiectasis, which may be the only presenting symptom in the "dry" form, as seen following tuberculous scarring. The amount of expectorated blood and frequency of bleeding are very variable and unpredictable. Occasionally, hemoptysis may be massive and life threatening.

Besides chronic indolent infection in bronchiectasis, recurrent acute respiratory infection, especially pneumonia, is common. Pneumonia in bronchiectasis tends to recur at the same location. With the progression of bronchiectasis and the development of airway obstruction, patients will have increasing dyspnea and may eventually develop respiratory failure. Chronic sinusitis is a frequently associated condition.

Physical findings in bronchiectasis vary with the degree of pathologic changes. In mild forms without complicating events, physical examination may be entirely normal. In more severe forms, rales and rhonchi may be heard over the involved area where breath sounds may be diminished. Clubbing of the fingers and toes is a common extrapulmonary manifestation of long-standing bronchiectasis. Fever is usually absent unless acute pulmonary infection supervenes.

Diagnostic Studies—Radiographic Examination and Laboratory Findings. Diagnosis of bronchiectasis, suspected by clinical presentation, is usually confirmed by radiographic examination. Standard chest x-ray films are almost always abnormal and may show certain changes that suggest bronchiectasis. They include increased lung markings due to peribronchial fibrosis, segmental atelectasis, and occasional multiple air–fluid levels. These changes are more frequent in the lower lung fields. CT of the chest may show the structural changes to better advantage.

The diagnosis of bronchiectasis, although strongly suspected from the history, physical examination, and chest radiographs without contrast, can only be made with certainty by bronchography. Since the advent of CT scanners, particularly by high-resolution computed tomography (HRCT), bronchography has rarely been necessary. With HRCT, various pathologic forms of bronchiectasis, both suspected and unsuspected, can be identified. Bronchographic study, which necessitates instillation of a radiopaque medium into the tracheobronchial lumen, demonstrates the extent of disease more clearly and gives a more detailed picture of saccular bronchiectasis (Fig. 10–2).

On sputum smear, large numbers of white blood cells and bacteria are usually seen. Both gram-positive and gram-negative organisms with various mixtures are frequently demonstrated. With sputum culture, both aerobic and anaerobic bacteria are identified. As in chronic obstructive pulmonary disease (COPD), the common organisms in bronchiectasis are *Haemophilus influenzae, Staphylococcus pneumoniae,* and *Moraxella catarrhalis.* Pseudomonas, a regular finding in cystic fibrosis, is also seen in some patients with bronchiectasis from other causes. *Mycobacterium avium* complex (MAC) is an-

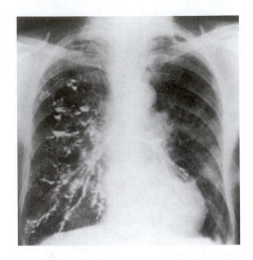

Figure 10–2. Bronchogram showing severe saccular bronchiectasis.

other organism increasingly recognized to be associated with this disease. It most likely represents colonization rather than having a pathogenic role. *Aspergillus* will be found in the sputum of patients with allergic bronchopulmonary apergillosis.

Many patients with mild to moderate bronchiectasis will have no abnormality detectable by routine spirometry and arterial blood gas (ABG) analysis. However, with advanced disease, patients may show marked derangement in lung volumes, ventilatory mechanics, distribution of ventilation, and gas exchange. Therefore, in severe bronchiectasis, both obstructive and restrictive ventilatory impairments are demonstrated. Associated chronic bronchitis and emphysema are the major causes of obstructive components; atelectasis and fibrosis result in restrictive changes. ABG abnormalities will depend on severity of the disease and other complicating factors. Hypoxemia is the most frequent blood gas abnormality.

Management. The principles of non-surgical management of patients with bronchiectasis are effective removal and reduction of bronchial secretions and prevention as well as treatment of infectious complications. These principles are also effective in preventing the disease progression, as discussed earlier in pathogenesis. Detection and treatment of the underlying cause, such as bronchial obstruction, should be adequately pursued for possible cure. Bronchodilator therapy may be beneficial in some patients, especially with pulmonary function test (PFT) evidence of obstructive ventilatory impairment.

In patients with cylindrical bronchiectasis, cough is usually effective in clearing the airways, as the caliber of bronchi reduces normally, and there is no collapse of the outflow tract of these bronchi with the forced expiration of coughing. In contrast, saccular and varicose bronchiectasis show disproportionate collapse of the lobar bronchi on coughing, without change in the bronchiectatic spaces (Fig. 10–3). The cough in patients with the latter forms of bronchiectasis will, therefore, be ineffective in emptying the dilated bronchi of their contents. Expectoration in these patients is usually the result of overflow or gravitational flow of secretions to more proximal bronchi, where they are expulsed by coughing. Thus, the bronchiectatic spaces, mostly those in dependent portions of the lungs, retain their secretions, facilitating infection and resulting in further bronchopulmonary damage.

The importance of emptying the dilated bronchi of the accumulated secretions cannot be overemphasized. This is done by *postural drainage* using gravitational force. The anatomic distribution and location of the involved bronchi should be known. The therapist should have adequate knowledge of bronchopulmonary segmental anatomy for selection of the optimal position of the patient for maximal drainage of the involved bronchi (Figs. 10–4 through 10–10). The patient or the family should be instructed by demonstration of the proper positionings for effective drainage, which should be followed regularly. The frequency and duration of drainage sessions will depend on severity of disease and the amount of secretions; however, every patient with bronchiectasis should follow this simple, inexpensive, but important measure *at least* twice daily, on arising in the morning and at bedtime. The evacuation of secre-

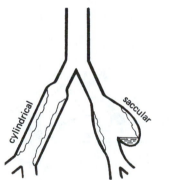
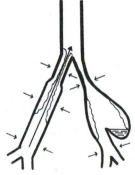

Figure 10–3. Effectiveness of cough in clearing bronchial secretions in two forms of bronchiectasis. Although cough is usually effective in clearing the secretions in cylindrical bronchiectasis, it is ineffective in emptying the contents of saccular bronchiectasis.

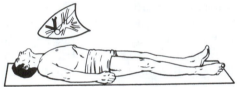

Figure 10–4. Postural drainage. Optimal position for drainage of anterior and superior segments of the upper lobes.

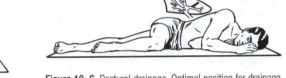

Figure 10–6. Postural drainage. Optimal position for drainage of posterior segment of the right upper lobe.

tions is facilitated by intermittent deep breathing and coughing. The use of humidification and bronchodilators may be helpful. The addition of chest percussion by cupping or mechanical devices is recommended for dislodging the thick and tenacious secretions. During an acute respiratory infection, the need for more vigorous and frequent postural drainage is increased.

Although with adequate postural drainage the frequency of respiratory infection is diminished, sometimes antimicrobial drugs will be necessary. There is no question of their usefulness in treating an acute intercurrent bacterial infection; however, continuous antibiotic "prophylaxis," advocated by some, is controversial. Nevertheless, patients who show episodic change in the quantity and the characteristics of their sputum, particularly when it becomes grossly purulent, usually benefit from a short course of antibiotic therapy. Bronchoscopy is indicated when an obstructing process, espe-

cially by a foreign body, is suspected to be the cause of bronchiectasis.

Patients with bronchiectasis, as with COPD, should avoid smoking and exposure to dust, noxious fumes, and other respiratory irritants. Adequate humidification of their rooms during the cold months is important. Sinusitis, a frequently associated condition with bronchiectasis, should be properly treated.

The decision for surgical treatment of bronchiectasis should not be made without a trial of intensive medical management as discussed previously. The condition then should be assessed in regard to the response to therapy, clinical severity, distribution of disease, form of bronchiectasis, associated pulmonary and extrapulmonary conditions, respiratory function, and other factors. Surgical resection is usually indicated when there are significant symptoms or complications in patients who fail to respond to conservative therapy, who have anatomically limited disease, and who have adequate cardiopul-

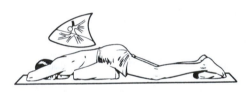

Figure 10–5. Postural drainage. Optimal position for drainage of superior segments of lower lobes.

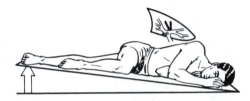

Figure 10–7. Postural drainage. Optimal position for drainage of the right middle lobe.

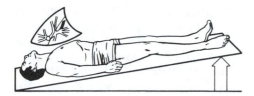

Figure 10–8. Postural drainage. Optimal position for drainage of the anterior basilar segments.

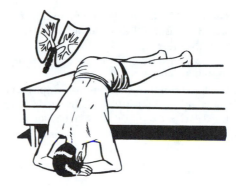

Figure 10–10. Postural drainage. Optimal position for drainage of the trachea.

monary reserve. Significant symptoms and complications include copious and foul-smelling sputum production, recurrent hemoptysis, and frequent pneumonia. Saccular bronchiectasis is often localized and more suitable for surgery. Cylindrical bronchiectasis, however, is usually not localized and thus is not amenable to surgical therapy.

The result of surgery in proper candidates is generally good. Although some patients may develop bronchiectasis in certain parts of the remaining lungs that were judged to be free of disease before surgery, the removal of the involved area may prevent spread of disease to the remaining lungs. When surgery is contemplated, intensive preoperative medical management is important in preparing these patients and preventing operative and postoperative complications.

Course and Prognosis. Variation in the severity and the extent of the disease and other associated factors affect the

prognosis to a great degree. Patients with mild bronchiectasis may have a normal life span; patients with extensive bilateral disease usually succumb within several years to respiratory and/or infectious complications. Except for a certain degree of natural improvement during adolescence in children with bronchiectasis, the course of this disease is usually one of slow deterioration interspersed by episodes of exacerbation. The progression, however, is quite variable. Obviously, proper management will have significant effect on the course and prognosis of bronchiectasis.

BIBLIOGRAPHY

Afzelius BA. A human syndrome caused by immotile cilia. *Science.* 1976; 193:317–319.

Barker AF, Bardana EJ Jr. Bronchiectasis: update of an orphan disease. *Am Rev Respir Dis.* 1988; 137:969–978.

Currie DC, Pavia D, Agnew JE, et al. Impaired tracheobronchial clearance in bronchiectasis. *Thorax.* 1987; 42:126–130.

de Iongh RU, Rutland J. Ciliary defects in healthy subjects, bronchiectasis, and primary ciliary dyskinesia. *Am J Respir Crit Care Med.* 1995; 151:1559–1567.

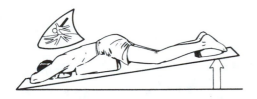

Figure 10–9. Postural drainage. Optimal position for drainage of the posterior basilar segments.

McGuinness G, Naidich DP, Leitman BS, et al. Bronchiectasis: CT evaluation. *AJR.* 1993; 160:253–259.

Nicotra MB. Bronchiectasis. *Semin Respir Inf.* 1994; 9:31–40.

Rubin BK. Immotile cilia syndrome (primary ciliary dyskinesia) and inflammatory lung disease. *Clin Chest Med.* 1988; 9:657–668.

Stanford W, Galvin JR. The diagnosis of bronchiectasis. *Clin Chest Med.* 1988; 9:691–699.

Stockley RA. Bronchiectasis: new therapeutic approaches based on pathogenesis. *Clin Chest Med.* 1987; 8:481–494.

Swensen SJ, Hartman TE, Williams DE. Computed tomographic diagnosis of *Mycobacterium avium-intracellulare* complex in patients with bronchiectasis. *Chest.* 1994; 105:49–52.

11.

Cystic Fibrosis

Cystic fibrosis (CF) or *mucoviscidosis* is a hereditary disease characterized by dysfunction of the exocrine glands and manifested by chronic pulmonary disease, pancreatic insufficiency, abnormally high electrolyte concentration in sweat, and sometimes abnormalities of other organs. Although characteristically a disease of early childhood, CF is seen more and more in adolescents and young adults because of improvement in early diagnosis and management.

With early recognition and institution of proper treatment, pancreatic insufficiency rarely constitutes a serious problem, whereas the pulmonary complications of CF remain very grave despite great progress in this area. Rarely does a patient with CF escape pulmonary involvement, and most patients eventually succumb to it.

Etiology and Incidence. CF is a hereditary disease transmitted as a *Mendelian recessive* trait. Various mutations of a single gene located in the long arm of chromosome 7 are now recognized to be the cause of CF. A normally functioning gene produces a protein by epithelial cells, which is named *CF transmembrane conductance regulator* (CFTR). The most common mutation, known as ΔF508, results in deletion of the amino acid phenylalanine at position 508 of CFTR protein. This mutation accounts for about 70% of CF cases. There are numerous other mutations that have been identified in other CF cases. As with the 508 mutation, the result is production of abnormal CFTR protein, which is the cause of a defect in chloride transport by epithelial cells (see later in this chapter). Carriers of a single defective gene (heterozygotes) have no clinical disease. If both parents are carriers of such a gene, children who inherit one abnormal gene from each parent will be homozygous and thus develop CF. Regardless of their sex, the children of two carrier parents will have a 25% chance of having the disease and 50% chance of being carriers (Fig. 11–1).

CF is much more common in Caucasians than in blacks. Its incidence has been estimated to be 1 in 2500 live births

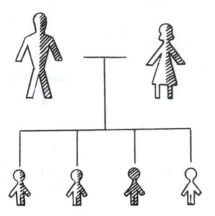

Figure 11–1. Mode of inheritance in cystic fibrosis. Both parents are carriers; one out of four children has CF and two out of four children are carriers.

in Caucasians and 1 in 17,000 live births in blacks. About 5% of Caucasians are heterozygous for CF. It is the most frequent lethal hereditary disease in this population.

Pathogenesis and Pathology. An increased concentration of sweat electrolytes and an abnormality of mucous secretion and elimination are the two distinct and well-recognized pathologic conditions in CF. These apparently separate disorders have a common basic pathogenetic mechanism, which is defective transport of chloride and sodium across the epithelial cell membrane as a result of abnormal CFTR protein production. Normally this protein, acting as a chloride channel, maintains the permeability of these cells to chloride ion.

Increased salt concentration of sweat, a hallmark of CF, is from defective absorption of ions by the epithelial lining of the sweat gland ducts. Sweat produced at the base of glands initially has a high salt concentration. Normally, as it traverses the ducts, chloride and consequently sodium escape into the epithelium, leaving the final sweat only slightly salty. In CF, however, because of the inability of epithelial cells to absorb ions from the ducts, the final sweat retains its high chloride and sodium concentration. Determination of sweat electrolyte concentrations continues to be a valuable diagnostic tool in CF. The clinical consequence of this abnormality has not been of significance, except for excessive and sometimes dangerous salt loss with prolonged exposure to heat and vigorous exercise (heat exhaustion).

The abnormality of mucus, its secretion and elimination, and the resultant obstruction cause most of the pathologic changes, in structures with mucous glands, such as bronchi, pancreatic ducts, intestines, and bile ducts. Reduced chloride movement from the epithelial tissue into the lumen of these structures is the basic defect.

The term *cystic fibrosis* was originally intended to describe the pathologic changes in the pancreas, where dilated glands and ducts, fibrosis, and degeneration of parenchyma are characteristic features. Pancreatic insufficiency, causing inadequate digestion and absorption of food, may result in severe malnutrition in these patients, mostly when they are not properly treated. Plugging of small biliary ducts affects the liver function in the minority of patients. Intestinal obstruction may occur as a result of the accumulation of thick stool, especially in the newborn (meconium ileus).

The lungs are involved to varying degrees in virtually all patients with CF. Diminished epithelial transport of chloride into the bronchial lumen and enhanced sodium uptake by the epithelium alters the mucosal fluid composition. This in turn results in the formation of thick and dehydrated mucus and impairment of mucociliary function, thus causing airway obstruction and a wide variety of pathologic changes in the lungs. Atelectasis, pneumonia, bronchiectasis, bronchiolectasis, bronchitis, peribronchitis, emphysema, abscess, and fibrosis are seen in various combinations. Obstruction and retained secretions pave the way for bacterial infection, which plays a major role in the development, perpetuation, and progression of most of these pulmonary complications. Although earlier in the course of CF mucous obstruction is the primary pathologic event, chronic infection appears to be an even more important contributor to progressive reduction of lung function and eventual death. Breakdown of inflammatory cells releases their DNA, which increases the viscoelasticity of mucus further, making its removal even more difficult. Although various organisms may be involved, *Staphylococcus aureus* and *Pseudomonas aeruginosa* are the most common pathogens infecting the lungs in CF. Patients with this disease are extremely susceptible to chronic infection with these organisms, especially the mucoid strain of *P aeruginosa*. The latter bacteria can be isolated from the sputum of almost all adult patients with CF. Normally, CFTR seems to be important in lung defense against *P aeruginosa* infection. Defective CFTR protein in CF, therefore, may be one of the contributing factors in increased susceptibility of CF patients to infection with this organism.

Clinical Manifestations. Pancreatic insufficiency is the cause of most gastrointestinal manifestations of cystic fibrosis, which include abdominal distension, abnormal stools, and malnutrition despite good appetite. Sometimes obstructive complication of the gastrointestinal tract may occur. *Meconium ileus* is due to plugging of the distal end of the small intestine by putty-like meconium in the new-

born. The intestinal obstruction in this condition is usually present at birth. There are other extrapulmonary manifestations, including hepatobiliary disease and reproductive system malfunction. Ninety-five percent of male patients are infertile, and the pregnancy rate in female patients is significantly diminished.

Pulmonary involvement, which results in the most important and potentially fatal manifestations of cystic fibrosis, eventually occurs in all patients. The time of onset of clinical pulmonary manifestations is quite variable; they may be apparent within a few weeks of birth or may occur years later. Cough is the earliest and the most common symptom, which is initially nonproductive, but may shortly become productive of thick and tenacious sputum. Repeated bouts of respiratory tract infection cause frequent exacerbation of these symptoms. With progressive and irreversible damage to the lungs, dyspnea is soon added to the clinical picture. Dyspnea may become quite severe with advancing disease. Some patients may present with episodic breathlessness and wheezing suggestive of asthma. Recurrent exacerbation of respiratory tract infection in the form of bronchitis and/or pneumonia is a typical feature of CF. Hemoptysis, which may be massive, is not uncommon in these patients. Spontaneous pneumothorax, a common occurence in CF, should be suspected when a sudden exacerbation of dyspnea occurs.

On *physical examination,* in addition to the evidence of malnutrition and poor body development, signs of pulmonary involvement are frequently present. The chest may be barrel-shaped and hyperresonant to percussion. Changes in breath sounds with varying adventitious sounds are often detected. In the advanced stage the patient may be in respiratory distress, using the accessory respiratory muscles.

Cyanosis and other signs of respiratory failure, including cor pulmonale, eventually occur. Clubbing of fingers and toes, a common finding in CF, is almost always present in adult patients. Chronic sinusitis and nasal polyps are frequently present, especially in older patients.

Diagnostic Studies. CF is usually suspected from family history, clinical presentation, and radiographic findings. Chest x-ray film in patients with pulmonary involvement usually shows evidence of diffuse hyperinflation, increased lung markings, and irregular densities (Fig. 11–2). Mucoid impaction and areas of atelectasis may be demonstrated. Frequent pulmonary infection usually manifests radiographically by new infiltration and occasionally by abscess formation. Pneumothorax and/or mediastinal emphysema may be manifest in some patients. Imaging by computed to-

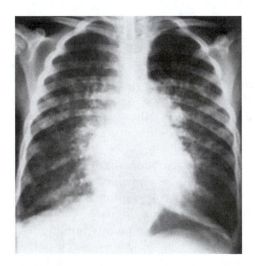

Figure 11–2. Chest radiograph of a child with severe CF. Bilateral irregular parenchymal infiltration and hyperinflation are demonstrated.

mography (CT), especially high-resolution computed tomography (HRCT), may be necessary to demonstrate more subtle changes. As demonstrated in Figs. 11–3 and 11–4, bronchiectatic changes and mucous impactions are clearly defined by this imaging technique. Sinus x-ray films are almost always abnormal in adults with CF.

Sweat test is the simplest and most reliable method for the diagnosis of CF. If performed properly, a positive test (ie, a sweat chloride concentration of more than 60 mEq/L) is diagnostic in an appropriate clinical setting. Because of a somewhat higher concentration of sweat electrolytes in normal adults and because of their increase in conditions other than CF, the diagnostic specificity of the test in adults is less than that in children. Its results should, therefore, be interpreted with caution, especially when the clinical presentation is atypical. A small number of patients have been described who have incomplete expression of their disease, which may be limited to pulmonary manifestations with normal or borderline sweat electrolytes. With a wider availability of CF gene detection it may become the diagnostic test of choice. Tests for CF gene detection are especially useful for identification of its carriers and for genetic counseling among the family members of a patient with known disease.

Pulmonary function tests in CF usually show evidence of obstructive ventilatory impairment and hyperinflation. Airway hyperreactivity, a common occurrence in CF, contributes to airway obstruction. Vital capacity is markedly diminished, while residual volume is increased up to several times the predicted normal. Blood gas abnormalities in CF occur in late stages of the disease.

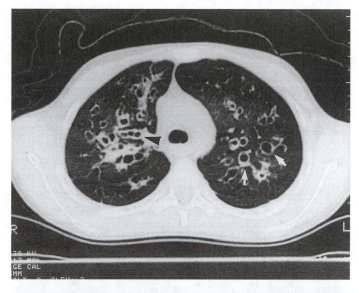

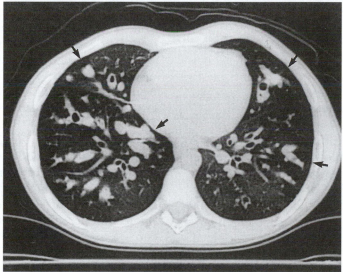

Figures 11–3 and 11–4. HRCT in two adult patients with advanced CF. Arrows point to some of the changes of severe bronchiectasis and mucous impaction.

Management. The greatest challenge in management of patients with CF is related to pulmonary complications. Gastrointestinal manifestations are usually controlled by proper diet, vitamins, and pancreatic enzymes. Despite significant advances in knowledge and understanding of pulmonary problems in CF and availability of effective therapeutic measures, lung disease accounts for most deaths from CF.

The treatment of these patients should be started very early in the course of their disease before the development of irreversible pulmonary damage. As indicated earlier, the common denominator of lung lesions is obstruction of airways due to bronchial secretions. Therefore, the principle of management will center around removal of these secretions and alleviation of obstruction. The role of antibiotics in treatment of these patients is evident from the importance of bacterial infection in causing many of the pulmonary complications.

In considering the measures for removal of mucopurulent secretions, it should be recalled that these secretions are thick and very tenacious; therefore, the importance of proper humidification and other methods for their loosening should be emphasized. Dry air and respiratory irritants should be avoided. Expectorants such as glycerol guaiacolate and mucolytic agents such as acetylcysteine have not been clinically useful to any significant degree. However, recombinant human deoxyribonuclease (rhDNase, Pulmozyme) delivered with a nebulizer is effective in reducing the viscoelasticity of thick purulent secretions by cleaving their DNA molecules. As a result of easier expectoration of such secretions, frequency of infectious exacerbations is diminished. This treatment is not recommended for patients younger than 5 years of age.

Effective cough is most important for removing secretions and should always be a part of the patient's daily routine. The effectiveness of time-honored postural drainage is proved by recent clinical studies. It should be carried out systematically, as discussed and illustrated in Chapter 10. Gentle chest tapping, cupping, or use of mechanical devices may help the effectiveness of postural drainage. Proper exercise is also known to improve the tracheobronchial clearance.

Antibiotic therapy is one of the most important aspects of management of patients with CF. The antibiotic is usually given therapeutically and, occasionally, prophylactically. Staphylococcal infection, which is the most common bacterial infection earlier in the course of CF, should be treated with a proper antibiotic. *Pseudomonas aeruginosa* is isolated from the sputum of these patients with increasing frequency as the disease advances. Once established, this organism is rarely, if ever, totally eradicated despite the use of potent antibiotics. However, with infectious exacerbations or development of Pseudomonas pneumonia, it should be vigorously treated with appropriate antimicrobial agents. It seems that aerosolized aminoglycosides, especially tobramycin, is effective in reducing the frequency of exacerbations resulting from infection with this organism.

Lung lavage with normal saline solution has resulted in variable success in some patients with severe and life-threatening pulmonary involvement. Surgery has been rarely considered for resection of localized lesions or control of massive hemoptysis. Nutritional support is an important part of comprehensive management of patients with CF. Gene therapy appears promising although it remains investigational. Patients with advanced disease are being considered for lung transplantation in increasing numbers.

Course and Prognosis. In most cases of CF, the severity of pulmonary complications determines the outcome. The degree of pancreatic insufficiency has no significant effect on the ultimate outlook if properly treated with adequate nutrition and replacement therapy. The increase in average life expectancy since the early 1950s from less than 2 years to about 30 years is the result of early diagnosis, availability and use of effective antibiotics, comprehensive management plan, and recognition of milder cases. Although some patients die in infancy or early childhood, an increasingly large number survive to ages of 30 to 40 years, occasionally even longer. Death from CF beyond the neonatal period is due to pulmonary complications such as overwhelming infection or respiratory failure. For some unknown reason(s), female patients with CF tend to have more rapid decline in their pulmonary function than do male patients. Recurrent pneumothorax denotes a poor prognosis.

BIBLIOGRAPHY

Aitken ML, Fiel SB. Cystic fibrosis. *Dis Mon.* 1993; 39:1–52.

Berger HA, Welsh MJ. Electrolyte transport in the lungs. *Hosp Pract.* 1991; 26(3):53–59.

de Boeck C, Zinman R. Cough versus chest physiotherapy: a comparison of the acute effects on pulmonary function in patients with cystic fibrosis. *Am Rev Respir Dis.* 1984; 129:182–184.

Davis PB, Drumm M, Konstan MW. Cystic fibrosis. *Am J Respir Crit Care Med.* 1996; 154:1229–1256.

Egan TM. Lung transplantation in cystic fibrosis. *Semin Respir Crit Care Med.* 1996; 17:137–147.

Fiel SB. Aerosol delivery of antibiotics to the lower airways of patients with cystic fibrosis. *Chest.* 1995; 107:61S–64S.

Fuchs HJ, Borowitz DS, Christensen DH, et al. Effect of aerosolized recombinant human DNase on exacerbation of respiratory symptoms and on pulmonary function in patients with cystic fibrosis. *N Engl J Med.* 1994; 331:637–642.

Hudson ME. Aerosolized dornase alfa (rh DNase) for therapy of cystic fibrosis. *Am J Respir Crit Care Med.* 1995; 151:S70–S74.

Kotloff RM, Zuckerman JB. Lung transplantation for cystic fibrosis. *Chest.* 1996; 109:787–798.

Marshall BC. Pathophysiology of pulmonary disease in cystic fibrosis. *Semin Respir Crit Care Med.* 1994; 15:364–374.

Marshall SG, Ramsey BW. Aerosol therapy in cystic fibrosis: DNase, tobramycin. *Semin Respir Crit Care Med.* 1994; 15:434–438.

Ramsey BW. Management of pulmonary disease in patients with cystic fibrosis. *N Engl J Med.* 1996; 335:179–188.

Rommens JM, Iannuzzi MC, Kerem BS, et al. Identification of the cystic fibrosis gene. *Science.* 1989; 245:1059–1080.

Rosenfeld MA, Collins FS. Gene therapy for cystic fibrosis. *Chest.* 1996; 109:241–252.

Spector ML, Stern RL. Pneumothorax in cystic fibrosis. *Ann Thorac Surg.* 1989; 47: 204–207.

Welsh MJ, Smith AE. Cystic fibrosis. *Sci Am.* 1995; 273(6):52–59.

Williams MT. Chest physiotherapy and cystic fibrosis. *Chest.* 1994; 106:1872–1882.

IV

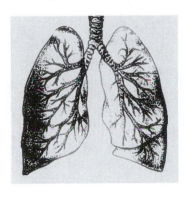

RESTRICTIVE LUNG DISEASES

12.

Chronic Diffuse
Infiltrative Diseases

Chronic diffuse infiltrative diseases of the lung, also known as *chronic interstitial lung diseases,* include many heterogeneous pathologic conditions with common clinicoradiologic features that justify their discussion under one heading. In contradistinction to chronic obstructive pulmonary disease, they are characterized by reduced lung volumes with *normal* expiratory flow rates and are, therefore, also referred to as *chronic restrictive lung diseases.* They are radiographically recognized by diffuse, bilateral, and more or less persistent densities that are predominantly interstitial. Gas transport abnormality, reflected in reduced diffusing capacity and manifested by arterial hypoxemia, is one of their main features. Their course is chronic, and diffuse fibrosis is the ultimate pathologic process in most of these conditions. Because

many conditions resulting in pulmonary fibrosis have known causes, including exposure to inhaled agents and certain drugs, adequate history is essential for evaluation of patients who present with evidence of diffuse infiltrative lung disease. Special attention should be given to environmental and occupational exposure, history of intake of drugs known to cause lung damage, and extrathoracic conditions known to be associated with this disorder.

This chapter begins by discussing the idiopathic pulmonary fibrosis as the prototype of this group of pathologic conditions. It is followed by a concise version of the differential diagnosis of chronic diffuse infiltrative diseases. In Chapters 13–15, some of the more common and better-defined entities in this category of diseases are considered.

■ IDIOPATHIC PULMONARY FIBROSIS

Idiopathic pulmonary fibrosis (IPF) is a chronic diffuse lung disease of unknown cause characterized clinically by chronic, slowly progressive dyspnea; radiographically, by widespread interstitial infiltrate; physiologically, by restrictive ventilatory impairment; and pathologically, by chronic inflammation and progressive fibrosis. It is also known by various other names, of which *cryptogenic fibrosing alveolitis* is most descriptive. The disease begins insidiously, apparently long before the onset of overt symptoms and the establishment of diagnosis. IPF is differentiated from other conditions presenting with a similar picture by its lack of causative relation with known diseases or etiologic agents.

Pathogenesis and Pathology. Although the cause of IPF is unknown, the chronic inflammation at the alveolar level (alveolitis), which precedes fibrosis, suggests continuous or repeated insult to the lung tissue. There seems to be a genetic predisposition for the development of pulmonary fibrosis. Initial injury most likely occurs at the alveolar epithelium followed by inflammatory response. Alveolar macrophages have a central role in maintaining the alveolitis by recruiting other inflammatory cells, especially the polymorphonuclear leukocytes and lymphocytes. Different substances released from inflammatory cells cause further lung damage and thus perpetuate inflammation. They include cytokines, enzymes, and oxidants. Toxic oxygen radicals, generated by granulocytes, are considered to play an important role in this process. By releasing certain mediators, especially growth factors, macrophages also increase the number of fibroblasts that are essential for the development of fibrosis by depositing collagen and other components of connective tissue.

Pathologic examination in the early stage of IPF shows evidence of patchy alveolitis with cellular infiltration predominantly by neutrophils and macrophages, and also including small numbers of lymphocytes and eosinophils. The alveolar walls are somewhat distorted and thickened with edema. With progression of the disease, there is derangement and loss of thin type I alveolar epithelial cells with proliferation of cuboidal type II cells. Proliferation of fibroblasts and deposition of fibrous tissue result in further thickening and distortion of the alveolar walls. Based on the preponderance of cell types, several pathologic forms of idiopathic interstitial pneumonitis have been described. Whether they are due to varied cellular responses to the same disease process or representative of different diseases is not determined.

Pathophysiology. Restrictive functional impairment, a characteristic feature of diffuse pulmonary fibrosis, is the result of the increased elastic recoil of the lungs (decrease in compliance) and their reduced volumes. Despite higher mechanical work against greater elastic recoil of the fibrotic lungs, there is increased minute ventilation from a faster respiratory rate. Higher respiratory frequency is primarily the result of an increase in afferent respiratory impulses from the receptors of the lungs and the thoracic wall. Diffusing capacity is almost always reduced. Mismatching of ventilation and perfusion is mostly responsible for arterial hypoxemia commonly seen in patients with diffuse pulmonary fibrosis. Because of the maintenance of an increased alveolar ventilation, arterial P_{CO_2} is frequently low. Hypercapnia is unusual in patients with diffuse interstitial lung disease. Increased pulmonary vascular resistance and eventual cor pulmonale are secondary to long-standing hypoxemia and reduced pulmonary vascular bed from extensive fibrosis.

Clinical Manifestations. IPF is mostly a disease of middle-age, with a 2:1 male-to-female ratio. Dyspnea, a cardinal symptom in patients with advanced pulmonary fibrosis, may be absent or mild in the early stage. Its onset is insidious and initially related to physical activity. Once developed, dyspnea is relentlessly progressive. A nonproductive cough is often present. Common complaints of weakness and easy fatigability are difficult to distinguish from exertional dyspnea.

Findings on physical examination depend on the stage of the disease. In advanced disease there is limitation of chest expansion. Rapid and somewhat shallow breathing is the usual pattern of respiration in patients with restrictive pulmonary disease. Fine crackles are very common findings on auscultation of the lungs, especially over the lower lung fields. The breath sounds may seem louder as a result of their enhanced transmission. Digital clubbing is often present. Cyanosis is common in more severe disease.

Roentgenographic Findings. Interstitial reticular and nodular density is the typical x-ray picture, which may involve both lung fields diffusely (Fig. 12–1). However, frequently it may be more severe in certain areas, such as the lower lungs, perihilar regions, or some other parts. In the early stages, the chest x-ray film may be normal, but usually the lungs appear hazy, like ground glass; a reticulonodular pattern develops later. Coarse trabeculation, mimicking honeycomb,

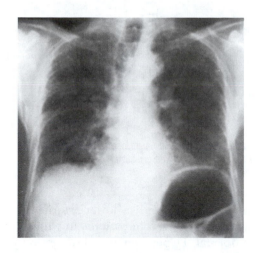

Figure 12–1. Advanced diffuse IPF. Lung volumes are reduced.

usually is indicative of long-standing fibrosis. Progressive reductions in lung volumes can be appreciated better by comparing serial x-ray films. The computed tomography (CT) scan of the chest, especially when performed with a high-resolution computed tomography (HRCT), is more sensitive in detecting early changes and for defining the lesions in detail.

Pulmonary Function Tests. Pulmonary function abnormalities in IPF, as in most cases of diffuse infiltrative lung diseases, have a restrictive pattern. The vital capacity, functional residual capacity, and total lung capacity are diminished. Unless there is concomitant airway obstruction, flow rates are normal. The FEV_1:FVC ratio is usually higher than predicted. A schematic presentation of a typical spirographic tracing is seen in Fig. 12–2. Reduction of diffusing capacity usually occurs earlier than changes in lung volumes. Arterial blood studies show a variable degree of hypoxemia and hypocapnia. Hypoxemia is usually made worse by

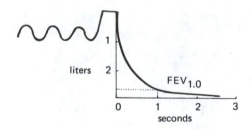

Figure 12–2. Forced spirogram in restrictive pulmonary disease. Vital capacity is reduced but flow rates are normal.

exercise. Exercise may lower arterial P_{O_2} significantly, even in patients in whom it is normal. Hypercapnia is observed only in the terminal stage of pulmonary fibrosis and when associated with obstructive changes.

Diagnosis. Although the clinical picture and radiographic findings are often suggestive, a lung biopsy is necessary for demonstration of characteristic histologic changes of fibrosis. Even then, the diagnosis of IPF cannot be made without proper exclusion of conditions in which similar clinical, radiographic, and pathologic changes may occur. This necessitates a thorough history taking, careful physical examination, and performance of necessary laboratory tests. The biopsy may be obtained by the transbronchial method through a bronchoscope or percutaneously by a cutting needle. Thoracotomy and open lung biopsy are often required, however, for a better representative sampling and a more thorough pathologic study.

Bronchoalveolar lavage has been proposed as an alternative to biopsy. It is particularly useful for the detection of the early inflammatory stage of the disease when the treatment is more effective. Unfortunately, the study lacks diagnostic specificity. Among other tests that

may help to determine the disease activity, radionuclide scanning with gallium-67 is commonly used.

Management. There is no known effective therapy for established pulmonary fibrosis. Patients with IPF are most often treated with systemic corticosteroids, which may only benefit patients with active disease. Because it is not usually possible to determine with certainty the presence or absence of ongoing inflammation, practically every patient with a diagnosis of IPF is treated with corticosteroids and/or other immunosuppressive drugs, at least on a trial basis. Therapeutic benefit from these drugs, even with evidence of active disease, is variable and unpredictable. Several promising therapeutic approaches, based on pathogenetic mechanism of chronic inflammation and ensuing fibrosis, are being currently investigated. These novel and still experimental approaches involve the use of inhibitors of certain cytokines, antioxidants, antiproteases, growth factor inhibitors, and other antifibrotic agents.

In well-established pulmonary fibrosis, the treatment is mostly supportive and symptomatic. Prevention and prompt treatment of infection and avoidance of respiratory irritants, smoking, and other noxious inhalants should be recommended, as for any patient with chronic pulmonary disease. In patients with severe hypoxemia, continuous oxygen therapy is indicated. Lung transplantation is the only effective treatment for end-stage disease. Unfortunately, the use of strict selection criteria, lack of availability of suitable donor lungs, and high cost limit the routine use of lung transplantation.

Course and Prognosis. IPF has a variable course. Some cases progress rapidly, resulting in severe hypoxemic respiratory failure in a short period of time, whereas other patients may have the disease for years, even decades, before becoming incapacitated. Approximately 50% of patients live 5 years or longer from the time of diagnosis. Because most patients are already symptomatic at the time of diagnosis, they live an increasingly difficult life, especially from breathlessness, before succumbing to their disease.

■ DIFFERENTIAL DIAGNOSIS OF CHRONIC DIFFUSE INFILTRATIVE DISEASES

An increasing number of patients who were thought to have IPF are being recognized in recent years as having additional pathologic changes of obliterating bronchiolitis with some areas of organizing pneumonia. Known as *bronchiolitis obliterans organizing pneumonia* (BOOP), this condition usually has no identifiable etiology, thus it is referred to as *idiopathic*. There are, however, several known causes of BOOP, which include connective tissue disease, certain drugs, acquired immunodeficiency syndrome (AIDS), and transplantation. Pulmonary infiltrates on radiographic examination are often patchy and may be migratory. Because of fever and other findings suggestive of respiratory tract infection, BOOP is often mistaken for pneumonia and treated with antibiotics without response. Diagnosis can be usually made by transbronchial biopsy. Response to corticosteroid therapy is considered to be a characteristic feature of BOOP.

In patients with clinical, radiographic, and pulmonary functional abnormalities suggestive of diffuse pulmonary fibrosis, other diagnostic possibilities should also be considered. More than 100 clinical entities have been described that have many of these characteristic features. They usually fall into the following categories of lung diseases:

1. Immunologic
2. Sarcoidosis
3. Environmental and occupational
4. Drug-induced
5. Circulatory
6. Neoplastic
7. Aspiration related
8. Related to physical agents
9. Infections
10. Miscellaneous

Immunologic disorders as a cause of diffuse infiltrative lung disease include several heterogeneous diseases, which are discussed in Chapter 13. Extrinsic *allergic alveolitis* and *connective tissue diseases* are the most common disorders in this category. They are usually suspected and may be diagnosed by history and characteristic clinical features. Certain laboratory studies, with or without tissue biopsy, are often necessary for their definitive diagnosis.

Sarcoidosis of the lung, which is discussed in Chapter 14, is a granulomatous disease of unknown cause with a propensity for pulmonary fibrosis. Increasing evidence indicates that immunologic alteration is involved in its pathogenesis. The diagnosis is usually established by transbronchial lung biopsy.

Environmental lung diseases are discussed in Chapter 15. Diffuse infiltrative diseases among them include inorganic dust pneumoconioses and lung lesions from inhalation of noxious gases. An adequate occupational history, including information on the nature of dust or gas exposed to and severity and duration of exposure, is necessary for proper diagnosis.

Drug-induced diffuse parenchymal disease is a well-known complication of some of the therapeutic agents. Anticancer drugs are by far its most common causes. Bleomycin, busulfan, methotrexate, and carmustine (BCNU) are the major offenders. Numerous other chemotherapeutic agents may occasionally result in lung injury. Nitrofurantoin (an antibacterial drug used for urinary tract infection) and amiodarone (an antiarrhythmic drug) are among other agents known for their significant pulmonary side effects. Pulmonary oxygen toxicity, discussed in Chapter 15, is another cause of diffuse lung injury and fibrosis.

Chronic pulmonary congestion from heart failure may appear as diffuse lung disease and is diagnosed by clinical presentation and its response to appropriate treatment. *Primary* or *metastatic lung cancer* may occasionally manifest as widespread pulmonary infiltration or interstitial density. Tissue biopsy is always diagnostic.

The *chronic aspiration* of gastric acid in patients with a predisposing condition, discussed in Chapter 17, has been implicated in causing pulmonary fibrosis. Among the physical agents, *x-radiation* is well known to cause lung injury in the form of pneumonitis and fibrosis. Radiation therapy for intrathoracic or extrathoracic malignancies is its cause. The areas of pulmonary reaction often coincide with the port of radiation, but occasionally other areas may also be affected. Use of certain anticancer drugs may potentiate the effect of radiation.

Diffuse infiltrative lung disease due to *infection* is often acute in its pulmonary and systemic manifestations; thus, it is usually diagnosed with little difficulty.

Chronic lung infiltration from infection with mycobacteria and fungi is identified by proper bacteriologic and/or pathologic examination.

There are a number of other conditions in which diffuse lung infiltration and fibrosis may occur. These uncommon diseases include histiocytosis X (esosinophilic granuloma of the lung), alveolar proteinosis, pulmonary hemosiderosis, and certain rare heredofamilial diseases. For a more detailed and comprehensive discussion of the differential diagnosis of diffuse infiltrative lung diseases, consult the review articles listed in the Bibliography.

BIBLIOGRAPHY

Chrétien J. Interstitial lung disease—clinical presentation. *Postgrad Med J.* 1988; 64(suppl 4):8–16.

Corrin B. Pathology of interstitial lung disease. *Semin Respir Crit Care Med.* 1994; 15: 61–76.

Crouch E. Pathophysiology of pulmonary fibrosis. *Am J Physiol.* 1990; 259:L159–184.

DePaso WJ, Winterbauer RH. Interstitial lung disease. *Dis Mon.* 1991; 37:67–133.

du Bois RM. Idiopathic pulmonary fibrosis. *Annu Rev Med.* 1993; 44:441–450.

Epler GR. Bronchiolitis obliterans organizing pneumonia. *Semin Respir Inf.* 1995; 10(2): 65–77.

Goldstein RH, Fine A. Potential therapeutic initiatives for fibrogenic lung diseases. *Chest.* 1995; 108:848–855.

Hansell DM, Kerr IH. The role of high resolution computed tomography in the diagnosis of interstitial lung disease. *Thorax.* 1991; 46:77–84.

Müller NL, Miller RR. Computed tomography of chronic diffuse infiltrative lung disease. *Am Rev Respir Dis.* 1990; 142:1206–1215.

Panos RJ, Mortenson RL, Niccoli SR, King TE Jr. Clinical deterioration in patients with idiopathic pulmonary fibrosis: causes and assessment. *Am J Med*. 1990; 88:396–404.

Posiello RA. Radiation-induced lung injury. *Clin Chest Med*. 1990; 11:65–71.

Raghu G. Interstitial lung disease: a diagnostic approach. *Am J Respir Crit Care Med*. 1995; 151:909–914.

Rosenow EC III, Limper AH. Drug-induced pulmonary disease. *Semin Respir Inf*. 1995; 10:86–95.

Sheppard MN, Harrison NK. Lung injury, inflammatory mediators, and fibroblast activation in fibrosing alveolitis. *Thorax*. 1992; 47:1064–1074.

13.

Immunologic Diseases of the Lung

The importance of immunology in various diseases is well recognized. It seems that, in a broader sense, the immune system is involved in almost every pathologic condition of the lung regardless of its cause. As discussed in Chapter 12, diffuse infiltrative lung diseases are mediated, at least partly, by immunologic reactions. In this chapter, following a brief discussion of immune responses and the basic immunologically mediated lung injuries, some of the infiltrative diseases in which immunology plays the major role are considered.

■ THE IMMUNE RESPONSE

Most biologic agents, as well as many foreign substances, when introduced into the lungs or any other organ of the body, elicit a set of highly regulated reactions that vary according to whether or not there was prior exposure to such agents. These agents are called *antigens,* and the reaction to them is known as the *immune response.*

The immune response is mediated by a complex interaction of several groups of specialized cells, which together with various organs and tissues involved with their formation, differentiation, and localization, make up the *immune system.* The principal cells in this system are macrophages and different classes of lymphocytes, which with the help of their chemical products of immunoglobulins (antibodies) and cytokines are primarily responsible for protecting the body against environmental pathogens. Other cells, such as granulocytes (including mast cells) and certain enzymatic proteins known as *complements,* play essential parts in immunologic reactions. They help and expand the function of immunologically active lymphocytes and macrophages.

The initial introduction of an antigen into the body results in activation and proliferation of the lymphocytes that bear membrane receptors specific for that antigen and in the production of specific antibodies. On a repeat encounter of the sensitized lymphocytes with the same antigen, a faster and greater response occurs. The two major groups of lymphocytes in the immunologic system are *T cells* (thymus-dependent) and *B cells* (bone marrow–derived). T lymphocytes have both regulatory and effector functions, which are mediated by their separate subpopulations. With the help of their mediators and certain other cells, the effector cells are responsible for induction of inflammatory responses, including delayed hypersensitivity reaction (cell-mediated immunity). Regulatory cells (memory cells) recognize specific antigens and regulate the functions of both effector T cells and B cells. Dependent on their membrane markers, T cells are also divided into two major groups of CD4-positive (T4) and CD8-positive (T8) cells. The CD4-positive cells include most of the regulatory cells that have helper function. On the other hand, CD8-positive cells include most of the regulatory cells with suppressor function and also cytotoxic cells.

The B lymphocytes are the precursors of antibody-producing cells known as *plasma cells*. With their surface markers, B cells are capable of reacting to specific antigens that stimulate them to manufacture specific antibodies. The regulatory T lymphocytes affect the extent of antibody production.

Macrophages, by presenting antigens to lymphocytes, play an important role in induction of the immune response. They are also important effector cells: they phagocytize microorganisms, attack the neoplastic cells, and remove foreign particles. Organisms coated by antibodies are phagocytized much easier by macrophages. With the mediation of some of the cytokines, macrophages have an essential role in cell-mediated immunity and delayed hypersensitivity.

Immunologic response is therefore divided into two broad categories of humoral and cell-mediated immunities, depending on the mechanism involved. In humoral or antibody-mediated immunity, the B lymphocytes are the primary cells involved, whereas in cell-mediated immunity, the T cells and macrophages play the central role. However, these two types of immune response may occur together.

Although the immunologic response is one of the most important mechanisms of the body's defense against different pathogenic agents, this response, because of abnormal regulation of the immune system, can be detrimental and may lead to immunologically mediated pathologic conditions. Allergic asthma is an example in which immunologic reaction to an inhaled antigen results in an asthmatic attack. One of the important characteristics of the immune response is its ability to distinguish between the body's own substances and foreign antigens. The lack of discrimination between self and nonself in certain disorders results in production of antibodies (autoantibodies) and sensitized lymphocytes against self-antigens. This pathologic response is the basis of conditions known as **autoimmune disorders,** such as systemic lupus erythematosus (see later in this chapter).

■ IMMUNE MECHANISMS OF LUNG INJURY

Immunologic reactions involved in pathogenesis of different lung diseases are varied and often not precise enough for their satisfactory classification. However, four standard types of immunologically mediated tissue injury seem to be operative in the pathogenesis of most of the allergic and immunologic pulmonary disorders, including different infiltrative lung diseases.

Type I, or immediate hypersensitivity, is the basic immunologic reaction in common allergic diseases. This type of immune response is the result of interaction between an antigen and its specific antibody (IgE) on the surface of mast cells and basophilic leukocytes causing the release of several mediators such as histamine and leukotrienes from these cells. Allergic asthma is a good example of this type of reaction (Chapter 9).

In *type II,* or antibody-dependent cytotoxic reaction, the circulating antibody reacts with a component of the cell or tissue that acts as an antigen, resulting in cellular or tissue damage. Goodpasture's syndrome (pulmonary hemorrhage with nephritis) is considered to represent a hypersensitivity reaction of this type. In this disease, circulating antibodies are directed against the alveolar as well as the glomerular basement membranes.

Type III, or immune complex reaction, is due to the presence of antigen–antibody complexes in tissues. These complexes, which result from a combination of antigens with their specific antibodies, are either deposited from the circulation or are formed locally. The tissue injury results from the activation of the complement system, which in turn attracts phagocytic cells. In the process, inflammation and necrosis of small blood vessels also develop. Pulmonary vasculitis may be part of the picture of certain systemic immunologic disorders of this type, such as systemic lupus erythematosus and allergic vasculitis. It is also suggested that

part of the immunologic process in extrinsic allergic alveolitis is related to this type of hypersensitivity reaction.

Type IV, cell-mediated or delayed hypersensitivity, is mediated by sensitized lymphocytes to various agents, mostly infectious. The effect of antigen on the sensitized T lymphocytes is their proliferation and release of lymphokines that affect macrophages and other cells, resulting in characteristic inflammation in which both of these effector cells predominate. The basis of the tuberculin test and other similar tests is a delayed hypersensitivity reaction. This type of reaction plays a major role in immunity against many infections. It is also the cause of basic pathologic changes in sarcoidosis and certain infectious diseases such as tuberculosis and fungal diseases. In extrinsic allergic alveolitis, type IV reaction seems to be an important feature. It plays a major part in organ transplantation and is responsible for graft rejection.

■ HYPERSENSITIVITY PNEUMONITIS (EXTRINSIC ALLERGIC ALVEOLITIS)

Hypersensitivity pneumonitis (HP) is an immunologically mediated, diffuse inflammatory lung disease resulting from the inhalation of antigenic and, mainly, organic dust. It may be acute, subacute, or chronic, depending on the severity and the duration of exposure.

Etiology and Pathogenesis. HP was originally described in workers who stripped bark from maple logs; in the same year, similar illness was observed in farmers exposed to moldy hay. Since then, numerous other occupations have been implicated in causing acute or chronic lung disorders, which later have been shown to be due usually to inhalation of certain organic dusts of animal, fungal, or bacterial origin.

These conditions have usually been named according to the occupations associated with them. Table 13–1 includes some of the known types of HP according to the sources of exposure and the causative agents. The complete list is longer and continues to grow. As shown in Table 13–1, the antigens causing these various conditions are mostly the spores of certain molds, particularly *thermophilic actinomycetes,* but sometimes they may be bacteria or animal proteins. The particle sizes are small enough to reach the alveoli, where they evoke immunologic reaction.

Because of their common pathogenetic mechanism, indistinguishable pathologic and radiographic changes, and similar clinical manifestations, these various diseases should be considered as a syndrome due to multiple causes.

Immunologic features of HP indicate the involvement of both type III (immune complex–mediated) and, more significantly, type IV (cell-mediated)

mechanisms. The elevation of specific serum antibody titers, characteristic skin reaction to the antigen, time interval between exposure and symptoms, and demonstration of antibodies in the lung tissue are strongly suggestive of a type III reaction. Inflammatory changes of alveolitis are the result of the immunologic response, which includes granuloma formation. Sometimes a nonspecific reaction also plays a part in inflammation. Type I reaction may develop in atopic individuals, resulting in allergic asthma.

Depending on the intensity, duration, and frequency of exposure to the antigen, two different forms of HP may develop. The acute form is usually secondary to heavy exposure of short duration, whereas the chronic form is the result of light but prolonged or repeated exposures. A subacute form has also been described. It should be emphasized that there is a significant variation in individual susceptibility for the development of HP, as is true with other immunologic diseases. Only about 10% of persons exposed to high levels of antigens known to cause HP develop this disease.

TABLE 13–1. TYPES OF HYPERSENSITIVITY PNEUMONITIS*

Disease	Source of Exposure	Main Antigen
Farmer's lung	Moldy hay	*Micropolyspora foeni*
Humidifier lung	Humidifier	*Thermoactinomyces vulgaris,* amebas, *Penicillium* spp
Bird-breeder's lung	Pigeons, other birds	Avian protein
Maple bark–stripper's lung	Moldy maple bark	*Cryptostroma corticale*
Bagassosis	Moldy sugar cane	*T vulgaris, T sacchari*
Mushroom-worker's lung	Mushroom compost	*M foeni* or *T vulgaris*
Suberosis	Moldy cork dust	*Penicillium* spp
Sequoisis	Redwood sawdust	*Pullularia* spp, *Graphium* spp
Wood pulp–worker's lung	Wood pulp	*Alternaria* spp
Malt-worker's disease	Moldy barley	*Aspergillus clavatus*
Cheese-worker's lung	Moldy cheese	*Penicillium caseii*
Detergent-worker's lung	Detergents	*Bacillus subtilis*

*Partial list.

Pathologic Changes. Pathologic changes depend on the stage of the disease at the time of examination. In the acute stage, there is interstitial pneumonitis with infiltration of the alveolar walls by various cells, including lymphocytes and macrophages. Granuloma formation with epithelioid cells, lymphocytes, and multinucleated giant cells, resembling sarcoid reaction, can be demonstrated in some sections. Bronchioles may show evidence of obstruction with organizing endobronchial exudate. Acute vasculitis of the alveolar capillaries has also been described. Bronchoalveolar lavage (BAL) fluid shows a markedly increased number of lymphocytes, which are predominantly CD8-positive cells. In the subacute stage, interstitial thickening with beginning fibrosis and changes of chronic bronchiolitis are demonstrated. In the chronic form, the basic pathologic feature is interstitial fibrosis, indistinguishable from diffuse pulmonary fibrosis of other causes or of unknown etiology.

Clinical Manifestations. The clinical picture depends on the degree and mode of exposure as well as the responsiveness of the individual. In susceptible persons, several hours after usually heavy exposure to organic dusts, symptoms resembling those of a respiratory tract infection will develop. Chills, fever, malaise, cough, dyspnea, and chest tightness are the usual presenting symptoms. Wheezing is not a feature of allergic alveolitis unless the patient also develops a type I hypersensitivity reaction and responds with concomitant asthma. In the acute form, the symptoms resolve spontaneously within a few days, only to recur following another exposure. Physical examination in this stage may reveal fever, tachypnea, cyanosis, and bibasilar pulmonary rales.

Some patients have a more insidious presentation, with slowly progressive cough, dyspnea, weakness, and weight loss. This form of onset is seen in patients with prolonged but light exposure. The patient is not usually aware of the relationship of symptoms to occupation. Repeated or prolonged continuous exposure to organic dusts is one cause of diffuse pulmonary fibrosis. At this stage, the symptoms are related to respiratory insufficiency.

Radiographic Findings. In the acute stage, the chest roentgenogram may show diffuse nodular or patchy infiltration. These changes usually clear with discontinuation of exposure. In the chronic form, reticular pattern of pulmonary fibrosis is the predominant radiographic finding. High-resolution computed tomography (HRCT) scan will show parenchymal changes more distinctly, which may help to differentiate chronic HP from other chronic interstitial lung diseases.

Pulmonary Function Tests. Pulmonary function studies will indicate restrictive impairment with reduction in vital capacity, diminished compliance, and low diffusing capacity. These abnormalities are reversible in acute form. In the chronic stage, in addition to restrictive ventilatory impairment, a certain degree of obstructive defect may be demonstrated.

Diagnosis. The most important source of information for the diagnosis of HP is from a thorough and accurate history. Because of the multiplicity of antigens that can result in this disease, the variation in the duration and the severity of exposure, and the time delay between the exposure and the occurrence of symptoms, a detailed occupational history, including the exact nature of work and hobby, should be obtained. The subacute and chronic forms are particularly difficult to diagnose.

Abnormality of serum proteins and presence of certain antibodies, particularly precipitating antibody against a suspected antigen, are common findings in HP. A positive precipitin test, however, is not diagnostic, as it may also be positive in healthy individuals who have been exposed to antigens without developing the disease. The value of positive skin reaction to suspected antigen is also limited. The most specific test of inhalation challenge with a suspected antigenic material is used primarily for research purposes. The demonstration of a positive response with development of symptoms, radiographic changes, and pulmonary functional abnormalities will be diagnostic. BAL, by showing predominance of CD8-positive lymphocytes, may be suggestive, but not diagnostic.

Management. As is true with all preventable diseases, the most effective measure is the avoidance of exposure to pathogenic agents. The acute symptoms usually subside spontaneously and require no treatment in mild cases. In more severe forms, corticosteroids will hasten the resolution and give symptomatic relief. Avoidance of further exposure to the responsible organic dust should be emphasized. In more chronic forms, removal of patients from the contaminated environment will prevent further progress of the disease.

■ GOODPASTURE'S SYNDROME

Goodpasture's syndrome is a relatively rare condition but is the only pulmonary disease known to be due to type II or cytotoxic hypersensitivity reactions. It is an autoimmune disorder in which circulating autoantibodies against renal glomerular basement membrane are directed also against the alveolar basement membrane, causing both glomerular and alveolar damage.

This syndrome is manifested by episodic pulmonary hemorrhage from diffuse injury to the alveolar capillary wall and renal impairment. Patients are usually young males. Pulmonary hemorrhage occurs more often in smokers than in nonsmokers. Virtually all smokers with Goodpasture's syndrome develop alveolar hemorrhage, whereas nonsmoking patients do so less commonly. This probably is due to increased lung permeability in cigarette smokers in general. It seems that the underlying lung injury from other causes, such as viral infection, may also predispose to alveolar hemorrhage in Goodpasture's syndrome. Common manifestations are hemoptysis, dyspnea, anemia, diffuse pulmonary infiltrate, and signs of kidney disease. Goodpasture's syndrome is a typical example of pulmonary–renal syndrome, which has several other causes and is characterized by alveolar hemorrhage and glomerular disease.

Radiographic study during an acute episode shows a pattern of patchy airspace consolidation distributed unevenly throughout the lungs. In several days, a reticular pattern replaces the consolidation, which may clear further until the next episode of pulmonary hemorrhage. The radiographic changes are due to intra-alveolar accumulation of blood and fibrotic reaction. Antibasement-membrane antibody can be demonstrated in the serum of most patients. The diagnosis is usually confirmed by the demonstration of immunopathologic changes in a kidney or lung biopsy. Spuriously increased CO diffusing capacity (DL_{CO}) in Goodpasture's syndrome is due to uptake of carbon monoxide by the blood retained in the alveolar spaces.

The prognosis of Goodpasture's syndrome is generally poor, and death usually results from progressive kidney failure. Treatment with corticosteroids and immunosuppressive agents has been of some benefit in a few patients. Plasmapheresis (plasma exchange) is currently the treatment of choice. By removing circulating antibodies, it results in fairly rapid improvement of pulmonary hemorrhage and renal impairment. To inhibit further antibody formation, this procedure is followed by therapy with corticosteroids and immunosuppressants.

A closely related condition involving the lungs but without kidney lesion or evidence of antigen–antibody reaction is referred to as *idiopathic pulmonary hemosiderosis,* which is primarily a disease of young children.

■ PULMONARY MANIFESTATIONS OF CERTAIN SYSTEMIC IMMUNOLOGIC DISEASES

Under this heading, important systemic immunologic disorders that commonly involve the respiratory system are discussed. Although the exact etiology of these diseases is unknown, there is ample evidence to believe that an immune mechanism is playing a major part in their pathogenesis. Because of the presence of certain antibodies against some of the body proteins or cell constituents in several of these conditions, they are sometimes referred to as *autoimmune disorders.* As connective tissue and blood vessels are involved, they are also recognized under the appellation of *collagen vascular disease.*

Systemic Lupus Erythematosus

Lupus erythematosus (LE) is a systemic autoimmune disease with varied clinical manifestations. Vascular and connective tissue lesions are the major pathologic changes, involving primarily the skin and serous membranes, but almost any organ in the body may be affected. This disease is more common in women of childbearing age. The clinical course is usually chronic, with frequent remissions and exacerbations. The major immunologic reaction is type III or immune complex–mediated, and vasculitis is an important pathologic change in systemic lupus. Autoantibodies are formed against different cell constituents, particularly cell nuclei and their proteins. Most common antibodies are against single- or double-stranded DNA. The diagnostic studies are based on demonstration of these antibodies and LE cell phenomenon. The latter consists of demonstration of neutrophilic white blood cells that have engulfed a homogeneous material derived from the nuclei of other cells.

Involvement of the lung and the pleura is a common feature of systemic lupus erythematosus (SLE); as many as 70% of patients have been reported to show such involvement. Pulmonary involvement may be acute or chronic. The acute form, known as *lupus pneumonitis,* manifests by symptoms and signs mimicking bacterial pneumonia both clinically and by radiographic examination. It may have a rapidly progressive course resulting in severe respiratory failure. Alveolar hemorrhage is another pulmonary manifestation of SLE that is due to inflammation of pulmonary capillaries (capillaritis). Because of susceptibility of patients with SLE to infection, respiratory tract infection should always be suspected and differentiated from changes directly related to lupus.

Chronic pulmonary disorder in SLE has an insidious onset that often remains unrecognized. It may be present without symptoms or abnormal physical findings. Slowly progressive fibrosis may cause dyspnea in the later stage. Standard radiographic examination usually shows increased interstitial changes with reduced lung volumes and basilar atelectasis. Bilaterally elevated diaphragm is the result of increased lung recoil from fibrosis and a weakened diaphragm. Pleural reaction with effusion is a characteristic manifestation of this disease. Pleural effusions are frequently bilateral and small. Pleuritis may be associated with chest pain. Patients with SLE have increased incidence of pulmonary thromboembolism.

Pulmonary function tests in SLE are often abnormal even without clinical or radiographic evidence of pleuropulmonary involvement. The most common findings include reduced vital capacity, diffusing capacity, and pulmonary compliance, indicating restrictive impairment. Arterial blood studies may show varying degrees of hypoxemia, usually with hypocapnia. In acute lupus pneumonitis, these abnormalities are severe and rapidly progressive.

Although treatment of SLE is also applicable to its pulmonary complications, they may require additional therapeutic measures, especially in acute lupus pneumonitis and alveolar hemorrhage. High-dose corticosteroids with or without other immunosuppressant drugs are the mainstay of treatment. Adequate respiratory management, including oxygen therapy and mechanical ventilatory support, may be needed depending on respiratory status.

Rheumatoid Disease

Rheumatoid disease, best known for its involvement of joints and related structures as rheumatoid arthritis, is a systemic disorder that may affect many other tissues and organs. Subcutaneous nodules, vasculitis, eye lesions, and pleuropulmonary manifestations are fairly common in patients with rheumatoid arthritis. Although its cause remains unknown, there is enough evidence to implicate an immune mechanism. Demonstration of antibodies against gamma globulins in serum and joint fluid supports the concept of autoimmunity in the pathogenesis of rheumatoid disease. The antibodies are generally known as *rheumatoid factors.*

Pulmonary and pleural lesions in rheumatoid arthritis are probably the result of immune complex–mediated reaction and are associated with high titers of circulating rheumatoid factor. The incidence of pleuropulmonary involvement in rheumatoid disease is quite variable in the reported series. In some, more than 50% of patients have been reported to show radiographic changes in the lung or pleura consistent with rheumatoid involvement. Although rheumatoid arthritis is much more common in women than men, pleuropulmonary manifestations are more prevalent among men.

Pleural involvement is probably the most common intrathoracic lesion in rheumatoid disease. A variable amount of pleural effusion, which has the features of an exudate, may be demonstrated. Very low glucose content of this fluid is characteristic of rheumatoid effusion.

Common pulmonary parenchymal lesions in rheumatoid disease are either nodular or diffuse. Nodular lesions of variable size and number usually cause no symptoms. Known also as *necrobiotic nodules,* they are identified by radiographic examination. Diffuse lung lesions are similar to changes seen in idiopathic pulmonary fibrosis (IPF) with the same clinical and radiographic manifestations. Bronchiolitis obliterans organizing pneumonia (BOOP) may also be diagnosed in some patients with rheumatoid disease. An increasing number of patients with rheumatoid lung disease have been shown to have bronchiectasis by HRCT scanning. Lung lesions may also occur as a result of pulmonary toxicity from certain drugs used for treatment of difficult cases of rheumatoid arthritis, such as gold preparations, methotrexate, and penicillamine.

Rheumatoid arthritis, on rare occasions, may be the cause of upper airway obstruction from the involvement of the larynx. Abnormality of the mandible from long-standing rheumatoid arthritis may be the cause of obstructive sleep apnea syndrome.

A closely related condition is ankylosing spondylitis, which characteristically involves the spine and causes fixation of the thoracic cage. In advanced cases, the chests of these patients show overinflation and marked restriction of move-

ment. Occasionally, apical lesions with fibrosis suggestive of tuberculosis may be seen on chest x-ray film. Although only a few patients may have respiratory symptoms, pulmonary function studies usually show a pattern of restrictive impairment with hyperinflation.

Progressive Systemic Sclerosis (Scleroderma)

Progressive systemic sclerosis is a disease that primarily involves the blood vessels and connective tissue and results in vascular insufficiency and progressive fibrosis of various organs. Its incidence is three times higher in females than males. There is increasing evidence that autoimmunity plays a major role in its pathogenesis. The resultant regulatory defect in the activity of fibroblasts with an uncontrolled collagen fiber formation seems to be the basic pathologic abnormality. The skin, musculoskeletal system, gastrointestinal (GI) tract, lungs, heart, and kidneys are frequently involved. Characteristic skin changes, especially of the face, may be diagnostic in typical cases. Scleroderma is a progressive disease and generally has a poor prognosis. Death is usually due to pulmonary complications, heart failure, or renal insufficiency.

Pulmonary manifestations are very common in progressive systemic sclerosis. Morphologic changes have been reported in up to 90% of autopsy cases. The usual pathologic findings are interstitial fibrosis, bronchiolar dilatation, pleural fibrosis with adhesions, and vascular changes. Clinical manifestations include progressive dyspnea, cough, basilar rales, and evidence of cor pulmonale. Some patients may have significant pulmonary hypertension and cor pulmonale with little or no clinical or radiographic evidence of lung disease. This is due to primary involvement of pulmonary vessels resulting in their narrowing and occlusion, which may occur without significant parenchymal disease. There is frequent association between pulmonary hypertension and Raynaud's phenomenon. The latter is characterized by intermittent attacks of blanching and cyanosis of fingers or toes in response to cold or emotion.

Radiographic findings in scleroderma lung are similar to changes due to pulmonary fibrosis from other causes. The earlier fine reticular pattern may progress to marked honeycombing, mostly in the lower lung fields. Changes in pulmonary hypertension may be noted, with or without increased parenchymal density.

As in other forms of chronic interstitial lung disease, pulmonary function tests show a pattern of restrictive impairment, including reduced diffusing capacity. Sometimes a functional defect may be present without radiographic abnormality. Hypoxemia, mostly with exercise, and hypocapnia are common blood gas abnormalities.

In addition to the primary involvement of the lung, patients with progressive systemic sclerosis are prone to develop other pulmonary complications, particularly pneumonia. Esophageal abnormalities, very common manifestations of scleroderma, may also predispose these patients to aspiration. There is no satisfactory treatment for pulmonary fibrosis secondary to scleroderma. Because of increasing evidence that autoimmunity is the basis for pathogenesis of systemic sclerosis, immunosuppressive drugs are often used.

Polymyositis

Polymyositis (*poly*, many, + *myositis*, inflammation of muscle) is a chronic inflammatory disease of striated muscles of unknown etiology. When the skin is also involved, it is referred to as *dermatomyositis*. Other organs, such as the heart, lungs, and GI tract, also may be occasionally affected. Based on pathologic evidence and the presence of autoantibodies in the serum of patients with polymyositis, cell-mediated autoimmunity is considered to be its underlying pathogenetic mechanism.

Clinical manifestations are mostly related to involvement of the skeletal muscles, resulting in progressive weakness of proximal muscles of the extremities as well as the cervical, pharyngeal, and trunk muscles. Pulmonary lesions may also develop in this disease, which is usually in the form of chronic interstitial pneumonitis and fibrosis. BOOP occurs more commonly in polymyositis than in other collagen vascular diseases. The most frequent respiratory complications of polymyositis, however, are the result of involvement of the muscles of respiration and deglutition. Indeed, bronchopneumonia, with or without respiratory failure, is the most common cause of death in polymyositis. Frequent use of large doses of corticosteroids and immunosuppressive drugs in the treatment of this disease has increased the infectious complications. Difficulty in swallowing predisposes the patient to frequent episodes of aspiration. Respiratory muscle weakness impairs the effectiveness of cough and other forced respiratory maneuvers, increasing the risk of pulmonary infection. Furthermore, severe inspiratory muscle weakness results in ventilatory failure, which is frequently precipitated by an intercurrent bronchopulmonary infection.

A condition in which the clinical features of more than one of the aforementioned entities coexist is known as *mixed connective tissue disease*. Pulmonary manifestations, which are mainly due to diffuse interstitial fibrosis, are very common in this disorder. There are many other rather uncommon systemic diseases due to immunologic disorders that may involve the lungs. These include *polyarteritis nodosa, Sjögren's syndrome, Wegener's granulomatosis*, and other related conditions. Due to the limitation of the scope of this book, they are not discussed. Interested readers are referred to other texts on pulmonary diseases and articles mentioned in the Bibliography.

BIBLIOGRAPHY

Anaya JM, Diethelm L, Ortiz LA, et al. Pulmonary involvement in rheumatoid arthritis. *Semin Arthritis Rheum.* 1995; 24:242–254.

Bienenstock J. The lung as an immunologic organ. *Annu Rev Med.* 1984; 35:46–62

Corley DE, Winterbauer RH. Collagen vascular diseases. *Semin Respir Inf.* 1995; 10:78–85.

Cortet B, Flipo RM, Remy-Jardin M, et al. Use of high resolution computed tomography of the lungs in patients with rheumatoid arthritis. *Ann Rheum Dis.* 1995; 54:815–819.

Dickey BF, Myers AR. Pulmonary disease in polymyositis/dermatomyositis. *Semin Arthritis Rheum.* 1984; 14:60–76.

Hoffman GS, Kerr GS, Leavitt RY, et al. Wegener granulomatosis: an analysis of 158 patients. *Ann Intern Med.* 1992; 116:488–498.

Kelly PT, Haponik EF. Goodpasture syndrome. *Medicine.* 1994; 73:171–185.

Legerton CW III, Smith EA, Silver RM. Systemic sclerosis (scleroderma). Clinical management of its major complications. *Rheum Dis Clin North Am.* 1995; 21(1):203–216.

Martens J, Demedts M, Vanmeenen MT, Dequeker J. Respiratory muscle dysfunction in systemic lupus erythematosus. *Chest.* 1983; 84:170–175.

Mills JA. Systemic lupus erythematosus. *N Engl J Med.* 1994; 330:1871–1879.

Orens JB, Martinez FJ, Lynch JP III. Pleuropulmonary manifestations of systemic lupus erythematosus. *Rheum Dis Clin North Am.* 1994; 20:159–193.

Owens GR, Follansbee WP. Cardiopulmonary manifestations of systemic sclerosis. *Chest.* 1987; 91:118–127.

Reynolds HY. Immunologic lung diseases. *Chest.* 1982; 81:626–631, 745–751.

Selman M, Chapela R. Hypersensitivity pneumonitis: clinical manifestations, diagnosis, and therapeutic strategies. *Semin Respir Med.* 1993; 14:353–364.

Sharma OP, Fujemura N. Hypersensitivity pneumonitis. *Semin Respir Inf.* 1995; 10:96–106.

Steen VD, Conte C, Owens GR, Medsgar TA Jr. Severe restrictive lung disease in systemic sclerosis. *Arthritis Rheum.* 1994; 37:1283–1289.

Sullivan WD, Hurst DJ, Harmon CE, et al. A prospective evaluation emphasizing pulmonary involvement in patients with mixed connective tissue disease. *Medicine.* 1984; 63:92–107.

Urbano-Márquez A, Casademont J, Grau JM. Polymyositis/dermatomyositis: the current position. *Ann Rheum Dis.* 1991; 50:191–195.

14.

Sarcoidosis

Sarcoidosis is a systemic granulomatous disease of unknown etiology that may involve almost any body organ, particularly the lymph nodes, lungs, liver, spleen, skin, and eyes. The characteristic histologic appearance of epithelioid granulomas with little or no necrosis is not diagnostic by itself. The diagnosis is considered established when consistent clinical and radiographic features are supported by the histologic changes. Diseases of known causes with similar histologic features should be excluded.

Pulmonary involvement is perhaps the most important manifestation of sarcoidosis. Hilar and mediastinal lymphadenopathy, which is readily identifiable by chest x-ray, is present in most patients.

Etiology and Pathogenesis. Although sarcoidosis is widespread throughout the world, its prevalence is variable in different countries and even in different areas of the same country. It is much more common among blacks than Caucasians in the United States. Sarcoidosis is rare in Native Americans, Eskimos, and Chinese. Sarcoidosis is seen in all age groups, but the most common age at the time of diagnosis is in the 20- to 30-year range. It occurs slightly more frequently in females than in males, especially among blacks.

Although several theories on its etiology and pathogenesis have been proposed, and numerous attempts at identifying a causative agent have been made, the cause of sarcoidosis and the exact mechanism of its development have remained undetermined. Because there is a significant variation in its incidence among different groups according to their ethnic background as well as their geographic location, both genetic makeup and environmental factors seem to be involved in its etiology. Whatever the elusive cause may be, a special reactivity to the causative agent(s) is necessary for the expression of sarcoidosis in an individual. A unique and rather specific reaction of sarcoidosis patients to a product prepared from a sarcoid tissue is indicative of their special reactivity: an intradermal injection of such a product, known as *Kveim antigen,* to a patient with active sarcoidosis results in the development of granulomas at the site of injection, whereas a similar injection to an individual without sarcoidosis does not produce granulomas. This phenomenon suggests that sarcoidosis results from an interaction between this particular tissue reactivity and certain, as yet unknown, factor(s).

In recent years, studies of the cells obtained with the help of bronchoalveolar lavage (BAL) have provided new information helpful in understanding certain aspects of the pathogenesis of sarcoidosis. These cells consist mainly of macrophages and lymphocytes. The latter are predominantly CD4-positive helper T cells. It has been shown that both macrophages and T lymphocytes are in an *activated* state, capable of producing different chemical mediators (cytokines). As the disease becomes less active, the number of CD4-positive cells diminishes and suppressor CD8-positive lymphocytes predominate.

Each of these cell lines, when activated, is able to stimulate the replication and the activation of the other with the help of the mediators. In addition to their mutual effects on the resident cells, they also recruit circulating lymphocytes and monocytes and direct their participation in granuloma formation. Macrophages seem to have a central role in initiating the cellular response and in setting the stage for granuloma formation of sarcoidosis. The inciting event in this process is unknown, although an antigenic stimulation is strongly suspected. It is the lack of modulation that, after the initial response, is responsible for perpetuating the reaction and producing more granulomas characteristic of sarcoidosis. It is, therefore, plausible that sarcoidosis is a state of enhanced immunologic reaction in which responses to antigenic stimuli are uncontrolled.

Pathologic Findings. Various organs may be the site of sarcoid reaction, but the lungs and the intrathoracic lymph nodes are among the most commonly involved. Sarcoid lesions in the lungs consist of disseminated nodules and variable fibrosis, although in the early stage alveolitis with or without granulomas may be present. Marked scarring with fibrosis and hyalinization, cystic formation, honeycombing, and emphysematous changes are indicative of advanced disease. The histologic hallmark of sarcoidosis is the presence of numerous, closely similar granulomas composed mostly of macrophage-derived epithelioid cells and occasional giant cells. In the lungs, the granulomas typically develop in peribronchial and subpleural interstitial tissues. Sometimes they are present in the bronchial mucosa. Fibrosis frequently accompanies the granulomas, some of which may be replaced by a relatively acellular mass of hyaline material. Significant necrosis is rare in sarcoid granulomas. It is interesting to note that histologic changes are frequently demonstrated in the lungs of patients with sarcoidosis who have no clinical or radiographic evidence of pulmonary involvement.

Clinical Manifestations. Symptomatology in sarcoidosis is quite variable because of differences in mode of onset, diversity of individual response, and involvement of various organs of the body. Different organs may be affected singly, in combination, or in sequence. Approximately one-half of the patients are asymptomatic or have minimal symptoms at the time of diagnosis. These are usually the patients with radiographic evidence of bilateral hilar lymphadenopathy (BHL). A more acute form of BHL is sometimes accompanied by fever, joint pains, and a purplish-red indurated rash on the extensor surface of legs and sometimes forearms (erythema nodosum). This type of onset occurs most often in young females.

In the chronic form of sarcoidosis, symptoms, if present, can be divided into two categories: those related to the involvement of specific organs and those due to constitutional manifestations. The latter symptoms include generalized weakness, fatigue, weight loss, malaise, and fever.

Although histologic involvement of the lungs can be demonstrated in the majority of patients, significant pulmonary symptoms develop in only about one-fourth of patients. These frequently include cough and dyspnea. Chest pain is not common and hemoptysis is rare. Dyspnea may be mild and only exertional, but it may progress to become extremely severe in advanced cases when pulmonary fibrosis develops.

Full description of other symptoms due to the involvement of other organs is beyond the scope of this book. It should be mentioned, however, that sarcoidosis may involve almost any organ in the body. The most frequent complaints, besides the respiratory symptoms, are related to the eye and skin. Symptoms due to musculoskeletal, neurologic, cardiac, hepatic, and renal involvement may sometimes be present.

The physical examination may be entirely normal in many patients or it may reveal evidence of abnormality in various organs depending on their involvement. Enlargement of peripheral nodes, various skin lesions, enlargement of liver or spleen, signs of eye lesions, swelling of joints, and abnormal neurologic findings are among the extrapulmonary manifestations that sometimes can be detected in these patients. Physical examination of the chest usually is not rewarding even when there are gross changes in the radiographic films. In some patients, a few scattered rales and rhonchi may be heard. In more advanced cases, when fibrosis has settled, physical findings of pulmonary fibrosis will be present.

Radiographic Findings. Radiographic changes in intrathoracic sarcoidosis may be due to lymph node enlargement, parenchymal pulmonary lesions, or combination of the two. Lymph node enlargement is characteristically localized in the hilar regions bilaterally in a more or less symmetrical fashion (Fig. 14–1). Enlargement of the right paratracheal nodes at the angle of the trachea and right main stem bronchus is also characteristic. Unilateral hilar node involve-

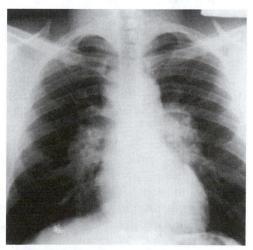

Figure 14–1. BHL of sarcoidosis. Mediastinal nodes are also enlarged.

ment is unusual. In most cases, lymph node enlargement subsides within 2 years. The enlarged lymph nodes may, however, persist and become calcified.

Radiographically demonstrable pulmonary lesions may occur without, accompany, or follow, but almost never precede, hilar lymphadenopathy. Pulmonary involvement is frequently diffuse and more or less evenly distributed throughout the lung fields. It usually has a reticulonodular pattern, but sometimes it may be predominantly alveolar. Sarcoidosis is commonly staged on the basis of findings on the standard chest radiographic films. In Stage 0, chest radiograph is normal. Stage I indicates BHL with or without mediastinal node enlargement but absence of parenchymal infiltrates. Stage II denotes a combination of parenchymal infiltrates with lymphadenopathy. In Stage III, there is pulmonary infiltrates without lymphadenopathy. It should be noted that these stages do not necessarily develop in sequence. Some patients present with pulmonary infiltration as the first demonstrable evidence of sarcoidosis, and some may develop lung lesions later in the course of the disease. Even in patients with sarcoidosis who have no infiltrates on the standard chest x-ray film, high-resolution computed tomography (HRCT) may show parenchymal changes, and lung biopsy often shows typical sarcoid lesions.

Most of the pulmonary infiltration slowly resolves, either completely or leaving only minor fibrotic residue. In some patients, however, fibrosis replaces the parenchymal infiltration, resulting in irregular and coarsely linear strands extending from the hili. Fibrosis is usually uneven in its distribution and may involve only certain portions of the lungs, particularly the upper lobes, distorting the normal hilar and vascular patterns. Retraction of fibrotic regions may accompany hyperinflation of the others. Sometimes air-containing cysts or cavities are formed, which may harbor a fungus ball. Pleural effusion is an uncommon feature of sarcoidosis. Gallium-67 is usually taken up by active sarcoid lesions. Scanning with this radioisotope is helpful in defining the disease activity, as well as in following the response to therapy.

Pulmonary Function Tests. Pulmonary function tests (PFTs) are frequently abnormal in sarcoidosis, even in patients with no radiographically demonstrable lung involvement. Ventilatory impairment usually has a *restrictive* pattern, although reduction in flow rates may occasionally be present. Lung compliance is commonly decreased. One of the most frequent abnormalities is low diffusing capacity. Arterial blood gas (ABG) analysis may show variable degrees of hypoxemia, which become more evident with exercise. Arterial blood P_{CO_2} is frequently low.

Other Laboratory Findings. Increased urinary calcium excretion and/or high blood calcium level may be demonstrated in some patients. Elevated serum gamma globulin levels are common. An interesting finding in most patients with sarcoidosis is a high level of an enzyme that converts angiotensin I to angiotensin II (angiotensin-converting enzyme, or ACE). It is due to the increased production of this enzyme by the cells of sarcoid granulomas.

Diagnosis. Diagnosis of sarcoidosis is considered established by consistent clinical and radiographic features together with histologic evidence from tissue biopsy. Sometimes the clinicoradiologic picture is so characteristic that the diagnosis of sarcoidosis can be made with reasonable accuracy without biopsy. The tissue for histologic examination may be obtained from a number of sites, but commonly mediastinal lymph nodes or lungs are preferred. With the advent of fiberoptic bronchoscopy, transbronchial biopsy has become the procedure of choice. Occasionally, an open-lung biopsy may be necessary. Biopsy of peripheral nodes and liver may have a high yield, but has not been considered to be quite satisfactory for definitive diagnosis, particularly in atypical cases. Because of the lack of commercial availability of necessary antigen, Kveim test is no longer used as a diagnostic test in sarcoidosis.

Other laboratory tests are available whose results may affect the diagnostic probability. Lacking specificity and sensitivity, however, these tests cannot be used for making or excluding the diagnosis of sarcoidosis. Measurement of serum ACE level, analysis of BAL fluid, and gallium-67 scanning are among such tests. They seem to be more useful for determination of disease activity and, sometimes, for assessment of therapeutic response.

Management. Most patients with sarcoidosis require no treatment. Corticosteroids and sometimes other immunosuppressive drugs are the only agents known to suppress the active process in sarcoidosis. Because of the significant side effects of these drugs, however, patients should be carefully selected for this type of therapy. The expected benefit of these agents should outweigh their potential harm to justify their use. Certain manifestations of sarcoidosis are definite indications for steroid therapy. These include progressive respiratory impairment, involvement of the eyes, cardiac sar-

coidosis, central nervous system (CNS) involvement, disfiguring skin lesions, and persistent elevation of serum calcium. The question of steroid therapy in less severe pulmonary involvement without significant respiratory symptoms has not been entirely settled. As most of these patients will have spontaneous remission, they may be observed closely and treated only when their disease shows progression.

Other anti-inflammatory drugs and immunosuppressive agents are rarely used in treatment of sarcoidosis. Management of respiratory insufficiency and failure due to far-advanced disease with fibrosis are discussed in other sections of this book (see Chapters 12 and 26).

Course and Prognosis. The frequency of limited forms of sarcoidosis and common spontaneous remissions make the prognosis favorable in the majority of patients. A fairly acute onset with BHL has excellent prognosis. More insidious disease involving the lungs may progress to pulmonary fibrosis. It is almost impossible, however, to predict accurately the long-term outcome. It has been estimated that about 65% of patients recover completely or have only minimal residual disease, and the remaining will have some degree of permanent disability due to pulmonary fibrosis or involvement of the eyes, kidneys, heart, or CNS. A small percentage of these patients may succumb to their disease early in life, mostly from respiratory failure.

Residual cystic or cavitary lesions from sarcoidosis not uncommonly may become the site for *Aspergillus* infection, resulting in the development of a fungus ball (page 101). The cause of significant hemoptysis in sarcoidosis is usually from this complication.

BIBLIOGRAPHY

Abe S, Munakata M, Nishimura M, et al. Gallium-67 scintigraphy, bronchoalveolar lavage, and pathologic changes in patients with pulmonary sarcoidosis. *Chest.* 1984; 85:650–655.

Brauner MW, Grenier P, Monpoint D, et al. Pulmonary sarcoidosis: evaluation with high-resolution CT. *Radiology.* 1989; 172:467–471.

Chesnutt AN. Enigmas in sarcoidosis. *West J Med.* 1995; 162:519–526.

Crystal RG, Roberts WC, Hunninghake GW, et al. Pulmonary sarcoidosis: a disease characterized and perpetuated by activated T-lymphocytes. *Ann Intern Med.* 1981; 94: 73–94.

DeRemee RA. Sarcoidosis. *Mayo Clin Proc.* 1995; 70:177–181.

Johns CJ, Scott PP, Schonfeld SA. Sarcoidosis. *Annu Rev Med.* 1989; 40:353–371.

Peckham DG, Spiteri MA. Sarcoidosis. *Postgrad Med J.* 1996; 72:196–200.

Sharma OP. Sarcoidosis. *Dis Mon.* 1990; 36:474–535.

Thomas PD, Hunninghake GW. Current concepts of the pathogenesis of sarcoidosis. *Am Rev Respir Dis.* 1987; 135:747–760.

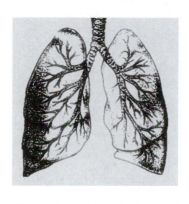

ENVIRONMENTAL AND INHALATIONAL LUNG DISEASES

15.

Environmental Lung Diseases

Environmental lung diseases are pathologic conditions of the respiratory tract that result directly from the inhalation of various gaseous or particulate matters in the air. Most, but not all, of these conditions are job related and, if so, are known as *occupational lung diseases.*

■ ENVIRONMENTAL EXPOSURE

The lungs are continuously exposed to a variety of external pathogenic agents in the form of fine particles and gas suspended in or mixed with atmospheric air. This atmospheric contamination is mainly man-made in populated areas of the world and, for the most part, is related to industrial development. These environmental pulmonary pathogens of various origin and composition enter the lungs as an aerosol or in gaseous form, or as a mixture of the two. The deposition and absorption of these substances on the airways or gas-exchanging membranes are related to their physical and chemical characteristics, the anatomic arrangement of air passages, and the rate of air flow.

Particle size is a major physical factor in determining the site where the aerosolized materials will deposit. The anatomic structures of the airways and changes in direction of airflow through the continuously dividing air passages result in *inertial impaction,* which is the principal mechanism of large particle deposition in the respiratory tract. Particles larger than 10 to 20 microns (μ) in diameter are almost totally removed in the upper airways by this mechanism. Although some of the smaller particles are also deposited by inertial impaction, settling by *gravity* (*sedimentation*) is a more important mechanism for their deposition, especially in more distal airways where airflow velocity is low. Inertial impaction occurs particularly with angulation of airways and narrowing of their lumen, which is why airway bifurcations are favorite sites for deposition of aerosolized particles. Very small particles are deposited mainly by diffusion or Brownian motion. The majority of particles reaching the terminal airways and alveoli are less than 4 μ in diameter and are deposited by gravitational forces and Brownian action. Much smaller particles, which will have no appreciable deposition, will be exhaled. Although large particles do not reach the distal airways, asbestos fibers can be demonstrated in the lung parenchyma despite their sizable length (up to 100 μ). The very small diameter of these fibers, despite their length, is probably the reason for their slowed sedimentation and their ability to penetrate deeper into the lung tissue.

Pulmonary Defense Mechanisms

Gaseous agents entering the lungs encounter little, if any, resistance. This is understandable considering the main function of the lung, which is to draw in environmental gases and distribute them throughout the alveolar surface area. Some of these gases may also enter the bloodstream. The only defenses that the lung may exhibit are temporary cessation of breathing as a reflex on exposure to irritant gases, partial absorption of soluble gases on the moist surfaces of the airways, and detoxification by chemical combination. These defenses, however, are inadequate; with significant exposure, noxious gases will have their damaging effects.

Inhaled particulate matters, once deposited on different areas of the respiratory tract, are taken care of by several defense mechanisms. Particles deposited on the mucous surface of the nasal passages and other parts of the upper airways are readily disposed of by ciliary movements toward the pharynx, from where they are swallowed or coughed out. Sneezing and blowing the nose also help in expelling these particles mixed with nasal secretions.

The mucous blanket over the ciliated epithelium of the tracheobronchial tree is the major vehicle for particles deposited on its surface. Cilia are normally bathed in more serous fluid, called the *sol layer,* or periciliary fluid, which facilitates their rhythmic beating. The mucus, or *gel layer,* actually floats over the sol layer, and only its undersurface is contacted by the cilia, which propel it from beneath (Fig. 15–1). Particular viscoelastic behavior of the tracheobronchial mucus is very helpful in its movement. The speed of mucus movement and, therefore, the transport of particles deposited on it has been estimated to be between 10 and 20 mm per minute, so that 90% of the material settled on the airway mucosa is physically cleared in less than 1 hour.

The irritating effect of certain particles and gases increases airway secretions. With repeated and chronic exposure, the mucous glands will hypertrophy and will secrete more mucus in response to a variety of inhaled irritants. This is the basic pathologic change of chronic bronchitis, which is discussed in Chapter 8. *Cough* is

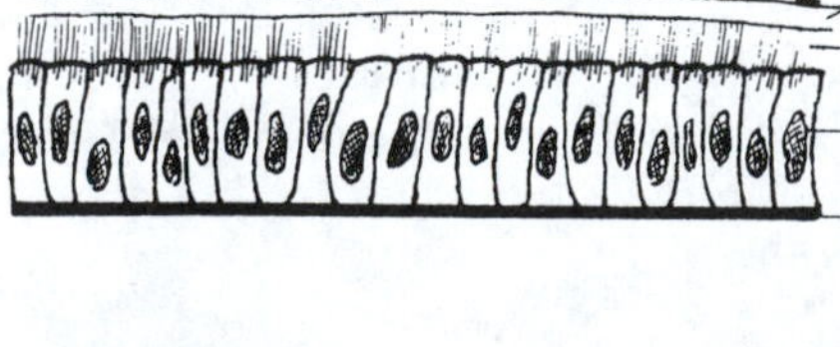

Figure 15–1. Mucous blanket on the ciliated epithelium.

particles
gel layer
sol layer and cilia
ciliated epithelium
basement membrane

an important mechanism by which secretions and foreign particles are expelled. Irritation of the nerve endings in the airway mucosa by these materials stimulates the cough reflex.

Distal airways (bronchioles) and alveoli have no ciliated epithelium, mucous glands, or goblet cells; therefore, particles deposited in their lumen are removed with more difficulty. Alveolar clearance involves more complex pathways of cellular and fluid transport. Phagocytic cells in the alveoli (macrophages) play the major role in disposing of the particles reaching this part of the respiratory tract. In addition, alveolar surfactant secreted by the type II alveolar cells and fluid originating from capillary transudation help in transporting the particles toward the mucociliary escalator or in draining into the interstitial space and, thence, to the lymph channels. Disposal of particles from the alveoli is a very slow process, and the respiratory membrane remains exposed to their harmful effects until the particles are removed. Coating of the particles by secretory materials such as surfactant and certain chemical reactions, as well as enzymatic action, diminish their injurious effects.

Once phagocytized, particles are processed by the metabolic and enzymatic apparatus of the alveolar macrophages. The phagocytic effectiveness of these cells is influenced by a variety of exogenous as well as endogenous factors. Sometimes the offending agents impair the function of these cells. For example, silica causes the death of macrophages, resulting in the release of their enzymes as well as the silica particles.

When these primary disposing mechanisms fail to control the pathogenic factors from exerting their harmful effects, the secondary cellular and humoral defense mechanisms are brought into action. These mechanisms result in inflammation, which consists of dilatation and increased permeability of capillaries, exudation of fluid, and infiltration of white blood cells. The immunologic system plays a major part in this process. Macrophages are involved in presenting antigenic substances to the immunocompetent lymphocytes and, therefore, in helping them to initiate an immunologic response. It seems, therefore, that the pathologic changes are, at least partly, the result of these secondary defense mechanisms.

Environmental pulmonary pathogens can be divided into four categories:

1. Infectious agents
2. Organic dusts
3. Inorganic dusts
4. Gases

Pulmonary diseases due to the agents in the first two categories, which include respiratory tract infection, asthma, and hypersensitivity pneumonitis, are discussed in separate chapters. Some of the common diseases known to be due to inorganic dusts and certain gases are reviewed in this chapter. Because of its importance in the pathogenesis of many pulmonary and extrapulmonary diseases, tobacco smoking is discussed separately in Chapter 16.

■ ENVIRONMENTAL DISEASES DUE TO INORGANIC DUSTS

Diseases due to inhalation of inorganic dusts are generally referred to as *pneumoconioses* (*pneumo,* lung; *konia,* dust; *osis,* condition). Several factors will determine the outcome of exposure to such particles. These include chemical nature, particle size, severity and duration of exposure, and host factors. The latter are related to individual susceptibility, including the immunologic response and local handling of dust by bronchopulmonary defense mechanisms. Thus it is not uncommon for two individuals with the same degree of exposure to the same agent and under similar circumstances to have two quite different responses; one may remain unharmed, whereas the other may show evidence of significant lung disease.

Almost all cases of inorganic dust pneumoconiosis are secondary to occupational exposure, particularly in the mining industry. There are other circumstances, however, in which exposure to such mineral dusts is possible. Only with a thorough and detailed *occupational* and *environmental history* will the exact nature of these diseases become recognized. There are few or no clinical or radiographic features that can identify the cause of specific occupational lung disease. With proper application of public health control measures and enforcement of existing laws on dust exposure limits, there has been steady reduction of new cases of pneumoconioses in the United States. However, there are still a significant number of patients with respiratory conditions related to inorganic dust exposure, and many of them have acquired their disease in recent years.

The most important inorganic dusts causing pneumoconiosis are silicon dioxide (silica), silicates (asbestos, talc, kaolin, mica, etc.), and carbon (coal, graphite, etc.). Pneumoconioses due to less common causes, such as beryllium, iron, tin, aluminum, cobalt, and several other metals, are not discussed.

Silicosis

Pneumoconiosis due to silica exposure is a chronic fibrosing disease of the lung that may occur in many occupations. Silica or silicon dioxide is a compound of the two most abundant elements of the earth's crust: oxygen and silicon. It is the

main constituent of more than 95% of the earth's rocks. It occurs in a variety of forms, but the most common form is crystalline quartz. It becomes harmful when small respirable particles (less than 5 μ in diameter) of crystalline silica are produced with its various industrial use. Sources of free silica dust include industries such as mining, quarrying, tunneling, stone masonry, road construction, sandblasting, stonecutting, abrasive industry, molding in foundries, pottery, and tile manufacturing. In many of these occupations, particularly in mining, the workers may be exposed to other particulate matters in addition to the silica dust, such as coal, asbestos, iron, and other minerals. Sandblasting, which is abrasive blasting with silica sand for industrial purposes, is notorious for causing silicosis in an accelerated fashion.

The development of silicosis depends on the particle size of the silica, its concentration in air, duration of exposure, and individual susceptibility. The particle size range that results in maximal alveolar deposition is 1 to 3 μ. The concentration of silica dust usually determines the rapidity of the onset of clinical manifestations of silicosis. Heavy exposure, sometimes seen in sandblasters, may result in a more acute form of silicosis after a relatively brief exposure. However, with a less heavy concentration, the disease requires many years of exposure to develop.

Pathogenesis and Pathology. Silica particles deposited in the alveoli are phagocytized by the macrophages. The interaction between these cells and silica seems to be pivotal in pathogenesis of silicosis. From in vitro studies, it is known that silica particles damage the macrophages and cause the release of intracellular enzymes as well as phagocytized silica. There is increasing in vivo evidence, however, that the release of inflammatory mediators (such as cytokines) from live macrophages is mainly responsible for pathologic changes of silicosis. Lymphocytes, neutrophils, and fibroblasts are all known to participate in the process. Immune mechanisms appear to have a significant role in silicosis. The impairment of function of macrophages is probably the cause of reduced defense of silicotic lungs against certain infections, especially tuberculosis (TB).

The characteristic pathologic changes in silicosis are *silicotic nodules,* which are whorled and densely packed fibrotic lesions. They measure 2 to 3 mm in diameter and are unevenly scattered throughout the lungs, mostly in the upper lobes and the perihilar regions. These nodules are usually surrounded by distorted lung tissue, which may show emphysematous changes. Silica particles may be demonstrated in these lesions as well as in hilar and mediastinal lymph nodes.

The coalescence of nodular fibrosis, particularly in the upper lobes, results in the formation of irregular masses, which may become quite large and occasionally may show evidence of central cavitation. These changes are characteristic of *progressive massive fibrosis* (PMF) and are indicative of *complicated* silicosis. Such lesions have been frequently attributed to concomitant TB, atypical mycobacterial disease, or other infections. With progressive massive fibrosis, the upper lobes may become contracted, and the lower lobes may show evidence of emphysema, sometimes with large bullous changes.

Clinical Manifestations. Silicosis is a chronic disease, usually with an insidious onset after prolonged exposure to silica dust. It is not uncommon for the symptoms to develop many years after cessation of exposure. With heavy exposure, as seen in sandblasting, the symptoms may develop more rapidly. The pulmonary lesions of silicosis and associated disability are often progressive, despite removal of the patients from their dusty environment. Patients with simple silicosis are often asymptomatic. The main symptom with *complicated silicosis* is dyspnea with or without cough. The severity of dyspnea is variable, but it is usually progressive. The history of cough and expectoration is often due to concomitant cigarette smoking. Other respiratory symptoms, such as hemoptysis or chest pain, are usually secondary to superimposed infection. Although TB and atypical mycobacterial infection are often implicated in the production of progressive massive fibrosis, clinical confirmation is difficult. Repeated bacteriologic studies are indicated, especially if the tuberculin test is positive. In more advanced complicated silicosis, respiratory failure may supervene.

Radiographic Findings. In the simple form of silicosis, multiple small nodular shadows can be demonstrated throughout the lung fields. For the development of radiographic changes, 10, 20, or more years of moderate exposure are necessary. However, with more heavy exposure, such as in sandblasting, roentgenographic changes may be demonstrated much earlier. In *complicated silicosis,* massive densities are seen in upper lung fields (Figs. 15–2 and 15–3). Progressive change from a simple nodular form to massive fibrosis may take place within 5 years. With the development of massive fibrosis, the upper lobes show evidence of volume loss, with eleva-

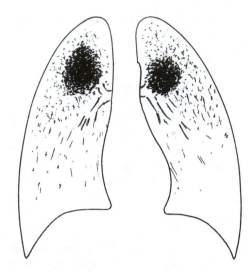

Figure 15–2. A diagrammatic demonstration of progressive massive fibrosis in complicated silicosis.

tion of the hili and emphysematous changes of the lower lobes. In a small percentage of patients, characteristic egg-shell calcification of hilar nodes may be present.

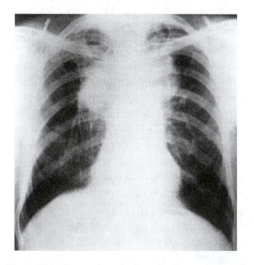

Figure 15–3. Chest radiograph of progressive massive fibrosis appearing as bilateral upper lobe masses. Both silicosis and CWP may cause this type of radiographic change.

Pulmonary Function Tests. There is no characteristic pattern of pulmonary functional abnormality in patients with silicosis. In simple silicosis, the routine spirographic study is usually normal. In more severe disease, restrictive, obstructive, or mixed patterns of impairment may be demonstrated. Diffusing capacity and pulmonary compliance are frequently reduced. Serial pulmonary function studies are very important in evaluating the course and progression of the disease.

Diagnosis. As is true in almost all environmental lung diseases, the diagnosis of silicosis is based primarily on history and radiographic findings. Exposure history has to be specific regarding the occupation, working conditions, and duration as well as intensity of exposure. Characteristic radiographic findings together with a history of adequate silica exposure are usually considered diagnostic of silicosis. Histopathologic confirmation is only needed when other treatable causes of chronic diffuse nodular lung disease cannot be excluded without lung biopsy. Therefore, there are three required criteria for diagnosis of silicosis: appropriate history of exposure, consistent radiographic findings, and absence of likely alternative explanation for similar clinico-radiographic presentation.

Management. There is no known effective treatment for any of the inorganic dust pneumoconioses, including silicosis. However, preventive measures are most effective against acquiring these diseases. Awareness of health hazards associated with various industries is the first step, which should be followed by efforts to eliminate or reduce the exposure of the lungs to these offending agents. Proper ventilation of the work area; use of wet techniques; wearing of special masks, hoods, or respirators; and other methods of controlling the environment would markedly diminish the occupational hazards of silica exposure.

The principles of management of diffuse pulmonary fibrosis discussed in Chapter 12 are equally applicable to well-established silicosis. Because of the increased risk of TB infection in patients with silicosis, necessary preventive and therapeutic measures should be taken against this complication. Patients with a positive tuberculin test without active TB are candidates for prophylaxis with isoniazid therapy.

Coal Workers' Pneumoconiosis

Coal workers' pneumoconiosis (CWP), commonly known as "black lung," is a chronic pathologic condition resulting from prolonged exposure to coal dust. The role of silica dust, often present with coal mining, is relatively small in CWP. There are occasional situations in coal mining, such as drilling operations in areas with significant rock strata, in which heavy silica exposure may result in silicosis. Although carbon is not considered to be fibrogenic, with massive and prolonged exposure the clearance mechanisms of the lungs are overwhelmed, and coal dust accumulates in terminal airspaces, resulting in pulmonary pathology.

As with other inorganic dust pneumoconioses, the severity and duration of exposure are among the major factors determining the pathologic changes due to coal dust inhalation. The area of mining at which coal is cut, known as the *coal face,* is the dustiest part of the mine.

Workers in this area are, therefore, exposed to a very high concentration of coal dust. The degree of exposure of workers in other areas of mining and transportation is variable. The incidence of pneumoconiosis in anthracite mining is much higher than in soft (bituminous) coal mining. It has been estimated that it takes at least 10 to 12 years of underground work for the development of CWP.

Pathogenesis and Pathology. The first reaction after the deposition of coal dust in the respiratory bronchioles and alveoli is phagocytosis of the particles by increasing numbers of macrophages. They move to the terminal bronchioles, from which they are removed by the mucociliary escalator. An excessive dust load results in overwhelming the pulmonary clearance mechanisms. Macrophages play a pivotal role in CWP by initiating inflammation and eventual fibrosis. Various cytokines, oxygen radicals, and enzymes are involved in the process. Fibroblasts lay a thin network of reticulin fibers without significant collagen formation. The aggregations of macrophages and dust particles enmeshed in reticulin fibers are known as *coal macules* (spots), as they appear as black dots on the lung sections. These spots are often associated with dilatation of respiratory bronchioles, called *focal centrilobular emphysema.* These changes are characteristic pathologic findings in *simple* CWP. The *complicated* form, as in silicosis, is characterized by massive fibrosis, involving mostly the upper lobes. However, in CWP, the lesions are black and, unlike silicosis in which the lesions consist of a conglomeration of silicotic nodules, they are amorphous and relatively homogeneous. They develop less commonly than in silicosis. Coal dust is also known to produce pathologic changes of chronic bronchitis. Cigarette smoking is, however, a much more important factor in causing bronchial mucosal changes than is coal dust in coal miners who are smokers.

Clinical Manifestations. Simple pneumoconiosis produces no significant symptoms or signs. Coal workers with simple pneumoconiosis or clear chest x-rays and who have significant symptoms, particularly dyspnea, usually have concomitant chronic bronchitis or emphysema probably unrelated to their exposure. In the complicated form, dyspnea, mostly with exercise, is often present. Expectoration of black material (melanoptysis) is common in coal workers, with or without pneumoconiosis. In the advanced and complicated form of disease, signs of respiratory failure, including pulmonary hypertension and cor pulmonale, may be present.

Radiographic Findings. Simple pneumoconiosis is characterized by reticular and nodular densities throughout the lung fields. The nodules are small and less defined than those of silicosis. Large shadows of 1 cm or more in diameter are indicative of complicated pneumoconiosis, known as *progressive massive fibrosis* (see Fig. 15–3). These lesions are almost always restricted to the upper lung fields. They may sometimes cavitate.

Pulmonary Function Studies. The majority of nonsmoking patients with simple pneumoconiosis have no significant abnormality on routine pulmonary function studies. Some increase in residual volume, however, has been demonstrated in many coal workers with simple

pneumoconiosis and sometimes without chest x-ray abnormalities. With special studies, evidence of small airway obstruction can be shown in most workers with significant coal dust exposure, even without radiographic abnormalities. Patients with complicated pneumoconiosis often have evidence of restrictive as well as obstructive impairment of pulmonary function. Diffusing capacity is often reduced. In most studies it has been demonstrated that in CWP, smoking is by far the most important factor in producing respiratory symptoms and reducing ventilatory functions.

Management. The measures mentioned in management of silicosis are relevant in prevention of CWP as well. Early detection of radiographic changes in the latter condition and cessation of exposure, however, prevents further progression of disease, in contrast to silicosis in which the lesions may progress despite removal of patients from their environment. Patients with simple CWP who have no symptoms need no treatment. The principles of treatment of complicated disease are similar to those discussed in chronic obstructive pulmonary disease (COPD) (Chapter 8) and pulmonary fibrosis (Chapter 12).

Asbestos-Associated Diseases: Asbestosis

Asbestos Exposure. Asbestos is a generic name applied to a family of fibrous hydrated silicates that have been widely used in industry because of their unique physical characteristics. Asbestos fiber is flexible, heat resistant, and extremely durable. Of the several forms of asbestos, chrysotile is most commonly mined and used in North America. Until recently, this mineral was extensively used in the construction industry in the form of asbestos cement products, such as pipes, tiles, shingles, and other roofing products. The risks of exposure not only occur during their manufacture, but also when they are being cut, drilled, or demolished. In addition, there are numerous other uses, including manufacture of insulation materials, car brake and clutch linings, air filters, fire-resistant clothing, ship building and repairing, and undercoating of cars.

Recent legislation has resulted in a significant reduction in the widespread use of asbestos in the manufacturing industry in the United States. Large amounts of asbestos, however, may still be released into the air during demolition and renovation of old buildings and ships, contributing to the atmospheric pollution. Moreover, many individuals are known who were exposed when asbestos use was uncontrolled. Asbestos carried in the clothing of workers has also been a source of exposure to other members of the household. Therefore, asbestos exposure occurs not only from work in mining, manufacturing, and use of its products, but also from neighborhood and other forms of contamination and general community asbestos air pollution. Although clinical asbestosis usually develops following more significant and prolonged exposure, the question of potential health hazards of low concentrations of asbestos and short duration of exposure, such as its carcinogenic effect, has remained unanswered. A long interval, sometimes up to 30 or 40 years, between the time of exposure and development of neoplasia makes the evaluation of the cause-and-effect relationship even more difficult.

Pathology and Pathogenesis. Pleuropulmonary complications of asbestos exposure are pulmonary fibrosis, bronchogenic carcinoma, pleural effusion, pleural fibrosis, and mesothelioma. They may develop singly or, often, in various combinations. The term *asbestosis* is applied to pulmonary parenchymal reaction to asbestos and development of fibrosis. The mechanism of production of pleuropulmonary lesion by asbestos fibers is not entirely understood. It seems that initial injury to the terminal airways, alveolar walls, and interstitial tissue causes inflammatory reaction, which leads to fibrosis. The inflammation is primarily the result of activation of the alveolar macrophages. The participation of other inflammatory cells, notably neutrophilic leukocytes, and the release of inflammatory mediators and oxygen radicals seem to be important in the progression of the pathologic process. Shorter asbestos fibers are readily phagocytized and removed. However, longer asbestos fibers remain in distal airways and alveoli and continue to stimulate unsuccessful phagocytic activity, perpetuating inflammation and fibrous tissue formation. The fact that the pathologic process continues long after the exposure has ceased is strongly supportive of this pathogenetic concept. Smoking enhances significantly the development of pulmonary fibrosis from asbestos exposure.

Fibrosis in asbestosis, unlike silicosis, is nonnodular, involves mostly the lower lung fields, and is often accompanied by fibrous pleural thickening. The extent of fibrosis is variable; in the mild form there is thickened alveolar septa; in severe fibrosis the alveolar spaces are hardly visible. Advanced asbestosis is one of the causes of honeycomb lung. Asbestos fibers can be identified in these lesions, sometimes enveloped in an iron-containing protein film, giving them a characteristic feature. They are referred to as *asbestos bodies* or, more appropriately, *ferrugenous bodies.*

Pleural reaction involving the parietal pleura, with fibrous thickening and plaque formation, is a common manifestation of asbestos exposure. Pleural calcification is a frequent finding. Pleural effusion, sometimes bloody, is a fairly common form of pleural reaction to asbestos.

Bronchogenic carcinoma is a frequent complicating event in asbestosis. However, the relationship is mostly due to the combined effect of asbestos and cigarette smoking. Whereas the incidence of lung cancer in nonsmoking asbestos workers is somewhat higher than in the nonsmoking general population, heavy smokers who are also exposed to asbestos have an 80- to 90-fold greater predisposition to bronchogenic carcinoma. Therefore, the combined effects of cigarette smoke and asbestos are more multiplicative than additive.

Another malignant disease associated with asbestos exposure is malignant pleural (sometimes peritoneal) mesothelioma. This cancer appears to develop almost exclusively in individuals with asbestos exposure, and smoking has no effect on its incidence. The risk of developing malignant mesothelioma reaches its peak 30 to 35 years after initial exposure.

Clinical Manifestations. Clinical manifestations of asbestosis are similar to those presented by pulmonary fibrosis in general. There is a various gradation of symptoms from the asymptomatic stage of early and mild cases to severe respiratory incapacity with advanced and severe fibrosis. The average period of exposure before developing symptoms is about 20 to 30 years. Symptoms rarely develop in patients with less than 10 years of exposure. Dyspnea, with or without cough, is the most common symptom. Physical examination often reveals basal pulmonary crackles. Digital clubbing is a common finding.

The presence of pleural disease may manifest by deformity and restriction of the chest, dullness to percussion, and reduced breath sounds. Most patients with pleural plaques have no symptoms unless there is concomitant asbestosis. The most common symptom of malignant mesothelioma is chest pain, which may be followed by dyspnea and systemic symptoms of malignancy. Physical findings of pleural effusion are usually present.

Radiographic Findings. Parenchymal lung disease manifests by interstitial markings with reticular density, predominantly involving the lower lung fields. The cardiac and diaphagmatic outline may appear indistinct and "shaggy." Sometimes a marked honeycomb pattern may be present. The lung volume is often diminished. Pleural changes are very common, including pleural thickening, plaques, calcification, and effusion. *Rounded atelectasis* is a characteristic radiographic finding that results from associated asbestosis with pleural effusion and fibrosis, in which a portion of the lung becomes trapped and atelectatic after the effusion is resorbed, and the trapped portion then assumes a round shape. It may mimic a neoplasm. Malignant mesothelioma frequently manifests with pleural thickening and effusion. Computed tomography (CT) scanning has proved to be very useful in studying patients with asbestos-associated pleural disease.

Pulmonary Function Tests. As in diffuse lung fibrosis in general, pulmonary function tests (PFTs) in asbestosis are indicative of restrictive ventilatory defect with reduced lung volumes and diffusing capacity. Flow rates are usually normal.

Management. Preventive measures and removal of patients from the contaminated environment at the first sign of disease are most important. Treatment of established asbestosis is the same as that of pulmonary fibrosis in general. In view of the marked increase in incidence of bronchogenic carcinoma and pulmonary fibrosis among cigarette smokers exposed to asbestos, they should be strongly urged to quit smoking.

■ ENVIRONMENTAL PULMONARY DISEASES DUE TO NOXIOUS GASES

As a result of the combustion of fuel for locomotion, heating, and power production in various industries and photochemical reactions in the atmosphere, the inspired air may contain small concentrations of certain noxious gases, such as sulfur dioxide, nitrogen oxide, carbon monoxide, hydrocarbons, and ozone. The injurious effects of these gases on the *healthy lung* at the concentration present in community air pollution have not been clearly demonstrated. However, many of these gases (as well as particulate matters), even in low concentrations, may play a contributing role in triggering and exacerbating symptoms from underlying bronchopulmonary disorders. Exposure to higher concentrations of these gases that may occur accidently or, rarely, intentionally is known to be always harmful.

Acute Exposure to Irritant Gases

Irritant gases are known to cause inflammation of mucous membranes on contact. They are irritating both to the eyes and to the mucous membranes of the respiratory tract, resulting in a burning sensation; itching, and watering of the eyes; sneezing and runny nose; and coughing. These irritating effects are usually severe enough to force the exposed victim to escape whenever possible; therefore, exposure time will be brief, and the amount of inhaled gas will be small. The degree of irritation of the eyes and the upper airway mucosa is proportional to the water solubility of these gases. The more soluble the gas, the more irritating it is to these areas; and thus, the less likely that it will produce a significant toxic effect on the distal airways and alveoli. It should, however, be noted that even the most soluble irritating gas can cause acute bronchiolar and alveolar damage if the victim is unable to escape and/or the inhaled dose is massive. The following is a list of some of the irritating gases that are known to cause respiratory tract injury:

- Ammonia (NH_3)
- Sulfur dioxide (SO_2)
- Chlorine (Cl)
- Nitrogen dioxide (NO_2)
- Ozone (O3)
- Phosgene ($COCl_2$)

They are listed according to their water solubility, ammonia being the most soluble and phosgene the least soluble. Because of their high solubility, the first three gases on the list cause intense irritation of the eyes and the upper airway mucous membranes and, therefore, they cannot be tolerated to any extent that would cause a significant harmful effect to the lower respiratory tract. Only with massive accidental exposure in a situation from which the victims are unable to escape will these gases result in serious bronchopulmonary injury. On the other hand, the last three gases on the list, which are much less water soluble and thus less irritating to the eyes and the upper airways, are better known for their injurious effect on the distal airways and alveoli.

The toxic effects of all of these gases to the respiratory tract are more or less similar. Hyperemia, edema, epithelial injury with mucosal sloughing, hypersecretion, and cellular reaction are usual tissue responses. Cough, increasing dyspnea, and cyanosis are common manifestations of heavy exposure to these agents. Radiographic changes of pulmonary edema become apparent within several hours. Hypoxemia may be severe and difficult to correct by oxygen administration.

A condition commonly known as *silo-filler's disease* is caused by exposure to a high concentration of NO_2, which is produced by fermentation of fodder in a silo. This gas and its polymer, being heavier than air, accumulate on top of silage as a reddish-brown "cloud." On exposure to this cloud, depending on the concentration of NO_2 and duration of exposure, various degrees of bronchopulmonary damage will ensue. Mild exposure may result in acute, self-limited bronchitis; heavy exposure may cause acute, sometimes fatal, pulmonary edema. There is a subacute form of clinical presentation in which the symptoms recur and persist after an apparent recovery.

Management of acute severe irritant gas injury is mostly supportive and symptomatic. As in hypoxemic respiratory failure from any cause, the first priority should be the correction of the hypoxemia. If oxygen administration by nasal cannula or mask does not correct the hypoxemia, or if there is progressive respiratory distress or inadequate spontaneous ventilation, mechanical ventilatory support will be needed as discussed in the management of respiratory failure (Chapter 26). The role of corticosteroids in the treatment of patients with irritant gas exposure is questionable. Complete recovery is the usual outcome in properly managed patients. However, sometimes residual functional impairment may be observed. Patients with pulmonary injury due to irritant gas exposure should have a close follow-up after their apparent recovery because of the possibility of recurrence.

■ CARBON MONOXIDE POISONING

CO has no *direct* injurious effect on the lungs. However, because of its ready absorption, its extreme affinity for hemoglobin, and, therefore, its interference with oxygen transport and delivery, poisoning with CO gas causes significant mortality and morbidity as a result of the impairment of tissue oxygenation.

Sources of Carbon Monoxide

CO is produced during incomplete burning of carbon or carbon-containing materials. Therefore, it can occur from the burning of fuels such as coal, wood, gasoline, or natural gas in an atmosphere in which sufficient oxygen is not available for their complete combustion. Automobiles characteristically burn gasoline incompletely; as a result, CO may reach highly toxic concentrations inside the car from a defective exhaust or in a closed garage within a short period of time. This has become an increasingly common cause of suicidal or accidental poisoning.

A low concentration of CO with air pollution may become significant during heavy traffic, particularly in places like toll booths, tunnels, and congested expressways. Use of charcoal grills indoors for cooking or heating, faulty gas refrigerators, and heaters or burners supplied with various fuels may cause accidental poisoning in houses and trailer homes. The combination of incomplete combustion and insufficient ventilation is the usual setup for such an exposure. Natural gas, as used in the United States, does not contain CO and has replaced the older manufactured gas, which had a significant concentration of CO. It is the incomplete combustion of presently used natural gas that produces CO. As discussed later in this chapter, the major cause of death from smoke inhalation is CO poisoning.

Tobacco smoke contains a high concentration of CO to which smokers are voluntarily exposed (see Chapter 16). Heavy cigarette smokers, as well as cigar smokers who inhale, have chronically high blood carboxyhemoglobin (COHb) levels. A small amount of CO is endogenously produced by the normal breakdown of hemoglobin. Carbon monoxide is also the metabolic by-product of methylene chloride, the main ingredient of most paint removers. Inhalation of this product after its application in a poorly ventilated space may result in a significant increase in serum COHb levels.

Toxic Effects of Carbon Monoxide

The most important effect of CO is related to its extremely high affinity for hemoglobin and the production of COHb, which impairs the ability of red blood cells to carry oxygen and deliver it to the tissues. CO and oxygen compete for the binding sites on hemoglobin molecules. The affinity for CO is about 240 times that for oxygen. Therefore, in competing for binding sites on hemoglobin molecules, CO is able to displace and readily replace O_2; to achieve an equal concentration of oxyhemoglobin and COHb with a P_{O_2} of 100 mm Hg at equilibrium, a Co tension of only 0.42 mm Hg will be necessary. A CO concentration of less than 0.1% in inspired air with long enough exposure time will be sufficient to cause such a high COHb level.

On exposure to CO, it is rapidly absorbed by diffusion via the alveoli until an equilibrium is reached, provided that an immediately fatal concentration is not inhaled. The COHb level at equilibrium is proportional to the CO concentration in inspired air (Fig. 15–4). The time required for equilibrium is inversely related to CO concentration. As in clinical situations the equilbrium is seldom reached, other factors in addition to inspired CO concentration and duration of exposure are important. They include metabolic rate, alveolar ventilation, and pulmonary blood flow.

In addition to reducing the oxygen-carrying capacity of hemoglobin, an equally important effect of CO on hemoglobin is the alteration in the position as well as in the shape of the oxyhemoglobin dissociation curve. The curve will be shifted to the left as the affinity of unoc-

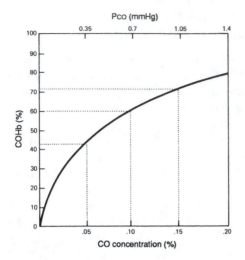

Figure 15–4. Relation of blood COHb levels and inspired CO concentration at equilibrium. Note that, at equilibrium, CO concentrations as low as 0.1% result in very high and even fatal COHb levels in blood.

cupied binding sites of hemoglobin for oxygen is increased; and the curve will tend to change from its normal sigmoid shape to a hyperbolic curve. Both of these changes have profound effects on oxygen unloading at the tissue sites.

The question of the significance of CO binding to other hemoproteins, such as cytochrome oxidase in mitochondria and myoglobin in cardiac and skeletal muscle cells, has not yet been satisfactorily answered. As these hemoproteins are important in oxygen metabolism, their putative involvement in CO intoxication would further impair cellular hypoxia. As pathophysiologic changes due to CO poisoning are all related to tissue hypoxia, the brain and the heart, which are highly sensitive to oxygen lack, are most affected.

Clinical Manifestations. The symptoms from CO poisoning depend on the blood level of COHb (measured as percent of total hemoglobin). A level of less

than 10%, as seen in heavy tobacco smokers, causes no significant symptom in otherwise healthy individuals. In patients with coronary artery disease, however, there is lowering of the threshold for exercise-induced angina. Patients are usually symptomatic with COHb concentrations of 20% and higher. Headaches, exertional dyspnea, dizziness, difficulty to concentrate, impaired judgment, incoordination, lethargy, and mental confusion are common manifestations. Nausea, vomiting, and other gastrointestinal (GI) symptoms may also be present. With higher concentrations of COHb, loss of consciousness, convulsions, and deep coma will supervene. Fatal cases show COHb levels of 60% to 80%. The symptoms develop more rapidly with exposure to higher concentrations of CO in air; sometimes CO is absorbed so fast that unconsciousness occurs suddenly and without warning symptoms.

Electrocardiographic changes indicative of myocardial hypoxia and various arrhythmias may be seen. Occasionally, there is evidence of acute myocardial infarction. Practically every organ may show functional impairment. Acute pulmonary edema, resulting from cardiac failure as well as from increased alveolar capillary leak, has been occasionally seen in severe CO poisoning. Various delayed neuropsychiatric manifestations are fairly common following severe CO intoxication. Chronic low-level CO poisoning, as commonly seen in heavy tobacco smokers, is a cause of increased red blood cells (polycythemia).

Diagnosis. Besides the history, there are very few clinical findings to help the diagnosis of CO poisoning. The cherry-red color of the skin and mucous membranes, frequently mentioned in most textbooks, is not a common finding in live victims. Once suspected, the diagnosis is readily made by measurement of the COHb level in the blood by one of the available methods. As there is an excellent correlation between the blood COHb level and expired CO concentration, the measurement of the latter by one of the CO analyzers may be used as a rapid screening test.

Arterial blood Po_2, as expected, is normal; however, oxygen *content* will be reduced proportional to the COHb level. If Po_2 and O_2 saturation studies are done independently, there will be a significant discrepancy between the calculated and measured O_2 saturation. Pulse oximetry usually overestimates arterial O_2 saturation by an amount equal to COHb level. Arterial Pco_2 is usually low. Metabolic acidosis may also be present due to lactic acid production of tissue hypoxia.

Management. Once the diagnosis of CO poisoning is suspected, treatment should be initiated immediately, before the results of laboratory studies are reported. The most important step in the treatment of CO poisoning is the removal of the victim from the contaminated atmosphere. In mild cases without significant symptoms, a few hours of bed rest, with or without added inspired O_2, will usually suffice. The factors that facilitate CO elimination include alveolar ventilation and inspired oxygen tension. From the therapeutic point of view, increasing alveolar O_2 tension is the most important and practical measure. CO elimination is exponential, the average half-life being inversely proportional to the alveolar Po_2. A half-life of 5 hours breathing room air is reduced to 1 hour by the administration of 100% oxygen at atmospheric (atm) pressure. The half-life will

be diminished further by the administration of oxygen in a hyperbaric chamber. The treatment goals in severe CO poisoning are to reverse tissue hypoxia and rapidly reduce the blood COHb level to less than 10%. Both are achieved by the administration of 100% oxygen. Patients with severe CO poisoning are treated in the hospital. Oxygen therapy should be continued until the COHb level is less than 10%. This usually takes several hours.

The precise role of hyperbaric oxygen in CO poisoning remains unsettled. However, more rapid CO elimination and a better tissue oxygenation by hyperbaric oxygen therapy makes it an attractive method for the management of CO poisoning. If a hyperbaric chamber is readily available, it should preferably be used for treatment of patients with severe poisoning and significant cardiac or cerebral dysfunction. Timely referral to a facility with a hyperbaric oxygen chamber is indicated for patients with a history of loss of consciousness, evidence of cardiac ischemia, or persistence of mental or neurologic deficit. Lack of improvement with 100% normobaric oxygen within 4 hours is also considered to be an indication for transporting patients to the nearest hyperbaric center. The importance of close monitoring of the patients and their supportive care cannot be overemphasized. The persistence of coma or other neurologic sequelae is indicative of hypoxic brain injury, which requires a more prolonged supportive care.

■ SMOKE INHALATION

Smoke inhalation is the most important cause of morbidity and mortality among fire victims and firefighters. The prognosis of most burns is often determined by the magnitude of concurrent smoke inhalation.

Pathogenesis and Pathology. Fire smoke is a complex mixture of gases, vapors, and particulate matter that result from combustion, evaporation, and pyrolysis. Pyrolysis is heat-induced decomposition of organic compounds in the absence of oxygen. The composition of smoke, therefore, varies not only because of the difference of the chemical makeup of substances that are burning, but also because of steady reduction in available oxygen that is being consumed by the fire. In addition to CO, which is the major cause of poisoning from smoke, many irritant and caustic gases may be generated. They include aldehydes (especially acrolein), hydrogen chloride, oxides of sulfur and nitrogen, and ammonia. They cause direct injury to the respiratory tract by their irritating and corrosive effects. With the increasing use of synthetic materials containing isocyanate compounds in buildings and furnishings, hydrogen cyanide has become an important component of smoke from fires. This gaseous form of cyanide exerts its toxic effect by binding to cytochromes, thus interfering with the oxidative metabolism at the cellular level.

In addition to inhaling the noxious gases, fire victims in enclosed spaces breathe an air with a steadily diminishing concentration of oxygen and increasing concentration of CO_2. Although inhalation of hot air may cause thermal injury to the upper air passages, distal airways and alveoli are spared. The pathologic changes in the respiratory tract are mainly from irritant gases. These changes are complex and quite variable. Tracheo-

bronchial mucosal edema, vascular congestion, and epithelial sloughing are often present. Alveolar edema is the result of leaky alveolar–capillary membrane. Bronchiolar damage may result in obliterative bronchiolitis. The pathologic changes begin to develop within several hours of exposure, but they may be delayed for 1 to 2 days, or even longer.

Clinical Manifestations. The clinical presentation varies considerably. The victim may be alert, drowsy, or unconscious, usually depending on the intensity of concomitant CO poisoning. Lack of evidence of external burns does not exclude the possibility of significant smoke inhalation. Upper airways may look inflamed. Cough, with expectoration of black phlegm, is often present. Tachypnea, stridor, grunting respiration, and other signs of respiratory distress may not appear until several hours later. With the development of pulmonary edema, severe dyspnea and signs of marked hypoxemia, including shock, will be evident. However, because of frequent association with CO poisoning, cyanosis may not be manifest, despite profound hypoxemia. Therefore, the patient may suffer from an extreme degree of tissue hypoxia due to combined effect of carboxyhemoglobinemia and respiratory failure.

The concomitant effect of cyanide on cytochromes impairs oxygen utilization further. Cyanide poisoning should be suspected in comatose victims of fires in which plastic or other synthetic materials are involved. It should, however, be noted that high blood cyanide levels are mostly seen in association with fatal COHb concentrations in the blood, especially when patients fail to recover after their blood COHb levels are lowered.

Diagnosis. Radiographic changes of smoke inhalation may be minimal or totally absent initially. Bilateral pulmonary edema, however, may appear later. Early bronchoscopy is often recommended when, despite high initial COHb levels in patients with smoke inhalation, there is no clinical or radiographic evidence of pulmonary involvement at the time of presentation. The presence of mucosal changes distal to the larynx is a good predictor of subsequent development of respiratory difficulty. Alternatively, radionuclide ventilation scan may be used for this purpose, which has a high negative predictive value; that is, a normal distribution with a normal clearance of the radioactive tracer virtually excludes the diagnosis of significant distal airway damage from smoke inhalation.

Management. In smoke inhalation, in addition to treatment for CO poisoning, patients with pulmonary injury will require appropriate management. Because both clinical manifestations and radiographic changes may be delayed, all patients exposed to smoke should be carefully observed, especially when the COHb levels are elevated. A patient with normal physical findings, a normal chest radiograph, and a safe level of COHb may be released after a short period of observation. If performed, a normal bronchoscopy or ventilation lung scan provides added assurance that late pulmonary complications will not develop. In view of frequent association with CO exposure, oxygen should be administered immediately while waiting for measurement of blood COHb level. Although many patients with smoke inhalation are exposed to hydrogen cyanide, poisoning is infrequent in fire fatalities, and when present it is associated with high blood COHb levels. Specific cyanide detox-

ification is rarely necessary in the treatment of victims of smoke inhalation.

Patients with evidence of bronchospasm are treated with inhaled bronchodilators and systemic corticosteroids if needed. Otherwise, there is no indication for corticosteroids in smoke inhalation. Prophylactic antibiotic therapy has not been proved to be effective in preventing pulmonary infections, which may develop in patients with severe lung injury. Such infections should be promptly and adequately treated once they occur.

With the development of progressive respiratory distress and persistent hypoxemia despite an adequate airway and oxygen therapy, mechanical ventilation will be necessary. Unless there is severe airway injury at the level of or proximal to the larynx, endotracheal intubation is preferred to tracheostomy. With severe pulmonary edema and intractable hypoxemia, positive end–expiratory pressure (PEEP) should be used, as discussed in management of acute respiratory distress syndrome (ARDS) (Chapter 27). Associated severe and extensive skin burn is known to increase the incidence and severity of ARDS with smoke inhalation.

■ AIR POLLUTION

In atmospheric air pollution, in addition to various gases, particulate matters in aerosolized form are also present. Chemical composition of these particulate pollutants varies, and usually includes carbon, metals, and other inorganic as well as organic compounds. Because of their very low concentrations, the lung defense mechanisms, discussed earlier, are normally quite adequate to prevent their harmful effects. However, in persons with underlying pulmonary disease and in individuals with hyperreactive airways or hypersensitivity states, the health hazard of air pollution with particulate matters may be significant. In mixed air pollution, particles are also important in their capacity for carrying noxious gases on their surface to distal airspaces, whereas such gases would have been removed by their solubility in the upper airways without carrying particles.

The effect of short-term exposure to noxious gases on healthy individuals at the concentration present in community air pollution has not been proved to be significant, and the respiratory consequences of long-term exposure in people without underlying chronic cardiopulmonary conditions, although suspected, have not been conclusively demonstrated. However, as with exposure to low concentrations of particulate matters, patients with chronic respiratory illness, such as asthmatics and persons with COPD, show evidence of significant deterioration of their symptoms and impairment of their respiratory function on exposure to noxious gases of air pollution.

Air pollution is, therefore, considered to be a relatively weak respiratory pathogen but an important aggravating factor on preexisting pulmonary disease. However, because of the unavoidable, involuntary, and continuous nature of exposure and uncertainty regarding its long-term effect, air pollution has deservedly received much attention and caused worldwide public concern about its potential health hazards.

■ OXYGEN TOXICITY

The toxic effect of a high concentration of oxygen has been suspected since the discovery of this gas in the eighteenth century. Only in recent years, however, has its clinical importance been fully recognized and its pathogenesis elucidated. Although the toxic effect of oxygen has been most extensively studied in relation to the respiratory system, it is also known that oxygen with high enough tension and sufficient duration of exposure may injure almost any organ system of the body through a complex biochemical reaction of cells. Its toxic effect on the retinal arteries of premature infants with development of a condition called *retrolental fibroplasia* is well known. Currently, with more judicious use of oxygen, monitoring arterial blood Po_2, and thus, avoiding unnecessarily excessive Po_2, this iatrogenic eye disease and blindness are rarely seen.

Neurologic toxicity, such as convulsions, is observed with a very high oxygen tension, which can only be reached in environments such as hyperbaric chambers in which O_2 at pressure greater than 2 atm is inspired.

The toxic effect of oxygen on any tissue is directly related to both its partial pressure and the duration of exposure. Without sufficient O_2 tension or sufficient time of exposure, injury will not result. Various effects of oxygen at high partial pressure are referred to as *hyperoxic syndromes.*

Pulmonary Oxygen Toxicity

As the lungs are exposed to higher partial pressures of oxygen than are other organs in the body, the primary toxic effect of a high Po_2 in the normobaric range is on the lung tissue. This effect is entirely separate from the ventilatory suppression of excessive oxygen administration in hypoxic patients with hypercapnia. Another nontoxic, but nevertheless harmful, effect of oxygen is *absorption atelectasis,* which is due to the lack of nonabsorbable gas in the lungs and, therefore, is a function of concentration (FIO_2) rather than PO_2 of the inspired gas, whereas pulmonary tissue damage of oxygen toxicity is related to the inspired oxygen tension rather than the FIO_2. A high concentration of oxygen is less damaging at a high altitude with low atmospheric pressures than it is at sea level. Moreover, astronauts who breathe 100% oxygen at a reduced ambient pressure show no evidence of toxicity.

The precise oxygen tensions and duration of exposure that result in toxic effects on the lungs have been difficult to establish. This is compounded by the fact that there is significant individual variation in susceptibility to oxygen toxicity. It is generally considered that clinically significant pulmonary toxicity occurs in individuals exposed to 100% oxygen at normobaric pressures when the exposure time is more than 24 to 48 hours; however, mild and reversible effects may develop with shorter exposures. An entirely safe partial pressure of oxygen for humans has not been agreed on by different investigators, but the likelihood of significant toxicity to the lungs at an inspired oxygen pressure below 0.6 atm is very small.

Pathogenesis and Pathology. Morphologic changes of oxygen toxicity with 100% oxygen and an exposure time of 6 to 24 hours occur in tracheobronchial mucosa, which can be demonstrated by bronchoscopy. However, studies by bronchoalveolar lavage (BAL) indicate that early changes may be an alveolar–capillary leak from injury to the endothelial and type I epithelial cells. With more severe damage that occurs with longer exposure, interstitial and alveolar edema

develops. When O_2 toxicity develops more insidiously, and following the acute exudative phase in surviving patients, the proliferative stage will occur. This stage is characterized by cellular infiltration, proliferation of type II alveolar epithelial cells, and beginning fibrosis.

Alveolar and capillary cell damage, therefore, appears to be the initial event in the pathogenesis of hyperoxic pulmonary toxicity. Cellular injury is not the direct effect of molecular oxygen, but is due to the toxic effect of highly reactive metabolites of molecular oxygen. These products, which are produced intracellularly, include free radicals, particularly superoxide anion, peroxides, and the hydroxyl radical. Normally, the cells are protected from the toxic effect of these products by antioxidant enzymes. One such enzyme, which is extremely efficient in detoxifying the superoxide radical, is superoxide dismutase. Glutathione is the primary intracellular antioxidant, which must be constantly reduced by special enzymes to maintain this function. Vitamin E, also an antioxidant, is known to have protective effects against these toxic agents. During exposure to hyperoxia, the production of free radicals and other oxidants overwhelms natural defenses against them, resulting in cell injury. Impairment of function of certain enzymes and inhibition of synthesis of DNA, protein, cellular lipid, and surfactant constitute the metabolic basis of tissue damage by these powerful oxidants. In addition, proinflammatory cytokines, produced mainly by alveolar macrophages, play an important role in oxygen toxicity.

Clinical Manifestations, Diagnosis, and Management. Persons exposed to 100% oxygen for less than 24 hours may develop tracheobronchitis manifested by a nonproductive cough and retrosternal pain that is aggravated by deep inspiration. In such patients, reduced vital capacity, low diffusing capacity, and changes in pulmonary compliance have been reported. Severe acute pulmonary oxygen toxicity manifests by symptoms and signs of respiratory distress syndrome.

In a practical setting, pulmonary oxygen toxicity should be suspected in patients receiving high concentrations of oxygen for several days and who develop unexplained diffuse pulmonary infiltration on radiographic examination, changes in pulmonary compliance, or increasing difficulty in oxygenating the arterial blood. These changes, however, are not specific for oxygen toxicity, and may well be due to other common disorders such as widespread pneumonia, heart failure, or other causes of alveolar–capillary leak. In most situations in which oxygen toxicity is suspected, there is significant hypoxemia requiring higher inspired O_2 tensions. In turn, the latter causes further lung damage and impairment of oxygen transport.

In view of the seriousness of hypoxemia in critically ill patients, withholding oxygen for fear of toxicity will be more disastrous in patients who are in need of prolonged oxygen support. However, the concentration of oxygen in these situations should not be more than what is needed for achieving an acceptable Po_2. Every effort should be made to improve oxygenation without increasing oxygen tension to potentially toxic levels. The correction of underlying pathophysiologic abnormalities, proper tracheobronchial toilet, control of heart failure, avoidance of excessive fluid administration, treatment of acid-base imbalance, optimal ventilation with adequate tidal volumes, and use of PEEP will diminish the requirement for high inspired oxygen tension for adequate oxygenation.

The role of antioxidants, such as glutathione, vitamin E, and superoxide dismutase, in the management of pulmonary oxygen toxicity in humans has not yet been established.

BIBLIOGRAPHY

Aberle DR, Balmes JR. Computed tomography of asbestos-related pulmonary parenchymal and pleural diseases. *Clin Chest Med.* 1991; 12:115–131.

Bascom R, Bromberg PA, Costa DA, et al. Health effects of outdoor air pollution. *Am J Respir Crit Care Med.* 1996; 153:3–50, 477–498.

Becklake MR. Asbestos-related diseases of the lung and pleura. *Am Rev Respir Dis.* 1982; 126:187–194.

Davis GS. The pathogenesis of silicosis. *Chest.* 1986; 89(suppl):166S–169S.

Davis WB, Rennard SI, Bitterman PB, Crystal RG. Pulmonary oxygen toxicity. *N Engl J Med.* 1983; 309:878–883.

Douglas WW, Hepper NG, Colley TV. Silo-filler's disease. *Mayo Clin Proc.* 1989; 64: 291–304.

Frank W, Loddenkemper R. Fiber-associated pleural disease. *Semin Respir Crit Care Med.* 1995; 16:315–323.

Green GM, Jakab GJ, Low RB, Davis GS. Defense mechanisms of the respiratory membrane. *Am Rev Respir Dis.* 1977; 115: 479–514.

Hampson NB, Dunford RG, Kramer CC, Norkool DM. Selection criteria utilized for hyperbaric oxygen treatment of carbon monoxide poisoning. *J Emerg Med.* 1995; 13:227–231.

Haponik EF, Crapo RO, Herndon DN, et al. Smoke inhalation. *Am Rev Respir Dis.* 1988; 138:1060–1063.

Hillerdal G. Rounded atelectasis. *Chest.* 1989; 95:836–841.

Ilano AL, Raffin TA. Management of carbon monoxide poisoning. *Chest.* 1990; 97: 165–169.

Jackson RM. Molecular, pharmacologic, and clinical aspects of oxygen-induced lung injury. *Clin Chest Med.* 1990; 11:73–86.

Morgan WKC, Lapp NL. Respiratory disease in coal miners. *Am Rev Respir Dis.* 1976; 113:531–559.

Peitzman AB, Shires GI III, Teixidor HS, et al. Smoke inhalation injury: evaluation of radiographic manifestations and pulmonary dysfunction. *J Trauma.* 1989; 29: 1232–1239.

Samet JM, Marbury MC, Spengler JD. Health effects and sources of indoor pollution. *Am Rev Respir Dis.* 1987; 136:1486–1508; 1988; 137:221–242.

Steenland K, Brown D. Silicosis among gold miners. *Am J Public Health.* 1995; 85: 1372–1377.

Stogner SW, Payne DK. Oxygen toxicity. *Ann Pharmacol.* 1992; 26:1554–1562.

Thom SR. Smoke inhalation. *Emerg Med Clin North Am.* 1989; 7:371–387.

Tibbles PM, Edelsberg JS. Hyperbaric oxygen therapy. *N Engl J Med.* 1996; 334: 1642–1648.

Vanhee D, Gosset P, Boitelle A, et al. Cytokines and cytokine network in silicosis and coal workers' pneumoconiosis. *Eur Respir J.* 1995; 8:834–842.

Wanner A, Salathé M, O'Riordan. Mucociliary clearance in the airways. *Am J Respir Crit Care Med.* 1996; 154:1868–1902.

Weill H. Occupational lung diseases. *Hosp Pract.* 1981; 16(4):65–80.

Weiss SM, Lakshminarayan S. Acute inhalation injury. *Clin Chest Med.* 1994; 15(1): 103–116.

16.

Tobacco Smoking

In several chapters of this book the role of tobacco smoking in causing or contributing to various respiratory disorders has been mentioned. This chapter focuses on the health consequences of tobacco smoking; it follows after a brief discussion of the physicochemical and biologic properties of cigarette smoke. As disease prevention is one of the primary responsibilities of health professionals, they should have a thorough knowledge and understanding of this man-made and entirely preventable health hazard. The unique position of providers of respiratory care affords them the opportunity and the obligation to inform their clients, as well as the general public, on the health effects of tobacco smoking and to help them stop their potentially dangerous smoking habits. Tobacco smoking is a very prevalent human behavior initiated by easily available psychosocial factors and continued by the addition of over-powering addictive forces. Although the avoidance of starting the habit is a relatively simple matter, smoking cessation after the establishment of psychological

and physical dependency becomes a most difficult and complex task. As discussed later in this chapter, one of the most challenging responsibilities of health care providers is to equip their smoking clients with enough incentive and encouragement that their desire for giving up smoking overcomes their desire for smoking. Knowledge of health consequences of smoking alone is not enough for this purpose. It also necessitates the understanding of the dynamics of smoking, both as an acquired behavior and as an illness.

Since the first report of the U.S. Surgeon General on smoking and health in 1964, follow-up reports and numerous scientific studies have reaffirmed the conclusion of the original report and also have provided data on various health problems related to both voluntary and involuntary (passive) smoking. It seems that, at least in the United States, most people are aware of many of the smoking-related diseases, yet the decline in cigarette consumption has been less than impressive, and teenagers and young adults continue taking up the habit in rather large numbers. However, development of new policies and legislation on the restriction of smoking in certain public places and work areas, steady decline of the social acceptability of smoking, and increasing public awareness of high-risk behaviors are some of the encouraging signs that the battle against smoking will eventually be won. Meanwhile, some 45 to 50 million Americans who are current smokers will need help for various health problems resulting from their smoking and for their struggle to give it up.

■ HARMFUL CONSTITUENTS OF CIGARETTE SMOKE

A lighted cigarette produces about 4000 known compounds and several thousand unidentified chemicals, some in gaseous form and most in aerosolized particulate form. Inhaled (mainstream) smoke is partly retained in, or absorbed from, the respiratory tract and partly exhaled. Sidestream smoke is the part that is released to the environment from the lighted end of the cigarette. The gaseous phase of the cigarette smoke includes carbon dioxide, carbon monoxide, oxides of nitrogen, hydrogen cyanide, aldehydes, ammonia, volatile nitrosamines, hydrocarbons, and free radicals. Carbon monoxide is the best-recognized harmful component of the gas phase. Its effects on hemoglobin and resultant impairment of oxygen delivery is discussed in Chapter 15. Most other components are known to be respiratory irritants, some (especially hydrogen cyanide and aldehydes) are toxic to the respiratory cilia, and a few have carcinogenic potential. Gaseous components of smoke have been considered to play a major role in the

pathogenesis of chronic obstructive lung disease. As respiratory irritants, they may provoke bronchospasm in individuals with hyperreactive airways.

Tar is the name given to the aggregate of the particulate matter in the cigarette smoke minus nicotine and moisture. In contradistinction to gases in the cigarette smoke, tar and nicotine are partly trapped in the filter tip. The amount of tar delivered in mainstream smoke in each cigarette constitutes its tar content. Therefore, it varies not only with the amount and brand of tobacco, but also the properties of the filter tip and the characteristics of the puffs. Tar contains numerous compounds known or suspected to be carcinogens, tumor promoters, or cocarcinogens. Among them, polynuclear aromatic hydrocarbons are the best-known carcinogens. The role of others such as nitrosamines, "tumorigenic" metals, and radionuclides in causing lung cancer in humans is less certain. Tar contents of American-made cigarettes have been reduced steadily during the past 35 to 40 years by processing and the reconstituting of tobacco brands, changing the cigarette papers, and introducing more effective filter tips. These changes, however, have not yet favorably influenced the incidence of lung cancer among cigarette smokers.

Nicotine

Nicotine is by far the most important pharmacologically active substance in every form of tobacco and its smoke. It is the principal cause of physiologic addiction to smoking. People who smoke cigarettes or use other tobacco products chronically do so mainly because of the nicotine content. The powerful addicting properties of nicotine are the cause of failure to quit smoking by most cigarette smokers who desire to quit and make numerous attempts to do so. Even the smokers who have tobacco-related illnesses and recognize the effects of smoking on their health have a very hard time giving it up. This type of behavior fits the definition of drug dependence, and the drug in question is nicotine.

Once in the bloodstream, nicotine readily crosses the blood–brain barrier and is distributed in various parts of the central nervous system (CNS). It has a variety of complex CNS actions through its binding to the brain receptors. Among many of its pharmacologic effects, autonomic ganglia are better-known targets. In small doses nicotine stimulates both sympathetic and parasympathetic ganglia; in large doses, it has an opposite effect. Catecholamines (epinephrine and norepinephrine) released from the activation of the sympathetic nerves and adrenal glands are the cause of several of nicotine's biologic responses. They include the effect on the heart rate, myocardial contractility, vascular resistance, and mobilization of fatty acids. An increase in the blood level of other hormones associated with cigarette smoking is probably related to the effect of nicotine. Tolerance to some of the effects of nicotine, which may develop quite rapidly, is well recognized. Unpleasant symptoms of dizziness, nausea, and vomiting in first-time smokers do not develop with repeat smoking, and other effects of nicotine are also attenuated. In habitual smokers, nicotine has a satisfying and pleasurable effect, which is at least partly the result of relief from unpleasant symptoms of abstinence. Arousal, relaxation, improved concentration and attention, and reduced anger and tension from stressful situations are some of the sub-

jective beneficial effects. Withdrawal symptoms that occur in about 80% of smokers include restlessness, irritability, anxiety, impatience, impaired concentration, and strong desire or craving to smoke a cigarette. Most of the symptoms are accounted for by the withdrawal of nicotine, as they also occur with the cessation of smokeless tobacco and nicotine preparations and are relieved by the administration of nicotine.

Nicotine is distilled from burning tobacco and carried on tar particles. The mainstream smoke of a filter-tipped cigarette on the average contains 15% of the nicotine in its tobacco, although it may vary depending on individual smoking characteristics. Most of the nicotine from cigarette smoke is absorbed through the wide surface of the alveoli after its inhalation. Its absorption from oral mucosa is negligible. However, nicotine in cigar and pipe smoke and in smokeless tobacco is absorbed from the oral mucous membrane. As drugs absorbed from sites other than the gastrointestinal (GI) tract bypass the liver, they are not detoxified and reach their target tissues or cells directly. Nicotine from the inhaled cigarette smoke reaches the brain within seconds of the first puff. The amount of nicotine that a smoker absorbs with each cigarette is determined not only by its nicotine content and the physical properties of its filter tip, but also by the puff volume, depth of inhalation, rate of puffing, and duration of breath holding after each inhalation. These smoking patterns also affect the amount of gaseous material and tar to which the individual smoker is exposed.

Interposition of an effective filter tip and reduction of tar and nicotine content of most cigarettes made in the United States are ostensibly positive steps in reducing user exposure to these harmful agents. Lack of significant effect on the risk of some smoking-related diseases in users of low-yield cigarettes, however, indicates that the degree of exposure to the agents has not been appreciably reduced. As smoking behavior in habitual smokers is primarily a response to the levels of nicotine in their system, they adjust their smoking pattern accordingly. Therefore, smokers of low-tar and low-nicotine cigarettes tend to increase the number of cigarettes smoked and to use a pattern of smoking that yields the maximum amount of nicotine from each cigarette in order to maintain their accustomed nicotine level.

■ RELATIONSHIPS OF SMOKING AND DISEASE

The mortality and morbidity statistics clearly demonstrate that smoking is associated with increased rates of death and illness. Despite a significant decline in the prevalence of cigarette use, smoking still remains the leading cause of preventable death in the United States. Life expectancy at any given age is significantly shortened by cigarette smoking. It is estimated that for each cigarette smoked, an average of 5½ minutes of life is lost: a 30- to 35-year-old man who smokes two packs of cigarettes daily has a life expectancy 8 to 9 years shorter than a nonsmoker of the same age. The excess mortality in both men and women who smoke is noted to be greatest for the 45- to 55-year-old age groups; therefore, smoking is associated with premature mortality. Judging from the prevalence of chronic illness and disability, the incidence of acute medical conditions, the number of days lost due to illness, and the frequency of hospitalization among smokers versus nonsmokers, there is a distinct and irrefutable correlation between smoking and morbidity. Smoking is also responsible for about 25% of all deaths and nonfatal injuries from fire. The following are some of the conditions known to be caused by or related to smoking.

Nonneoplastic Bronchopulmonary Diseases. The cause-and-effect relationship between smoking and chronic obstructive pulmonary disease (COPD) is well known. Although only about 10% to 15% of smokers develop clinically significant COPD, more than 80% of deaths from this disease are attributed to smoking. The etiologic role of smoking in chronic bronchitis and emphysema and its effect on precipitation and aggravation of asthmatic symptoms are discussed in Chapters 8 and 9. Cigarette smokers have a much higher frequency of respiratory symptoms. Both cough and expectoration are proportional to the amount and the duration of smoking. It has been demonstrated that even asymptomatic smokers have impaired ventilatory function when compared with nonsmokers of the same age. Current smokers have lower FEV_1 than nonsmokers, and it declines in more accelerated fashion with aging. In addition to changes in ventilatory function, smokers show evidence of impairment of pulmonary clearance, including ciliary and alveolar macrophage functions. Respiratory infections are more prevalent and severe among cigarette smokers, particularly heavy smokers, than among nonsmokers. Smoking plays a significant role in the severity of symptoms and disabililty in many patients with occupational lung disease, especially in coal miners. Postoperative pulmonary complications are seen more frequently in cigarette smokers than in nonsmokers.

Bronchogenic Carcinoma. Cigarette smoking is considered to be the most important causative factor in bronchogenic carcinoma. Its incidence is more than 10 times higher in smokers than in non-smokers. Certain histologic types are seen almost exclusively in smokers. The risk of developing lung cancer increases with the intensity and duration of smoking. Heavy and long-time smokers are the most likely victims, in whom the incidence may be as much as 70 times higher than in non-smokers. Although cigarette smoking is associated with lung cancer in women, this relationship, for some unknown reasons, appears to be stronger in men. However, lung cancer mortality rates in women are increasing more rapidly than in men, and this apparent difference in susceptibility may not hold much longer. There are certain indications that the tar content of cigarettes is the major factor in the carcinogenesis of smoking. The higher the level of tar in the smoke reaching the lungs, the more is the risk of developing lung cancer. The incidence of lung cancer appears to be higher among cigarette smokers with chronic bronchitis than without. Certain occupational exposures, particularly to asbestos, act synergistically with smoking in causing lung cancer. Host factors and genetic susceptibility affect the risk of lung cancer in smokers.

Laryngeal Cancer. Association between smoking and laryngeal cancer is as strong as in bronchogenic carcinoma. It has been estimated that about 84% of all the cases of laryngeal cancer are directly related to smoking. It seems that alcohol use has a synergistic effect with smoking. Higher incidence of cancer of the larynx in men as compared with women is at least partly due to higher alcohol consumption in men.

Other Malignant Neoplasms. Oral cancer is much more common in smokers of cigarettes, pipes, and cigars, especially among heavy smokers. Smokeless tobacco use (chewing and snuff dipping) has also been considered to be causally related. Carcinoma of the esophagus is also more prevalent among smokers. Alcohol use in smokers further increases the incidence of oral and esophageal cancers. Other malignancies associated with smoking include cancers of the pancreas, bladder, kidney, stomach, and cervix.

Coronary Artery Disease. The death rate from heart attack is much higher among smokers than among nonsmokers. It is estimated that about 25% of deaths from coronary artery disease are attributable to smoking. Cigarette smoking is considered to be one of the major risk factors for the development of coronary atherosclerosis. Smoking may also precipitate angina pectoris in patients with coronary artery disease. Both nicotine and carbon monoxide have been implicated in the development of these processes, as well as precipitation of coronary thrombosis. The incidence of myocardial infarction and sudden death in both men and women is much more prevalent among smokers. Smoking, together with any other risk factors such as hypertension, hypercholesterolemia, and diabetes, increases the risk of heart attack to an alarmingly high level. It has been demonstrated that the efficacy of some of the antianginal medications is reduced by cigarette smoking. Smoking is a readily controllable risk factor. Smoking cessation not only rapidly reduces the risk of coronary artery occlusion, but also influences the outcome following myocardial infarction and coronary artery surgery.

Cerebrovascular and Peripheral Vascular Diseases. Cigarette smokers have higher death rates from stroke than do nonsmokers. Women on oral contraceptives who smoke have a markedly increased risk for cerebrovascular accident. Heavy cigarette smoking is the most important recognizable risk factor for atherosclerotic peripheral vascular disease, which may result in progressive occlusion of arteries, especially of the lower extremities. Mortality from abdominal aortic aneurysm is two to three times higher in smokers than in nonsmokers.

Peptic Ulcer Disease and Other Gastrointestinal Disorders. Cigarette smokers have an increased prevalence of peptic ulcer and its complications as compared with nonsmokers. Smoking appears to reduce the effectiveness of standard ulcer treatment and to slow the rate of ulcer healing. "Heartburn," as a result of reflux of gastric juice to the esophagus, has been shown to increase with smoking.

Hematologic Disorder. Heavy smokers of cigarettes and cigars are known to develop secondary polycythemia, which is caused by chronically elevated blood carboxyhemoglobin (COHb) levels. Patients with chronic lung disease are particularly prone to develop this complication as a result of combined effects of chronic hypoxemia and high blood COHb levels on increased red cell production.

Pregnancy. Smoking during pregnancy has a retarding effect on fetal growth as manifested by low infant birth weight and an increased incidence of prematurity. In addition, it seems that women who smoke during pregnancy have significantly greater risk of an unsuccessful pregnancy than do women who do not smoke.

Smoking and Drug Metabolism. Cigarette smoking is known to alter the metabolism and pharmacologic effects of certain drugs. The best-known among drugs affected by smoking is theophylline. Smokers usually need a 50% increase in the maintenance dose of theophylline. It should also be noted that stopping smoking in chronic theophylline users, as during hospitalization, may result in theophylline toxicity if proper dosing adjustment is not made. Cigarette smoking and oral contraceptives may interact and increase the risk of thromboembolic events, such as stroke and coronary artery occlusion. Smoking reduces the effectiveness of histamine (H_2)-blocking drugs and antacids in peptic ulcer disease.

Involuntary Smoking

Involuntary or *passive smoking* is defined as the inhalation by nonsmokers of the products of tobacco combustion generated by active smokers. More descriptive terminology is *exposure to environmental tobacco smoke* (ETS). Smoke from the burning ends of cigarettes or other tobacco products (sidestream smoke) and the exhaled smoke not retained by the smoker (mainstream smoke) are the source of this special form of indoor air pollution. It contains all the constituents of tobacco smoke, although in a lower concentration.

In recent years, the subject of involuntary smoking, also known as *secondhand smoking,* has received an increasing amount of public attention and has resulted in more controversy and dispute than any other aspect of smoking. It also is having a greater impact on smoking practices than ever before. As a result of increasing public awareness and concern about involuntary smoking, a growing number of private policies and public ordinances are being enacted and enforced.

Unlike the health effects of active smoking, which are on solid scientific grounds, information on involuntary smoking is sparce and often disputed. Acute exposure by normal subjects to the environmental tobacco smoke may result in many subjective symptoms, although objective changes are unusual. Eye irritation, nasal symptoms, headache, cough, and throat irritation are often reported. Persons with allergic disorders are especially prone to these symptoms, which are mostly due to the irritating effect of tobacco smoke rather than from allergic response. True allergy to tobacco smoke is a very rare occurrence. In asthmatic subjects, however, it may, as with other bronchial irritants, nonspecifically precipitate or aggrevate an asthma attack.

The effect of long-term exposure to environmental tobacco smoke on the airways of normal adults is generally small or negligible. It is, therefore, doubtful that chronic exposure to secondhand smoke would increase the risk of chronic lung disease in nonsmoking adults. Several studies, however, have shown a significant association between parental smoking and prevalence of acute respiratory ill-nesses in infants and young children. These illnesses in turn have been implicated as a risk factor for developing COPD in older age. Childhood chronic exposure to household smoking may, therefore, play an indirect role in the pathogenesis of COPD. Numerous epidemiologic studies show increased incidence of lung cancer among nonsmokers chronically exposed to ETS, such as nonsmoking women living with their smoking husbands. Recently, the U.S. Environmental Protection Agency (EPA) has classified ETS as a Class A (known human) carcinogen.

■ CESSATION OF SMOKING

With a plethora of information on the impact of smoking on health in general, and on its harmful effects on specific organs, it is obvious that smoking cessation is one of the most important steps toward restoration of health, or at least in the prevention of its further deterioration. Unfortunately, once the habit is ingrained it is not easy to give up. The factors that result in the initiation of smoking are different from those that result in the establishment and maintenance of smoking behavior. The main causes of smoking initiation are social and familial. The dynamics of continuation of smoking, which include behavioral, psychological, and pharmacologic components, are much more complex. The importance of nicotine in tobacco smoke, as a highly addictive pharmacological substance, has been reemphasized in recent years. Genetic factors seem to play a part in smoking behavior. Some people are more susceptible to taking up the habit and have more difficulty in giving it up.

Certain social and familial environments are more conducive to perpetuation of smoking. To be successful, any smoking cessation program should consider and address all of these and other related factors. One of the most challenging, as well as rewarding, tasks of the health care professional is motivating a chronic smoker to stop smoking permanently. Although the majority of smokers would like to terminate their costly and unhealthy habit, and have tried more than once, their success rate is disappointingly small. Increasing emphasis on personal responsibility for individual health maintenance and disease prevention seems to have a significant impact on giving up the smoking habit.

In many instances there is a need for the use of one or more of the various smoking-cessation methods. They include participation in self-help groups, behavior modification, psychotherapy with or without hypnosis, and pharmacologic intervention. There are many stop-smoking programs that incorporate various interventions to assist smokers to go through the stages of decision, preparation, action, and maintenance of smoking cessation. The role of health care providers for motivating smokers to quit, especially when they have medical conditions related to their habit, is very important. They should be able to explain the health benefits to smokers and their non-smoking family members, to recommend a proper smoking-cessation program, and to provide information on how to obtain pamphlets and other materials from local and national organizations. The availability of pharmacologic aides has resulted in an increase in the importance of the role of clinicians in smoking cessation.

With the knowledge that the major factor in causing the smoking habit and making it difficult to quit is addiction to nicotine, replacement therapy with various nicotine preparations has become an important part of smoking cessation programs. Three methods of nicotine delivery systems are chewing gums, patches, and nasal sprays containing nicotine. These preparations, by providing nicotine, reduce withdrawal symptoms without exposing the users to other harmful constituents of cigarettes. It has been shown that the rate of successful smoking cessation is significantly increased with the use of these preparations, especially in smokers who depend heavily on nicotine. Because of the possibility of adverse effects of nicotine in certain individuals, nicotine replacement therapy should be under proper medical counseling and monitoring. Although nicotine therapy increases the likelihood of continuation of abstinence from smoking, other factors that are known to contribute to failure or relapse in smoking cessation should always be considered in any program. Other pharmacologic agents that have been tried as adjunctive therapy in smoking cessation, such as clonidine, have had limited success. Because of their significant side effects, they are not usually recommended.

Logically, smoking prevention should be addressed primarily to the persons most susceptible to the smoking habit, especially school-age children and adolescents. Although smoking cessation programs are generally helpful in reducing the number of smokers, without smoking prevention efforts, the goal of achieving a smoke-free society will not be possible.

Almost 90% of smokers start smoking before the age of 20, and every day more than 3000 youngsters in the United States become new smokers. As the start of smoking is promoted by psychosocial forces from peer pressure and misleading advertisements, these should be considered carefully in any public health measures addressing the issues of smoking.

BIBLIOGRAPHY

American Thoracic Society. Cigarette smoking and health. *Am J Respir Crit Care Med.* 1996; 153:861–865.

Bartecchi CE, McKenzie TD, Schrier RW. The human costs of tobacco use. *N Engl J Med.* 1994; 330:907–912; 975–980.

Belt WT Jr. Tobacco smoking, hypertension, stroke, and coronary heart disease: the importance of smoking cessation. *Semin Respir Med.* 1990; 11:36–49.

Benowitz NL. Pharmacologic aspects of cigarette smoking and addiction. *N Engl J Med.* 1988; 319:1318–1330.

Centers for Disease Control. *The health benefits of smoking cessation: a report of the Surgeon General, 1990.* Rockville, MD: U.S. Department of Health and Human Services, Public Health Service, 1990. DHHS publication no. (CDC) 90-8416.

Crofton J, Masironi R. Chronic airway disease: the smoking component. *Chest.* 1989; 96(suppl):349S–355S.

Fiore MC, Pierce JP, Remington PL, Fiore BJ. Cigarette smoking: the clinician's role in cessation, prevention, and public health. *Dis Mon.* 1990; 35:186–241.

Fiscella K, Franks P. Cost-effectiveness of the transdermal nicotine patch as an adjunct to physicians' smoking cessation counseling. *JAMA.* 1996; 275:1247–1251.

Fisher EB Jr, Haire-Joshu D, Morgan GD, et al. Smoking and smoking cessation. *Am Rev Respir Dis.* 1990; 142:702–720.

Griffith DE, Garcia JGN. Tobacco cigarettes, smoking, smoking cessation, and chronic obstructive pulmonary disease. *Semin Respir Med.* 1989; 10:346–371.

Health and Public Policy Committee, American College of Physicians. Methods for stopping cigarette smoking. *Ann Intern Med.* 1986; 105:281–291.

Henningfield JE. Nicotine medications for smoking cessation. *N Engl J Med.* 1995; 333:1196–1203.

Huber GL, Byrne B, Allen PG, Pandina RJ. The role of nicotine in smoking behavior. *Semin Respir Crit Care Med.* 1995: 16:134–154.

Idell S, Garcia JGN. Mechanisms of smoking-induced lung injury. *Semin Respir Med.* 1989; 10:345–355.

Kikendall JW, Evaul J, Johnson LF. Effect of cigarette smoking on gastrointestinal physiology and non-neoplastic digestive disease. *J Clin Gastroenterol.* 1984; 6:65–78.

Knudson RJ, Knudson DE, Kaltenborn WT, Bloom JW. Subclinical effects of cigarette smoking. *Chest.* 1989; 95:512–518.

Koop CE. Smoking and cancer. *Hosp Pract.* 1984; 19(6):107–132.

Krzyzanowski M, Sherrill DL, Paoletti P, Lebowitz MD. Relationship of respiratory symptoms and pulmonary function to tar, nicotine, and carbon monoxide yield of cigarettes. *Am Rev Respir Dis.* 1991; 143:306–311.

Law M, Tang JL. An analysis of the effectiveness of interventions intended to help people stop smoking. *Arch Intern Med.* 1995; 155:1933–1941.

Mahajan VK, Huber GL. Health effects of involuntary smoking. *Semin Respir Med.* 1990; 11:87–114.

Nemery B, Moavero NE, Brasseur L, et al. Changes in lung function after smoking cessation. *Am Rev Respir Dis.* 1982; 125:122–124.

Prochazka A. Medical approach to smoking cessation. *Semin Respir Crit Care Med.* 1996; 17:289–297.

Shafer DR, Nett LM. Medical consequences of cigarette smoking. *Semin Respir Crit Care Med.* 1995; 16:84–91.

Tager IB, Weiss ST, Muñoz A, et al.

Longitudinal study of the effects of maternal smoking on pulmonary function in children. *N Engl J Med.* 1983; 309:699–702.

Tashkin DP, Clark VA, Coulson AH, et al. Effects of smoking cessation on lung function. *Am Rev Respir Dis.* 1984; 130:707–715.

Tobin MJ, Suffredini AF, Grenvik A. Short-term effect of smoking cessation. *Respir Care.* 1984; 29:641–649.

U.S. Department of Health and Human Services. *Reducing the health consequences of smoking: 25 years of progress. A report of the Surgeon General, 1989.* 1989. DHHS publication no. (CDC) 89-8411.

VI

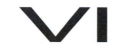

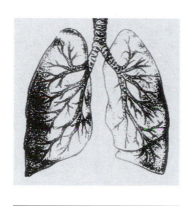

PULMONARY ASPIRATION-ATELECTASIS: POSTOPERATIVE PULMONARY COMPLICATIONS

17.

Pulmonary Aspiration

Inhalation of endogenously produced secretions or exogenous substances into the airways beyond the vocal cords is referred to as *aspiration*. Aspiration, even in normal individuals, is a common event that, in most instances, is mild, usually well tolerated, and often unrecognized. However, when clinically significant, it may have serious and sometimes fatal consequences. The development of respiratory complications depends on the amount and physicochemical characteristics of the aspirate, as well as the frequency and depth of aspiration.

■ MECHANISMS AND CAUSES OF PULMONARY ASPIRATION

Pulmonary defense mechanisms as related to respiratory tract infection and environmental lung diseases are briefly discussed in Chapters 3 and 15. The defense against aspiration depends mainly on proper function of supraglottic and glottic structures that, through a complex

yet coordinated interaction of muscles of deglutition and laryngeal reflexes, are capable of protecting the more distal airways. Predisposing factors for pulmonary aspiration are, therefore, the conditions that impair these important protective structures and their functions. Table 17–1 outlines the important and fairly common conditions in which pulmonary aspiration may occur. The dominant factor in most clinical situations associated with aspiration is impaired consciousness. Alcohol intoxication, seizure disorders, drug overdose, general anesthesia, cerebrovascular accident, head trauma, and other organic and metabolic brain dysfunction are frequent causes. Both nasogastric intubation and tracheostomy are known to predispose to recurrent pulmonary aspiration. Swallowing difficulty from neurologic disorders or structural lesions of the mouth, pharynx, larynx, and esophagus are other conditions associated with aspiration. Vomiting or regurgitation of gastric content together with almost any of the previously listed disorders makes pulmonary aspiration almost

TABLE 17–1. CONDITIONS PREDISPOSING
TO ASPIRATION

Altered level of consciousness
  Alcoholic intoxication
  Drug overdose
  General anesthesia
  Seizure disorders
  Cerebrovascular accident
  Head trauma
Conditions affecting neuromuscular function
  Polymyositis
  Muscular dystrophy
  Myasthenia gravis
  Guillain-Barré syndrome
  Amyotrophic lateral sclerosis
  Multiple sclerosis
  Syringomyelia
  Parkinson's disease
Locations of structural lesions that impair swallowing
  Mouth
  Pharynx
  Larynx
  Esophagus
Other contributing factors
  Cardiopulmonary resuscitation
  Nasogastric tube
  Tracheostomy
  Gastric dilatation, gastroparesis
  Gastroesophageal reflux
  Frequent vomiting

a certainty. It is not unusual for vomiting to occur with alcoholic intoxication, during cardiopulmonary resuscitation (CPR), with drug overdose, or following a head injury. Impaired cough reflex is a common finding in patients with chronic recurrent aspiration.

Aspirated material may be oropharyngeal secretions, vomitus, regurgitated gastric content, blood, food, drink, or other exogenous substances. When aspirated, these materials may result in pathophysiologic changes related to three different mechanisms, each causing distinctive clinical syndromes of infection, toxic reaction, and mechanical ob-

struction. These syndromes may develop alone or occur in various combinations. They may present as an acute single event or may manifest as a recurring and chronically debilitating condition. Infectious consequences of pulmonary aspiration are mentioned in Chapter 3 and, therefore, they are not discussed further here. In addition to bronchopulmonary diseases resulting from the aspiration of toxic fluids and mechanical effect of aspiration, a somewhat related subject of near-drowning is also discussed in this chapter.

■ ASPIRATION PNEUMONITIS

There are several exogenous chemicals that, under unusual circumstances, may be aspirated, resulting in inflammatory reaction in the lungs; however, the most common and important problem of aspiration in clinical practice is related to gastric acid. For the purpose of this discussion, the term *aspiration pneumonitis,* which is used interchangeably with the term *chemical pneumonitis,* refers to pulmonary complication of aspiration of acid gastric content.

Pathogenesis and Pathologic Changes. The main toxic effect of gastric juice stems from its high concentration of hydrochloric acid. The whole picture of aspiration pneumonitis can be produced by intratracheal injection of sterile hydrochloric acid in experimental animals. Its effect has been considered to be a chemical burn related to the very low pH of the aspirate. Data from animal studies indicate that a pH of less than 2.5 and a volume of at least 1 mL/kg of weight are necessary for an aspirate to cause a significant lung injury. However, in clinical situations other factors, such as distribution of the aspirated material and the presence of food particles, also affect the outcome of the aspiration of the gastric content. Chemical effect of gastric acid on the respiratory tract is almost immediate and, with enough volume, quite extensive, owing to its rapid distribution. Although the acid is neutralized within a few minutes, the damage has already occurred.

Pathologic changes usually consist of extensive acute inflammatory reaction, which, together with alveolar and capillary injury, results in exudation of fluid into and around the airspaces. The lungs are heavy and edematous with areas of hemorrhage. The early parenchymal changes are peribronchial, which become more diffuse in advanced stages. The mucosa of the bronchi are often destroyed. The lesions following pulmonary aspiration are more severe in dependent portions of the lungs (ie, lower lobes and posterior segments of upper lobes). The right lung is usually involved more so than the left because of its bronchus offering easier access to the aspirated material. In more severe cases, the entire lung fields are involved.

Reduction of pulmonary compliance, ventilation–perfusion imbalance, intrapulmonary shunting, and severe hypoxemia are the usual pathophysiologic consequences of aspiration pneumonitis.

Clinical Manifestations. Despite its frequent occurrence in various clinical situations, the diagnosis of aspiration pneumonitis without history or witness of vomiting and aspiration is almost impossible to make. Most often it is presumed or suspected in patients with the aforementioned predisposing factors and consistent clinical picture. Aspiration of small amounts of gastric content may cause no symptom or sign; however, if a sufficient volume of highly acid gastric secretion is aspirated, a distinct picture of acute respiratory distress develops. Usually within 2 to 5 hours following aspiration of liquid gastric content, there is abrupt onset of dyspnea, tachypnea, cyanosis, and tachycardia. Fever may or may not be present. Some patients become hypotensive and develop clinical shock. There is often evidence of bronchospasm with diffuse wheezing; frothy pink sputum and pulmonary rales are commonly present. The symptoms and signs become progressively worse unless appropriate treatment is instituted.

The most characteristic laboratory feature of aspiration pneumonitis is severe hypoxemia, which is often difficult to correct with increased FIO_2. Arterial blood PCO_2 is usually reduced unless there is significant ventilatory impairment. Blood gas abnormalities may be present right after aspiration, before development of a full clinical picture or radiographic changes. This may be an important clue in early diagnosis of aspiration pneumonitis.

Severe aspiration pneumonitis is one of the major causes of acute respiratory distress syndrome (ARDS) (see Chapter 27).

Radiographic Findings. The chest x-ray may show bilateral diffuse mottling, more marked in dependent lung regions (Fig. 17–1). The changes may be limited to a few segments or lobes in less severe cases, the location of which will depend on the patient's body position at the time of aspiration.

Management. Because of extreme seriousness of aspiration pneumonitis, which

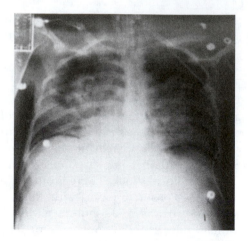

Figure 17–1. Chest radiograph of severe bilateral aspiration pneumonitis. There is diffuse interstitial and airspace infiltration in both lung fields (noncardiac pulmonary edema).

often has a fatal outcome, every effort should be made toward its prevention. Close observation of patients at risk of aspiration, such as patients with impaired consciousness; proper positioning of patients; appropriate preparation before general anesthesia; precautionary measures and immediate care of patients with seizure disorders; and close watch of patients with an indwelling nasogastric tube, mostly if they are being fed through the tube, are some of the important measures that help in reducing the incidence of aspiration. The administration of a water-soluble antacid or an H_2-receptor antagonist before general anesthesia, especially when there is a question about the gastric content, results in a significant reduction in the occurrence of serious aspiration pneumonitis. Because commonly used particulate antacids are known to produce pulmonary injury when aspirated, they should not be used for this purpose.

Once aspiration is witnessed, immediate proper positioning of patient and suctioning of the airways should be un-

dertaken. Tracheal lavage with saline solution or an attempt to neutralize gastric acid with bicarbonate solution may be more harmful than beneficial.

The most important aspect of treatment of aspiration pneumonitis is correction of hypoxemia by administration of oxygen. Bronchodilators, such as aminophylline or beta-adrenergic stimulating agents, may be tried. If hypoxemia cannot be corrected by simple means, intubation and mechanical ventilation, usually with positive end–expiratory pressure (PEEP), will be necessary. As is true with most cases of ARDS, the correction of hypoxemia is the most important part of management of aspiration pneumonitis.

The role of corticosteroids in the management of aspiration pneumonitis remains controversial. Once the full clinical picture has developed, their use has no demonstrable effect. Administration of steroids immediately following aspiration or within a few hours has been commonly practiced, despite a lack of conclusive evidence for their benefit. Antibiotic therapy for prophylaxis against bacterial infection is another unsettled question in the management of aspiration pneumonitis. However, because of a high incidence of pulmonary infection following aspiration, periodic bacteriologic examination of sputum as well as close clinical evaluation and follow-up radiographic studies should be performed for the early detection of infection and its proper treatment.

Chronic Recurrent Aspiration

In contrast to the acute dramatic clinical picture, aspiration, if mild but chronic and recurrent, may produce more insidious and protracted symptoms. Transient recurrent fever, chronic cough and wheezing, subtle radiographic changes, and even progressive pulmonary fibrosis may be due to chronic aspiration of gastric content in patients with esophageal disorder and/or impaired consciousness. The management of such patients is often difficult and usually unsuccessful because of the nature of the underlying predisposing conditions. Surgical interventions that are based on separating the airway from the alimentary tract necessitate a tracheostomy with or without the closure of the larynx. Supraglottic or glottic closure, laryngotracheal separation, and tracheoesophageal diversion are some of the surgical techniques for this purpose. The tracheoesophageal diversion procedure, in which the proximal tracheal segment is connected to the esophagus, is potentially reversible and easier to perform. It would allow secretions and oral intake that may pass into the larynx to enter the esophagus. The decision for any of these interventions requires the considerations of many factors, which include lack of response to simpler measures, patient acceptability, prognosis of the underlying chronic disease, and patient's life expectancy.

Hydrocarbon Pneumonitis

Hydrocarbon pneumonitis usually results from the aspiration of accidentally ingested hydrocarbons such as kerosene, gasoline, or certain household compounds (furniture polishes) containing hydrocarbons. It is most commonly seen in young children after inadvertent ingestion of such substances. In adults, it may occasionally occur with suicide attempts, industrial accidents, or siphoning of gasoline. Because of their low viscosity and very low surface tension, hydrocarbons, once aspirated, spread throughout the lungs. Being lipid solvents, they are directly toxic to the lung tissues, causing widespread injury and inflammation of the airways and alveoli. The clinical picture of hydrocarbon pneumonitis is one of rapidly progressive pulmonary edema with severe hypoxemia. The diagnosis is often suggested by the odor of the patient's breath.

The prevention of further aspiration is most important in the management of hydrocarbon pneumonitis. Measures that may cause vomiting should be avoided. Adequate oxygenation by supplemental oxygen, constant positive airway pressure (CPAP), or mechanical ventilation with PEEP, depending on the severity of the disease, will be necessary. The role of corticosteroids in its management has not been established.

■ MECHANICAL EFFECT OF ASPIRATION: FOREIGN-BODY ASPIRATION

Aspiration of solid or liquid material may cause ventilatory impairment and other pulmonary complications by mechanical airway obstruction. These materials may be inert or have limited toxic effect on the lungs.

Aspiration of foreign bodies can occur at any age, but it is most common in children between the ages of 1 and 3 years. The usual objects include nuts, seeds, pins, coins, and beads. Depending on the size and shape of solid material in relation to the airway, a variable degree of obstruction will result. Large objects will lodge in the larynx, causing upper airway obstruction. This is discussed in Chapter 7 along with other causes of upper airway obstruction. Smaller objects may lodge in one of the mainstem bronchi or more distally. The shape of the object will determine whether the obstruction will be complete from the beginning or will become complete secondary to tissue reaction to traumatic or toxic effect of the aspirated material. Because of the direction of the right mainstem bronchus, foreign bodies lodge in right lung bronchi twice as often as the left.

The initial symptoms of foreign-body aspiration are choking, cough, respiratory distress, and wheezing. A large body occluding the larynx results in suffocation; a smaller object in the larynx will cause hoarseness or complete loss of voice and croupy cough. As a result of laryngeal spasm and/or edema, obstruction may become complete if the object is not removed. Lodging of a foreign body in one of the bronchi will cause irritating cough and varying degrees of dyspnea, depending on the size of the obstructed bronchus and degree of obstruction. Localized wheezing or absent breath sounds may be detected.

Radiographic examination may show the aspirated object if it is radiopaque, or secondary changes may be demonstrated. Complete obstruction of a mainstem or a lobar bronchus results in atelectasis; incomplete blockage may behave as a check valve and cause overinflation of the involved lung or lobe. This can be demonstrated better by comparing inspiratory with expiratory films. *Bronchoscopy* is decisive in making the diagnosis and is essential for the removal of bronchial foreign bodies.

If untreated, the foreign body in a bronchus will result in late infectious complications, including pneumonia, lung abscess, empyema, and bronchiectasis. Frequently, the early symptoms of foreign-body aspiration are transient and may be forgotten; therefore, late complications may be its only manifestations. The importance of bronchoscopic examination in these situations cannot be overemphasized.

Aspiration of any liquid material in large enough volume produces abrupt suffocation by total obstruction of air passages. Sometimes aspiration of a massive amount of vomitus may be the cause of respiratory arrest. This is not an uncommon terminal event in certain debilitated patients, particularly with impaired cerebral or other neurologic functions. Only immediate tracheal suctioning may be lifesaving. In massive hemoptysis, the cause of death is often due to mechanical obstruction of the airways from inundation of blood. It is often said that the patient with massive hemoptysis may "drown in his (or her) own blood."

■ DROWNING AND NEAR DROWNING

Drowning is death from asphyxiation as a result of submersion, but in *near drowning* the victim survives at least temporarily following such an accident. Near-drowning victims may suffer from *secondary drowning*, which is death from delayed complications following apparent recovery. Despite declining death rate from drowning in the United States in recent years, more than 5000 individuals, mostly young, still die from drowning each year. This number is only a small fraction of annual submersion accidents in this country.

Causes of Drowning and Near Drowning. The sequence of events resulting in drowning (or near drowning) is quite variable. A commonly portrayed drowning scene in which a panic-stricken child or adult not able to swim struggles unsuccessfully to remain afloat is only one of the ways described by witnesses. Some of the victims of drowning or near drowning may be seen to become motionless in the water with no apparent reason; some, after diving into a pool, may never surface; and some may submerge and disappear without any evidence of thrashing in the water. Therefore, there is no typical set of circumstances that characterizes drowning or near drowning. Although in most cases drowning or near drowning is the cause of loss of consciousness, in some instances the victim may become incapacitated from other causes. They include head or neck injury from diving, vagally mediated bradycardia or cardiac arrest in cold-water immersion, seizure disorder, cardiac arrhythmia, myocardial infarction, and cerebrovascular accident.

Pathophysiology. In drowning or near drowning, initial reaction is most likely breath holding, which may last until increasing hypoxemia and hypercapnia force the victim to inhale. The entrance of water into the larynx causes intense laryngospasm. About 10% to 15% of drowning victims die from asphyxia due to glottic spasm without water entering into the lung; this is referred to as "dry drowning." The remaining victims aspirate the water into the tracheobronchial passages all the way to the terminal airways and alveoli. In either event, the essential problem is related to respiratory arrest, which results in severe hypoxemia, acidosis, and death unless the victim is rescued (near drowning).

Severe hypoxemia and respiratory acidosis may result in myocardial depression and reduced cardiac output. Marked impairment of tissue perfusion from peripheral vasoconstriction and low cardiac output, together with arterial hypoxemia, causes a profound tissue anoxia and lactic acidosis. Cerebral hypoxia, which is the cause of altered mental state and unconsciousness, may result in brain edema and

increased intracranial pressure. Irreversible hypoxic brain damage is the most feared sequela in near drowning.

Near-drowning victims, after being rescued, may have diminished or no respiration. Hypoxemia and respiratory acidosis from lack of ventilation are sustained or even worsened with the development of pulmonary edema, which may occur during and/or after the rescue. Aspirated water, alveolar capillary leak, loss of surfactant, and myocardial depression may contribute to the development of pulmonary edema. The amount of aspirated water varies, but most near-drowning victims do not aspirate more than 4 mL/kg of body weight. This amount of fluid cannot by itself result in significant pulmonary edema. Increased alveolar capillary leak, which plays a more important role, may be due to injury from hypertonic salt solution of seawater, severe hypoxia, neurogenic effect, and the presence of other dissolved or particulate matters in aspirated water. Loss of surfactant, especially with freshwater aspiration, enhances pulmonary edema and also causes atelectasis. In severe near drowning, therefore, a clinicopathologic picture of ARDS develops. Ventilation–perfusion mismatch and intrapulmonary shunting may persist until the victim's full recovery. In some patients, initial success in restoring adequate ventilation and oxygenation is followed by progressive respiratory distress and death (secondary drowning).

The distinction between freshwater and seawater near drowning is not clinically important. Although an occasional patient may have significant problems with water and electrolyte imbalance or other distrubances as a result of aspiration of hypotonic (fresh) or hypertonic (sea) water, the major clinical problems in all near-drowning victims, regardless of the nature of immersion medium, are related to hypoxia and acidosis. Immersion in cold water may be detrimental from its hypothermic effect, which makes the victim susceptible to drowning or near drowning by causing mental status change and resulting in vagally induced cardiac dysfuntion. However, in near-drowning victims, hypothermia is known to have a protective effect against permanent brain damage from anoxia (anoxic encephalopathy).

Clinical Manifestations. On rescue, a near-drowning victim is usually unconscious or agitated and confused, cold, and cyanotic. Respiration is often absent; otherwise tachypnea, cough, and frothy pink expectoration may be noted and rales and rhonchi may be heard. The pulse is often difficult to feel, and heart sounds are difficult to hear. Because of severe vasoconstriction, blood pressure is usually hard to measure. Neurologic examination shows varying degrees of cerebral dysfunction.

Chest radiograph in near drowning may be normal initially despite significant respiratory impairment. More often, patchy infiltrates or diffuse pulmonary edema are noted. These changes may develop later. Blood-gas abnormalities are always present; hypoxemia, hypercapnia, low serum bicabonate level, and very low blood pH are commonly seen. Varying patterns of electrocardiographic abnormalities can often be demonstrated. In seawater near drowning, serum sodium and chloride may be high.

Management. The primary objectives of treatment of near-drowning victims should be preventing brain injury by prompt restoration of ventilation, adequate oxygenation, and correction of aci-

dosis. The initial stage of therapy should be on-the-scene emergency care with usual diligent resuscitative procedures (ie, establishment and maintenance of an adequate airway, mouth-to-mouth breathing or use of a hand respirator with supplemental oxygen if available, and application of cardiac massage if there is no heartbeat). If near drowning is suspected to be the result of a diving accident, the possibility of head and neck injury should be considered and appropriate measures taken. Although the Heimlich maneuver has been advocated by some for on-the-scene removal of water from the lungs, it is only indicated after unsuccessful attempts at ventilation suggest upper airway obstruction by a foreign body. Whenever possible, endotracheal intubation should be performed if needed for airway maintenance and easier ventilatory support. Emergency care should be continued during the transportation of the victim to the hospital. At the hospital, the unconscious victim should be intubated, if not done in the field, and mechanically ventilated with adequate supply of oxygen. Positive expiratory pressure may be required for proper oxygenation. If the patient is conscious and breathes spontaneously, he or she should be kept in the hospital for observation and monitoring of clinical signs and blood gases while receiving supplemental oxygen. It is not uncommon that the near-drowning victim, after apparent initial recovery, develops progressive respiratory distress. Other therapeutic measures should include restoration of fluid, electrolyte, and acid-base balance. Under certain circumstances, ionotropic drugs and diuretics may be used. Although infectious complications involving the respiratory tract are common, prophylactic antibiotic use is not recommended. Such infections should be watched for and treated promptly once recognized. Corticosteroids have not been proved to be beneficial for prevention or treatment of pulmonary complications in near drowning. Their use, however, is sometimes recommended for treatment of cerebral edema and increased intracranial pressure (ICP), which occurs commonly as a result of prolonged brain anoxia.

Neurologic status after initial resuscitation is the best indicator of outcome in most patients. Near-drowning victims who breathe spontaneously and are conscious have a very good prognosis. However, it should be emphasized that many patients who remain comatose, even for a prolonged period, are known to recover, often with restoration of most of their neurologic functions. Therefore these patients should be maintained with proper intensive care during their unresponsive state and, later, be subjected to vigorous rehabilitative measures. The usefulness of "cerebral salvage" techniques, such as induction of hypothermia, ICP monitoring, and barbiturate coma, is not well established.

BIBLIOGRAPHY

Brin MF, Younger D. Neurologic disorders and aspiration. *Otolaryngol Clin North Am.* 1988; 21:691–699.

Bross MH, Clark JL. Near-drowning. *Am Fam Physician.* 1995; 51:1545–1551.

Burton EM, Brick WG, Hall JD, et al. Tracheobronchial foreign body aspiration in children. *South Med J.* 1996; 89:195–198.

DePaso WJ. Aspiration pneumonia. *Clin Chest Med.* 1991; 12:269–284.

Gonzalez-Rothi RJ. Near drowning: concensus and controversies in pulmonary and cerebral resuscitation. *Heart Lung.* 1987; 16:474–482.

Joyce TH III. Prophylaxis for pulmonary acid aspiration. *Am J Med.* 1987; 83(suppl 6A):46–52.

Karlson KH Jr. Hydrocarbon poisoning in children. *South Med J.* 1982; 75:839–840.

LeFrock JL, Clark TS, Davies B, Klainer AS. Aspiration pneumonia: a ten-year review. *Am Surg.* 1979; 45:305–313.

Limper AH, Prakash UBS. Tracheobronchial foreign bodies in adults. *Ann Intern Med.* 1990; 112:604–609.

Miller FR, Eliachar I. Managing the aspirating patient. *Am J Otolaryngol.* 1994; 15:1–17.

Modell JH. Drowning. *N Engl J Med.* 1993; 328:253–256.

Nelson HS. Gastroesophageal reflux and pulmonary disease. *J Allergy Clin Immunol.* 1984; 73:547–556.

Orlowski JP, Abulleil MM, Phillips JM. The hemodynamic and cardiovascular effects of near-drowning in hypotonic, isotonic, or hypertonic solution. *Ann Emerg Med.* 1989; 18:1044–1049.

Redding JS. Drowning and near drowning. *Postgrad Med.* 1983; 74(1):65–97.

Tietjen PA, Kaner RJ, Quinn CE. Aspiration emergencies. *Clin Chest Med.* 1994; 15(1):117–135.

Wolkove N, Kreisman H, Cohen C, Frank H. Occult foreign-body aspiration in adults. *JAMA.* 1982; 248:1350–1352.

18.

Pulmonary Atelectasis

Although *atelectasis,* in the strictest sense of the word (*ateles,* imperfect; *ektasis,* expansion), refers to incomplete expansion of the lung at birth, it is generally used in broad terms to include partial or complete collapse of lung tissue that has previously been expanded. Atelectasis may involve an entire lung or be limited to any portion of it, from a lobe to the smallest lung unit. It is one of the most common changes in the lung that can occur under numerous conditions.

Pathogenesis. To understand the development of atelectasis, it is important to consider the mechanisms that normally keep the lungs expanded. The natural tendency of the lungs to collapse is opposed by the tendency of the chest wall to expand. At the resting position (functional residual capacity [FRC]), these two forces are oppositely equal; as a result, there is a negative (subatmospheric) pressure between the lung and thoracic wall (pleural pressure). Once this negative pressure is eliminated as a result of conditions such as pneumothorax or pleural effusion, the underlying lung will collapse (Fig. 18–1).

The volume of individual alveoli is determined by an opposing negative intrathoracic pressure, which tends to expand them, and elastic recoil together with *surface tension* of the alveoli, which tend to collapse them (Fig. 18–2). The presence of surfactant reduces the surface tension of the alveoli. As the alveoli diminish in volume during expiration, reduction in surface area of the alveolar wall results in increased thickness and change in configuration of lipid–protein structure of surfactant layer; thus, alveolar surface tension is lowered (Fig. 18–3). This protective mechanism prevents collapse of the alveoli when they reach a certain volume, at which they would have collapsed without the presence of such a surface-tension–lowering agent. Reduction or absence of surfactant, which occurs in numerous pulmonary pathologic conditions, is one of the most important contributory factors in production of atelectasis.

There is a significant difference in

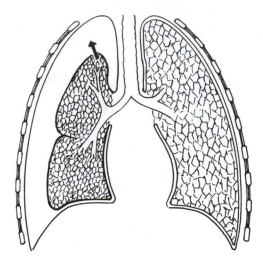

Figure 18–1. A diagram of the chest showing collapse of the right lung as a result of elimination of negative intrathoracic pressure with pneumothorax.

the volume of alveoli in various lung regions. At FRC, the alveoli in the upper lung zones are already expanded, whereas those in the lung bases have smallest volumes and, therefore, are capable of in-

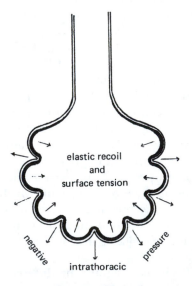

Figure 18–2. Forces determining the alveolar volume.

creasing their volumes much more during inspiration. The lower lung regions contribute much more to pulmonary ventilation than the upper ones, and they are, at the same time, more predisposed to atelectasis.

Continuous ventilation of the lung regions assures an adequate supply of air to the alveoli. The cessation of air replenishment, as may happen from the obstruction of the supplying bronchus, results in the resorption of air and, therefore, atelectasis (absorption atelectasis, Fig. 18–4). Complete obstruction of the bronchus of a lobe will result in absorption of its air within 24 hours. In contrast to small peripheral airways, alveoli with low surface tension cannot collapse completely by deflation without their gas content being absorbed. If the lobe is filled with oxygen, atelectasis will occur much more rapidly. Sometimes the obstructing lesion will act as a one-way valve, allowing the air to escape from a lobe during various expiratory efforts but preventing its entrance during inspiration. This results in more rapid development of collapse. However, the reversal of function of such a one-way valve causes hyperinflation.

The obstruction of airways more distal to a lobar bronchus may or may not result in collapse of a corresponding portion of the lung. The effect of obstruction then will depend on the presence and the function of *collateral communication* between adjacent alveoli (Figs. 18–5 and 18–6). The most significant collateral ventilation occurs through the *pores of Kohn,* which are openings or discontinuities of alveolar walls. Adequacy of collateral ventilation depends on the degree of inflation of the lungs; with partial deflation, the communications may close.

Normally the variation in depth of respiration with such acts as sighing, yawning, talking, laughing, crying, coughing,

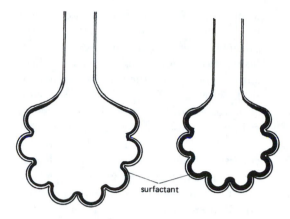

Figure 18–3. Reduction of alveolar surface tension during expiration, resulting from increased thickness of surfactant layer.

surfactant

exertion, and excitement ensures periodic expansion of the areas of the lungs that otherwise would collapse. In patients who are anesthetized, sedated, or obtunded from other causes, or when they are on a constant-volume ventilator, such periodic deep breathing does not occur. Although their ventilation may be adequate for gas exchange, they do not expand the lungs sufficiently for collateral

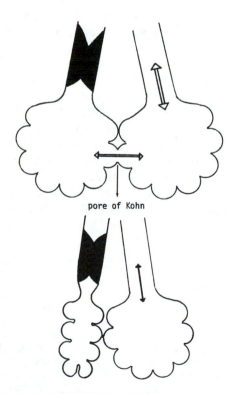

pore of Kohn

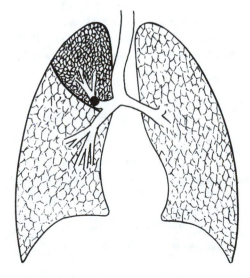

Figure 18–4. Diagrammatic demonstration of atelectasis of the right upper lobe as a result of the occlusion of its bronchus.

Figures 18–5 and 18–6. Schematic demonstration of collateral communication between the alveoli (pore of Kohn). Such a communication, when open, prevents alveolar atelectasis with distal airway obstruction (Fig. 18–5). Adequacy of collateral ventilation depends on the degree of alveolar inflation; with partial deflation, the communication may close (Fig. 18–6).

ventilation between the alveoli, some of which may have plugged airways, and atelectasis will result. It has been demonstrated that continuous ventilation at fixed and low tidal volumes causes reduction of lung volume (atelectasis). Preexisting bronchopulmonary disease will hasten this complication.

Regional reduction or cessation of pulmonary blood flow is usually followed by diminished ventilation to the corresponding region. Atelectasis in this situation is always incomplete.

In many clinical situations there is usually a combination of two or more of the previously mentioned pathogenetic mechanisms. In addition, atelectasis may result from compression of the lung (eg, by large tumors or cysts) and scarring.

Etiology. From the discussion on pathogenesis, it is clear that a varying degree of atelectasis may be seen under numerous circumstances (Table 18–1). Indeed, atelectasis is one of the most common complications that occurs in both medical and surgical patients, with or without preexisting pulmonary disease.

The presence of air or fluid in the pleural space will result in the collapse of underlying lung. Atelectasis is a common mode of presentation of patients with bronchogenic carcinoma due to airway obstruction. A foreign body in a bronchus, a mucous plug, or other endobronchial lesions may manifest by atelectasis. The compression of bronchi by lesions, such as enlarged lymph nodes or an abnormal blood vessel, may result in collapse of the corresponding part of the lung. Inadvertent intubation of the right mainstem or intermediate bronchus with an endotracheal tube causes atelectasis of the left lung and sometimes the right upper lobe. In many instances, a mucous plug may be the culprit, such as with asthma, chronic bronchitis, prolonged mechanical ventilation, and debilitated individuals with suppressed cough. Some degree of atelectasis is very common in patients with drug overdose. Atelectasis is part of the pathologic changes in bronchiectasis and cystic fibrosis. Pneumonia may result in some volume loss of the involved lung. Partial atelectasis is common in pulmonary embolism. One of the characteristic features of respiratory distress syndrome in infants and adults is pulmonary volume loss.

Impaired thoracic expansion from respiratory muscle paralysis or weakness,

TABLE 18–1. MECHANISMS AND CORRESPONDING COMMON CAUSES OF ATELECTASIS

Mechanisms	Causes
Elimination or reversal of negative pleural pressure	Pneumothorax, pleural effusion
Bronchial obstruction (absorption atelectasis)	Accumulated secretions, mucous plug, endobronchial neoplasm, foreign body, bronchial compression, intubation of right mainstem or intermediate bronchus
Lack or loss of surfactant	Respiratory distress syndrome, near drowning
Impaired diaphragmatic function	Phrenic nerve paralysis, high spinal cord injury, upper abdominal or thoracic surgery, abdominal distention, splinting from pain
Fixed and low tidal volume breating	Improper ventilation setting, unconsciousness, immobility
Reduced pulmonary blood flow	Pulmonary embolism
Scarring	Rounded atelectasis (asbestosis)
Compression of lung	Large intrathoracic tumor or cyst; tension pneumothorax or hydrothorax

certain intra-abdominal conditions, and splinting of the chest wall and diaphragm from pain are well-recognized causes of lung volume loss and atelectasis. Postoperative causes of atelectasis are discussed in Chapter 19. Chest trauma and other painful disorders of the thoracic wall or upper abdomen, by preventing deep breathing, may result in atelectasis. Acute chest syndrome in sickle cell crisis is partly from painful infarction of thoracic bones. Some of the pathophysiologic changes in this syndrome are the result of loss of lung volume from limitation of respiratory movement because of severe pain.

As mentioned in Chapter 15, rounded atelectasis in asbestosis is caused by collapse of a portion of the lung as a result of pleural effusion and fibrous pleural adhesion in which the trapped segment, unable to expand, rolls into a rounded mass. Although it may rarely result from various pleuropulmonary conditions, rounded atelectasis is a characteristic finding in asbestosis.

Pathophysiology. Atelectasis results in absent or reduced ventilation of the involved area of the lung and the proportional reduction of the lung volumes. Both FRC and vital capacity (VC) are diminished. Although as a result of pulmonary vasoconstriction, blood flow to the atelectatic region tends to diminish, ventilation–perfusion mismatching and intrapulmonary shunting are the usual pathophysiologic changes in atelectasis that cause hypoxemia.

Clinical Manifestations. Symptoms related to pulmonary atelectasis are frequently overshadowed by the presence of underlying pathologic conditions. Most patients with mild or small atelectasis have no symptoms referable to it. When present in more significant atelectasis, the symptoms are nonspecific. Dyspnea, cough, and chest discomfort may suggest atelectasis under certain circumstances, such as following major surgery. Changes in lung mechanics in patients on a mechanical ventilator or increasing oxygen requirement for adequate oxygenation may indicate atelectasis. Physical findings are usually present in patients with collapse of a lung or lobe. Flattening of the chest wall with reduction of its expansion, deviation of trachea to one side, elevation of diaphragm, dullness to percussion, and diminished or absent breath sounds are some of the signs of pulmonary atelectasis. With less extensive involvement, physical findings are less impressive and less suggestive. The presence of basal rales and diminished breath sounds are the most common findings in postoperative atelectasis. Contrary to the commonly held view, atelectasis without associated infection probably does not cause fever.

Pulmonary atelectasis is an important cause of ventilation–perfusion abnormality and hypoxemia. The latter may be the only manifestation of atelectasis.

Radiographic Findings and Diagnosis. Radiographic examination is most important in diagnosing atelectasis. Radiographic signs may be both direct and indirect. Direct radiographic signs include increased density and reduction of the volume of a whole lung or part of a lung. Increased density, however, does not appear until a significant volume of air is absorbed or expressed from the involved lung, except when there is other associated parenchymal disease. Displacement of interlobar fissures, eleva-

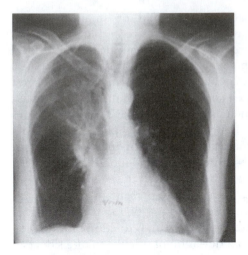 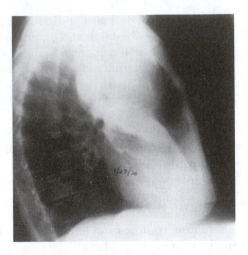

Figures 18–7 and 18–8. Lobar atelectasis. Posteroanterior (Fig. 18–7) and lateral (Fig. 18–8) chest radiographs showing atelectasis of the right upper lobe.

tion of the diaphragm, mediastinal shift, hilar displacement, alteration of bronchial and carinal angles, and changes in the chest wall are among the indirect signs of atelectasis (Figs. 18–7 and 18–8). Frequently, underlying pulmonary disease may be identified. There are known patterns of radiographic changes with various lobar and segmental atelectasis. Their description is beyond the scope of this book.

Platelike atelectasis is a radiographic term applied to linear shadows of increased density, mostly situated in the lung bases in a roughly horizontal position. They are due to atelectasis of the alveoli in lower lung fields not related to specific bronchial distribution. Platelike atelectasis is frequently due to diminished diaphragmatic movement as a result of intra-abdominal disease or surgery. As mentioned earlier, the combination of reduced ventilation, small airways obstruction due to secretion, lack of collateral ventilation due to inadequate inflation of the alveoli, and the presence of

fluid in alveoli will result in this type of atelectasis.

In many instances the diagnosis of the underlying cause of atelectasis, particularly when it involves a lung, a lobe, or a segment, will require bronchoscopic examination.

Management. The prevention and the treatment of underlying conditions are the most important and effective measures against pulmonary atelectasis. In view of the multiplicity of the causes of atelectasis, only certain principles of management are outlined here.

In some instances atelectasis is a corollary to a more important basic disease, the treatment of which will solve the problem. Withdrawal of air or fluid from the pleural cavity, removal of the foreign body from the bronchus, and resectional surgery for neoplasms are a few examples. However, in the majority of cases, as discussed earlier, there is a combination of several factors that should be considered for proper management.

Inadequate lung inflation from pain, sedation, mental obtundation, and many other causes should be prevented by encouragement of periodic deep-breathing and other lung-expansion maneuvers. Such maneuvers have proved useful for both prophylactic and therapeutic purposes. Incentive spirometry is the most commonly used technique. Chest physiotherapy and the use of dead-space rebreathing tubes, blow bottles, and continuous positive airway pressure (CPAP) by facial or nasal masks are other methods that can be effective in preventing and treating atelectasis. The use of intermittent positive pressure breathing (IPPB) has declined significantly in recent years, mainly because of the availability of simpler and more effective techniques. The choice of any of these methods depends on the circumstances in which atelectasis commonly occurs and on the patient's ability and willingness to cooperate. Nasal CPAP has proved particularly useful in poorly responsive patients. In cooperative and fully alert patients, simple deep-breathing exercises or incentive spirometry will suffice. Cough not only helps in clearing the airways, but also increases ventilation and lung expansion. Because bronchial secretion is a major factor in producing atelectasis, every effort should be made in its removal by cough, postural drainage, and suctioning. Adequate humidification with proper hydration and inhalation therapy will prevent drying of secretions and facilitate their removal. The presence of underlying chronic bronchopulmonary conditions increases the need for these measures.

Both critically ill patients and patients with tracheal intubation, on or off a ventilator, should be given special attention in treating or, better, in preventing atelectasis. Such patients are greatly handicapped by their inability to cough and clear their tracheobronchial tree. With their serious underlying problems with the lungs and other organs, the development of atelectasis, even in mild form, is poorly tolerated and will markedly impede recovery. Adequate bronchial hygiene and close monitoring of the ventilatory status, lung mechanics, blood gases, and chest radiographs are essential for prevention and early detection of atelectasis. The use of fiberoptic bronchoscopy in management of atelectasis in these patients has been rewarding. Kinetic therapy making use of rotating beds has shown to be beneficial in preventing pulmonary complications, including atelectasis, in critically ill patients, especially in those with head and neck injuries. The importance of the role of allied health professionals, particularly respiratory therapists, nurses, and physiotherapists, in the prevention and treatment of atelectasis in both surgical and medical patients cannot be overstressed. Prevention and management of postoperative atelectasis are discussed in Chapter 19.

BIBLIOGRAPHY

Bartlett RH. Respiratory therapy to prevent complications of surgery. *Respir Care*. 1984; 29:667–677.

Bateman JRM, Newman SP, Daunt KM, et al. Is cough as effective as chest physiotherapy in the removal of excessive tracheobronchial secretions? *Thorax*. 1981; 36:683–687.

Bellet PS, Kalinyak KA, Shukla R, et al. Incentive spirometry to prevent acute pulmonary complications in sickle cell diseases. *N Engl J Med*. 1995; 333:699–703.

Celli BR, Rodriguez KS, Snider GL. A controlled trial of intermittent positive pressure breathing, incentive spirometry, and deep breathing exercises in preventing pulmonary complications after abdominal surgery. *Am Rev Respir Dis.* 1984; 130:12–15.

Duncan SR, Negrin RS, Mihm FG, et al. Nasal continuous positive airway pressure in atelectasis. *Chest.* 1987; 92:621–624.

Engoren M. Lack of association between atelectasis and fever. *Chest.* 1995; 107:81–84.

Gentilello L, Thompson DA, Tonnesen AS, et al. Effects of a rotating bed on the incidence of pulmonary complications in critically ill patients. *Crit Care Med.* 1988; 16:783–786.

Hammon WE, Martin RJ. Chest physiotherapy for acute atelectasis. *Phys Ther.* 1981; 61: 217–220.

Mintzer RA, Sakowicz BA, Blonder JA. Lobar collapse: usual and unusual forms. *Chest.* 1988; 94:615–620.

Peruzzi WT, Smith B. Bronchial hygiene therapy. *Crit Care Clin.* 1995; 11:79–96.

Reines HD, Harris RC. Pulmonary complications of acute spinal cord injuries. *Neurosurgery.* 1987; 21:193–196.

Stiller K, Geake T, Taylor J, et al. Acute lobar atelectasis: a comparison of two chest physiotherapy regimens. *Chest.* 1990; 98: 1336–1340.

Voisin C, Fisekci F, Voisin-Saltiel S, et al. Asbestos-related rounded atelectasis. *Chest.* 1995; 107:477–481.

19.

Postoperative Pulmonary Complications

Postoperative pulmonary complications are defined as clinically identifiable structural or functional abnormalities of the respiratory system that occur following surgery and that adversely affect the clinical course or outcome. As is discussed in this chapter, minor clinical or radiographic changes or mild abnormalities of gas transport and other pulmonary function tests (PFTs) are expected occurrences following certain procedures. They are not included in this definition. However, it should be noted that such clinically insignificant changes may represent the beginning of true complications and therefore should not be overlooked. Despite remarkable advances in surgical techniques and significant improvement in postoperative care, pulmonary complications continue to occur as a result of the inclusion of high risk patients in complex and often prolonged surgical procedures.

There are several types of postop-

erative pulmonary complications (Table 19–1) that may develop singly; however, as many of them are interrelated, two or more frequently occur together. Because of their common occurrence and the importance of measures in their prevention and treatment, pulmonary atelectasis and pneumonia are the main focus of discussion in this chapter. Discussion of pulmonary complications following lung transplantation is beyond the scope of this book.

Pathogenesis and Pathophysiology. Pathogenesis and pathophysiology of postoperative pulmonary complications are discussed in connection with surgery and other related interventions. The individual complicating conditions are generically described in the appropriate chapters in this book (Chapters 3, 17, 18, 21, 22, and 26). Changes in lung function are known to occur as a result of *general anesthesia,* under which practically every

**TABLE 19–1. TYPES OF
POSTOPERATIVE COMPLICATIONS**

Atelectasis
Pneumonia
Pulmonary embolism (thromboembolism or fat embolism)
Pleural effusion
Respiratory failure
Pneumothorax
Hemothorax
Empyema
Bronchopleural fistula
Hemoptysis
Diaphragm paralysis

major surgical procedure is performed. Functional residual capacity (FRC) is almost always reduced following anesthesia. The diaphragm is positioned further inside the thoracic cavity, resulting in loss of volume and *atelectasis* of the basal portions of the lungs. These changes are known to persist to a certain extent during the postoperative period. Some of the anesthetic agents may inhibit hypoxic pulmonary vasoconstriction, causing continuation of perfusion in poorly ventilated areas. The result will be ventilation–perfusion ($\dot{V}/\dot{Q}$) mismatching, increased alveolar-arterial oxygen gradient, and hypoxemia. Application of positive end expiratory pressure (PEEP) during anesthesia has been demonstrated to reduce these changes. There is some evidence to suggest that the mucociliary function is diminished for several days following anesthesia. Narcotic analgesics and sedatives are well known to depress ventilatory drive and suppress the cough reflex; therefore, airway protective mechanisms are impaired.

Pulmonary changes from anesthesia in *upper abdominal* and *thoracic surgery* tend to persist or become more significant, whereas in other types of surgery these changes improve in a few days.

Upper abdominal or thoracic surgery may cause pulmonary changes besides those resulting from general anesthesia. Postoperative pain in the incision site is considered to be an important reason for preventing adequate lung expansion and consequent atelectasis. However, the fact that pain control does not eliminate the problem suggests that other factors are also involved. In upper abdominal surgery, stimulation of the visceral or somatic afferent nerve endings is known to have inhibitory effect on diaphragmatic function. There may be a shift of respiratory muscle activity from the diaphragm to other muscles. Paradoxical abdominal movement may occur as seen in patients with a weak diaphragm. An increase in abdominal muscle activity may tend to reduce lung volumes (especially FRC) further. In the postoperative period following upper abdominal and thoracic surgery, tidal volume usually is reduced and respiratory rate is increased. The maximum inspiratory pressure is also diminished. A shift from ventilatory activity from the diaphragm to other muscles results in a redistribution of ventilation from lower lungs to upper parts, which is another reason for atelectasis of lower lung fields. Cough mechanism is often impaired from pain as well as inadequate inspiratory volumes and reduced forces necessary for an effective cough. Cardiopulmonary bypass, especially when prolonged, may result in alveolar epithelial injury and reduced surfactant production.

Pneumonia in the postoperative period is the result of several factors; most of which are also the cause of atelectasis. They include abnormal mucus transport, impairment of an effective cough, and aspiration of upper airway secretions. Preexisting respiratory tract infections, which are often occult, may be an important factor in causing postoperative pneumonia. As with atelectasis, pneumonia occurs more commonly following thoracic and upper abnominal surgery. Pneumonias following surgery are considered to be *nosocomial*.

During the postoperative period, patients are predisposed to *pulmonary thromboembolism* as a result of deep-venous thrombosis (DVT). DVT is a common occurrence following a variety of surgical procedures. Immobility during and following surgery is the most important factor. There may also be a state of hypercoagulability as a result of the release of tissue procoagulants into the bloodstream. Orthopedic surgical procedures of the lower extremities are commonly associated with DVT. *Fat embolism* may also occur in orthopedic patients, especially in association with multiple trauma involving the large bones.

Pleural effusion following surgery has several causes. Small effusions (sympathetic effusions) after abdominal surgery are usually self-limited with no significant clinical consequence. Pleural fluid may develop as a result of cardiac failure and pulmonary thromboembolism or it may be parapneumonic.

Postoperative respiratory failure is a more common complication in patients with severe chronic obstructive pulmonary disease (COPD) who are subjected to thoracic or upper abdominal surgery. Obviously, resection of any functioning lung, as done in lung cancers, would increase the likelihood of respiratory failure in such patients. Other conditions, discussed in the section on risk factors, will predispose to this serious complication. In patients without preexisting cardiopulmonary or neuromuscular disorders, respiratory failure is a rare occurrence. Overwhelming pneumonia, large pleural effusion, pneumothorax, or airway obstruction may cause respiratory failure during the postoperative period. Following emergency surgery in patients with multiple trauma, acute respiratory distress syndrome (ARDS) may develop. Such a dreadful complication may also develop as a part of systemic inflammatory response from sepsis (see Chapter 27).

Paralysis of the diaphragm, especially the left hemidiaphragm, used to be a common occurrence following open heart surgery for coronary artery bypass. As a result of cardiac cooling with iced slush, the nearby phrenic nerve (usually the left) is subjected to hypothermic injury. With the development of newer techniques of insulating the pericardium during the myocardial cooling, the incidence of phrenic nerve injury has been reduced. Phrenic nerve injury also sometimes occurs when the internal mammary artery is used in coronary artery surgery. As discussed in Chapter 24, unilateral diaphragm paralysis in otherwise healthy individuals is well tolerated. However, it may result in significant impairment of respiration in compromised patients.

Resectional lung surgery may result in several other complications, which are the consequences of bleeding from inadequate hemostasis or air leak from a bronchial stump. Such complications manifest as hemothorax, hemoptysis, pneumothorax, hemopneumothorax, bronchopleural fistula, and empyema.

Risk Factors

Understanding risk factors for postoperative pulmonary complications is crucial for surgical decision making, for prognostication, for the modification of *modi-*

fiable factors, and for application of appropriate pre- and postoperative care. Risk factors are related to both patients and operative intervention (Table 19–2). It should be emphasized that two or more of these risk factors frequently coexist in the same patient.

Patient-Related Risk Factors. Preexisting clinically significant pulmonary disease is an important risk factor for patients undergoing major surgery. Although both obstructive and restrictive lung diseases increase the respiratory difficulty following major surgery, the former, especially obstructive chronic bronchitis, is a greater risk for postoperative pulmonary complications. Frequency and severity of such complications are proportional to severity of ventilatory impairment as determined by PFTs. The most feared complication is respiratory failure as well as the difficulty in taking the patient off mechanical ventilatory support. In asthmatic patients, the risk of

---

TABLE 19–2. RISK FACTORS FOR POSTOPERATIVE PULMONARY COMPLICATIONS

Patient-related risk factors
　Preexistent pulmonary disease
　Smoking
　Age
　Obesity
　Cardiovascular disease
　Neuromuscular disease
　Immunologic defect
　Other significant organ dysfunction and metabolic disorders

Risk factors related to anesthesia, surgery, and pre- and postoperative care
　Site of surgery and incision
　Lung resection
　Duration and type of anesthesia
　Duration and type of surgery
　Emergency versus elective surgery
　Number of blood transfusions
　Inadequate preoperative preparation and postoperative care

---

complications depends on adequacy of asthma control before, during, and following surgery.

Although the postoperative pulmonary complications related to cigarette smoking are often from the associated pulmonary and/or cardiovascular diseases, smokers without clinical or laboratory evidence of obstructive airways disease and with normal cardiac function are at higher risk for developing such complications. It seems that increased tracheobronchial secretions, impaired ciliary function, and the presence of pathogenic organisms in the airways of smokers are the reasons for their predisposition for pulmonary complications during the postoperative period.

In most clinical investigations, age has been found to be a significant risk factor. There is a slow but steady decline in pulmonary function with increased age. Forced expiratory flow rates, maximum voluntary ventilation (MVV), and elastic recoil of the lungs diminish. Alveolar–arterial oxygen tension difference increases and Pao_2 decreases. Older individuals are more prone to pulmonary infection and have difficulty in clearing their tracheobronchial secretions because of weaker respiratory muscles. There are also other associated age-related conditions that make the aged population more susceptible to pulmonary complications. With technical advancement in cardiothoracic surgery, increasingly larger numbers of elderly patients are being subjected to coronary artery bypass and resectional surgery for lung cancer. As a result, this subgroup constitutes a significant portion of patients with postoperative pulmonary complications.

Obesity is another significant risk factor for developing atelectasis following upper abdominal surgery. Hypoxemia, which is a fairly common finding in morbidly obese individuals, becomes more pronounced following major surgical procedures, especially when the patients are in supine position. It is caused by worsening $\dot{V}/\dot{Q}$ mismatch. When there is also reduced ventilatory drive, hypercapnia may also develop.

With preexisting heart disease, especially heart failure, there is an increased risk of pulmonary edema postoperatively whenever there is excessive fluid administration or occurrence of cardiac ischemic events or arrhythmias during or following surgery. Coronary artery bypass graft (CABG) is done in many patients with impaired myocardial function who are proved to have pulmonary edema of cardiac origin.

As indicated in Chapter 24, a variety of neuromuscular disorders affects respiration. Therefore, patients with such conditions will have further difficulty following surgical procedures that cause additional abnormality of lung mechanics and gas transport. Weak cough and immobility predispose these patients to atelectasis and pneumonia. Ventilatory failure may readily supervene if the respiratory muscles become weaker and/or the work of breathing increases.

Other systemic medical conditions, especially immunologic and metabolic disorders, dysfunction of other organs, and psychiatric problems, are other factors that may also adversely affect postoperative course and predispose to pulmonary complications and compound their prevention and management.

Risk Factors Related to Surgery and Other Pre- and Postoperative Interventions.
Among risk factors, the site of surgery and incision is better known. *Upper abdominal surgery* and *thoracic surgery*

result in more frequent and significant postoperative pulmonary complications, mainly atelectasis and pneumonia. As mentioned earlier, following such procedures FRC, VC, and flow rates are often diminished. These changes may persist for several days after surgery. Laparoscopically performed cholecystectomy, the most commonly performed upper abdominal surgery, results in significantly fewer pulmonary complications than open cholecystectomy. Resectional lung surgery increases respiratory complications beyond those related to thoracotomy. Depending on the preexisting lung disease and extent of lung resection, it may result in respiratory failure and difficulty in discontinuation of postoperative mechanical ventilation.

The further away the surgical procedure from the diaphragm, the fewer are the pulmonary complications. However, it should be stressed that the incidence of DVT and, therefore, pulmonary embolism are much more common in patients undergoing orthopedic surgery of the lower extremities, especially the hips and knees.

The duration of anesthesia, which usually depends on the duration of surgery, also has significant effect on the incidence of postoperative pulmonary complications. Emergency surgery is also known to increase such complications. There is a direct correlation between the amount of intraoperative blood transfused and the likelihood of postoperative complications, especially because of unstable circulatory and volume status and the complexity of surgical procedures.

Proper preoperative preparation and postoperative care will have significant effect on the incidence and severity of various complications as is discussed later in this chapter.

Clinical Manifestations and Diagnosis. Symptoms and signs of fully developed pulmonary complications during the postoperative period, such as pneumonia, atelectasis, pulmonary embolism, pleural effusion, and respiratory failure, are discussed in Chapters 3, 18, 21, 22, and 26. It should be noted, however, that most of these complications, especially in the early stage of their development, are quite subtle and often overshadowed by findings related to the surgery itself. A high index of suspicion, mostly in patients who have one or more risk factors for pulmonary complications, is crucial for detecting the complications earlier. Unexplained fever, change in respiration (tachypnea, dyspnea), alteration of breath sounds, disproportionate hypoxemia, and changes in peripheral white blood cell count are some of the clues that should be heeded and pursued by close follow-up and additional studies, such as chest radiography and sputum examination. X-ray films should be carefully reviewed for the presence of infiltrates, pleural effusion, pneumothorax, and signs of lung volume loss. The last may manifest by elevated diaphragm, shift of the heart and mediastinum, and change of position of lung fissures. Increased parenchymal density may be from atelectasis, pneumonia, or pulmonary infarction. Patients suspected to have thromboembolic disease should be studied for DVT (by compression venous ultrasound or impedence phlethysmography) and pulmonary embolism (by radionuclide lung scan).

Preoperative Evaluation

Except in emergency situations, patients considered for surgery, most often major surgery, are clinically evaluated prior to the intended operation. History and physical examination are most important for this purpose. A pertinent history, important for identification of risk factors for postoperative pulmonary complications, should include information on respiratory symptoms, smoking, treatment for cardiac or respiratory disease, chest pain, occupational or environmental exposure to noxious agents, level of activity, exercise tolerance, neuromuscular disorder, prior chest infection, and previous thromboembolic disease.

Physical examination should comprise the determination of body size (obesity), chest deformity, respiratory rate and pattern, use of accessory respiratory muscles, quality of breath sounds, duration of expiratory phase, presence of adventitious sounds such as rhonchi or crackles, force of cough, presence of digital clubbing, and peripheral edema. An observation of the patient's ability to walk and climb stairs with the examiner would give important information about the patient's cardiopulmonary reserve if it is in question. These simple and inexpensive ways of evaluating patients are usually sufficient for assessment of risk factors and identification of modifiable ones. They would also help in determining the necessity for additional studies.

Preoperative radiographic study of the chest is commonly done, especially when there is question of underlying cardiopulmonary disorder. Determination of arterial blood gases or pulse oximetry is usually part of preoperative evaluation of patients who are known to have chronic lung disease. In patients who are not considered for lung resection, pulmonary function studies are not usually necessary unless indicated by history or physical examination *and* when upper abdominal or thoracic surgery is planned. In such situations, a simple spirometry along with determination of MVV suffices. Although PFT cannot reliably predict postoperative pulmonary complications, it is useful for defining a subset of surgical patients who are at higher risk.

Except for thoracic surgery for lung resection and CABG surgery, an absolute contraindication for an elective surgery based on pulmonary function studies has not been identified. This is because with proper preoperative and postoperative care, including additional ventilatory support, most patients with markedly abnormal PFTs do reasonably well postoperatively. The decision for surgical intervention in these high-risk patients should, however, be made with careful consideration of the risk:benefit ratio.

Because of high postoperative mortality with CABG in patients with severe obstructive ventilatory impairment (defined as FEV_1 of less than 50% of predicted), such an operation is usually contraindicated. When resectional lung surgery is being contemplated, most commonly for lung cancer, pulmonary function studies are performed routinely not only for determination of risk of postoperative complications from thoracotomy, but also for estimation of the function of remaining lung tissue. Radiographic studies, including chest computed tomography (CT) and bronchoscopic findings, usually would provide information about the amount of lung tissue that will be necessary to remove, such as segmental resection, lobectomy, or pneumonectomy. However, a definitive decision about the extent of resection can sometimes be made only in the operating room after opening the chest. In these situations, it should be determined preoperatively whether the patient would be able to tolerate a pneumonectomy. In any patient considered for removal of a part of or a whole lung, it should be determined whether the candidate will be able to tol-

erate it without dying from respiratory failure or without becoming totally disabled with an unacceptable poor quality of life following surgery. Clinical, radiographic, and pulmonary function studies may be sufficient to eliminate certain patients from consideration for resectional surgery or to accept certain others without further investigation. Among routine PFTs used to screen patients, an MVV of less than 50% of predicted is commonly considered to be associated with a high postresectional mortality and disability. It should, however, be emphasized that the presence of other risk factors will influence the outcome despite acceptable preoperative PFT results.

Split-lung function studies to predict the effect of lung resection on postoperative pulmonary performance status usually is done by radionuclide lung scan (perfusion with or without ventilation scan). With this method, along with preoperative measurement of FEV_1 and DL_{CO}, the function of the remaining lung units can be more accurately predicted. From a pulmonary function point of view, a predicted postresectional FEV_1 should be at least 800 mL for most patients to be acceptable for lung resection. Such a requirement, however, may be too stringent for a small woman, and it may be too generous for a large man. Therefore, the decision for such an operation should be individualized and other factors besides the absolute PFT values should be carefully weighed.

Preoperative Prevention Measures

Although preoperative and postoperative preventive measures are discussed separately, they are interrelated and often include continuation of the same interventions. Moreover, preoperative patient instruction and practice of such measures would be more effectively implemented during the postoperative period. The risk factors outlined earlier in this chapter should be a guide in directing the preoperative interventions. *Modifiable factors* should be more vigorously pursued. They include smoking, obesity, reversible airway obstruction, cardiac decompensation, preexisting respiratory tract infection, and other treatable disorders. The importance of the complete cessation of smoking should be emphasized. Very obese patients should undergo a weight reduction program, especially before thoracic or upper abdominal surgery. Elective surgery should be postponed as long as possible to allow adequate weight loss. Patients with reversible airway obstruction, as demonstrated by PFTs, should undergo intensive bronchodilator therapy. Although antibiotic prophylaxis is routinely advised, patients with chronic bronchitis and bacteriologic evidence of infection may benefit from a short course of antibacterial treatment prior to planned surgery. Other recognized treatable conditions that are known to increase postoperative pulmonary complications, such as heart failure; fluid, electrolyte, and acid–base disorders; and metabolic abnormalities, should be appropriately treated.

Preoperative patient education and training centers around measures countering the causes of commonly occurring postoperative complications, namely atelectasis and pneumonia. These measures intend to preserve lung volumes and maintain clear airways. Deep-breathing exercises and effective cough are most effective for these purposes. The importance of these simple, but often overlooked, measures should be stressed to patients preoperatively, when they are attentive and not affected by sedatives or narcotics. Demonstration of deep-breathing methods by various techniques, such as incentive spirometry prior to surgery, makes their use easier and more effective postoperatively.

Prophylaxis against venous thromboembolism is often begun prior to surgery, especially in high-risk patients and when surgical interventions are known to be associated with high incidence of venous thrombosis and pulmonary embolism. The use of low dose heparin and/or mechanical means such as intermittent pneumatic compression devices are measures that are often begun preoperatively.

Postoperative Preventive and Therapeutic Measures

Depending on the respiratory status and nature of surgery, the patient may need ventilatory support beyond the usual anesthesia-related mechanical ventilation. This aspect of postoperative care is not much different from the care of nonsurgical ventilator patients. Therefore, the general principles of mechanical ventilation discussed in Chapter 28 are applicable to these patients. Once adequacy of spontaneous unsupported respiration and airway maintenance in conscious patients are assured, they are extubated and closely monitored. The importance of good nursing care in the prevention of pulmonary complications during this period cannot be overemphasized. Positioning the patient in a sitting or at least semirecumbent position is preferable for improving ventilation and oxygenation. The respiratory management objective at this time should be preventing or reducing atelectasis and, therefore, pneumonia. This objective is usually achieved by measures that increase lung volumes and clear the airways.

There have been various methods for the purpose of preventing and treating postoperative atelectasis (Table 19–3). Expiratory maneuvers against resistance such as the use of blow bottle or expiratory positive airway pressure (EPAP) are less effective than inspiratory maneuvers for lung expansion. Increasing minute ventilation by rebreathing methods (dead-space rebreathing tubes) is rarely used currently. Deep-breathing maneuvers, either voluntary or with the help of mechanical devices, are effective means for prevention as well as treatment of postoperative atelectasis. Judicious use of adequate pain control is necessary for

TABLE 19–3. METHODS FOR PREVENTING AND TREATING POSTOPERATIVE ATELECTASIS

Resistance breathing
  Blow bottle
  Blow glove
  EPAP

Increasing minute ventilation
  Dead-space rebreathing tube

Deep-breathing maneuvers
  Voluntary deep breathing
  Incentive spirometry (volume- or flow-oriented)
  Sustained maximum inspiration (breath stacking)
  IPPB

Increasing FRC
  CPAP

Maneuvers for clearing airway
  Cough
  Chest percussion (with or without postural drainage)
  Suctioning
  Bronchoscopy

Inhalation treatment
  Bronchodilators
  Humidity

Miscellaneous
  Body repositioning
  Kinetic bed
  Ambulation

proper use of, and patient compliance with, these techniques and for other interventions requiring the patient's active participation. In highly motivated and cooperative patients, intermittent deep breathing without any gadget will be adequate. However, incentive devices, by providing immediate feedback, would encourage patients further and allows objective assessment of their progress. There are numerous such devices on the market that are manufactured to demonstrate and encourage either inspiratory flow or inspiratory volume. Although the volume-oriented devices seem to be more appropriate for maximizing lung expansion, the flow-oriented spirometers can be equally effective if combined with adequate inspiratory time and may have the added advantage of conditioning inspiratory muscles. Several deep-breathing maneuvers are usually performed successively every 1 to 2 waking hours with or without supervision. Sustained maximum inspiratory maneuvers are a series of stacked inhalations from FRC to total lung capacity (TLC), at which time the breath is held for several seconds. Breath-stacking is performed with the use of a modified incentive spirometer equipped with a one-way valve. It appears that this method is more useful than standard incentive spirometry for the treatment of established atelectasis.

After being used extensively in postoperative patients, intermittent positive pressure breathing (IPPB) has fallen in disfavor because of lack of evidence for its advantage over simpler maneuvers in patients without neuromuscular disorders. As in such conditions, active lung inflation cannot be achieved even with patients' full cooperation. IPPB would be more effective.

Continuous positive airway pressure

(CPAP), applied either by a facial mask or nasal mask, increases FRC, and this is useful for prevention as well as improving atelectasis and for increasing O_2 transport. In patients with severe emphysema, it should be used, if ever, with extreme caution. CPAP may be used intermittently (for preventive purpose) or continuously (for treatment of established atelectasis). CPAP has the advantage of being used with only minimal patient cooperation if a tight facial or nasal mask is tolerated. This mode of respiratory therapy is being used increasingly in the United States. A tight-fitting face mask should not be used in patients who are prone to vomit or who have significant airway secretions. Because of the problem with adequate mask seal, the presence of a nasogastric tube is a relative contraindication for the use of CPAP in nonintubated patients.

For clearing the airways from excessive secretions, no maneuver is more effective than properly performed cough. When spontaneous cough is inadequate, it should be directed by a member of the health care team. Proper positioning with protection and splinting of incision site with application of gentle pressure over a pillow or folded towel is important for effective cough. Deep breathing, either spontaneous or following incentive spirometry, may induce cough. Coughing at lower lung volumes may help in moving secretions from distal to central airways. Chest percussion (cupping and clapping) or vibration with or without postural drainage is generally ineffective in postoperative patients for the purpose of clearing the airways. Tracheal suctioning and bronchoscopy may be necessary in some situations in which simpler maneuvers are ineffective for treatment of severe atelectasis.

Bronchodilator aerosol therapy, although frequently prescribed, has limited usefulness for the prevention or treatment of postoperative pulmonary complications, except in asthmatics and patients with COPD who have evidence of a reversible component to their airway obstruction.

Other interventions that are an important part of proper postoperative patient care also help in preventing pulmonary complications during the postoperative period. They include proper body repositioning at regular intervals, use of kinetic beds, and early patient mobilization and ambulation. These interventions are not only useful for prevention and treatment of atelectasis, they are also important as part of DVT prevention. As discussed earlier, prophylactic anticoagulation and use of mechanical devices such as intermittent pneumatic compression should be continued postoperatively in high-risk patients. If primary prophylaxis was not instituted prior to surgery, patients should be tested for venous thrombosis. Mechanical antithrombotic devices should be used only after exclusion of DVT in such patients.

High-risk patients and others with clinical indication or suspicion of any other postoperative pulmonary complications depicted in Table 19–1 should be properly investigated and treated as necessary.

BIBLIOGRAPHY

American Association for Respiratory Care (AARC). Clinical practice guidelines: directed cough. *Respir Care*. 1993; 38:495–499.

Baker WL, Lamb VJ, Marini JJ. Breath-stacking increases depth and duration of chest expansion by incentive spirometry. *Am Rev Respir Dis*. 1990; 141:343–346.

Brooks-Brunn JA. Postoperative atelectasis and pneumonia. *Heart Lung.* 1995; 24: 94–115.

Celli BR. Perioperative respiratory care of the patient undergoing upper abdominal surgery. *Clin Chest Med.* 1993; 14:253–261.

Engoren M. Lack of association between atelectasis and fever. *Chest.* 1995; 107:81–84.

Ephgrave KS, Kleinman-Wexler R, Pfaller M, et al. Postoperative pneumonia: a prospective study of risk factors and morbidity. *Surgery.* 1993; 114:815–821.

Ford GT, Rosenal TW, Clergue F, Whitelaw WA. Respiratory physiology in upper abdominal surgery. *Clin Chest Med.* 1993; 14:223–252.

Gunnarsson L, Lindberg P, Tokics L, et al. Lung function after open versus laparoscopic cholecystectomy. *Acta Anaesthesiol Scand.* 1995; 39:302–306.

Hall JC, Tarala RA, Hall JL, Mander J. A multivariate analysis of the risk of pulmonary complications after laparotomy. *Chest.* 1991; 99:923–927.

Hall JC, Tarala R, Harris J, et al. Incentive spirometry versus routine chest physiotherapy for prevention of pulmonary complications after abdominal surgery. *Lancet.* 1991; 337:953–956.

Johnson D, Kelm C, Thomson D, et al. The effect of physical therapy on respiratory complications following cardiac valve surgery. *Chest.* 1996; 109:838–844.

Johnson D, Kelm C, To T, et al. Postoperative physical therapy after coronary artery bypass surgery. *Am J Respir Crit Care Med.* 1995; 152:953–958.

Kearon C, Hirsh J. Starting prophylaxis for venous thromboembolism postoperatively. *Arch Intern Med.* 1995; 155:366–372.

Kroenke K, Lawrence VA, Theroux JF, Tuley MR. Operative risk in patients with severe obstructive pulmonary disease. *Arch Intern Med.* 1992; 152:967–971.

Marshall MC, Olsen GN. The physiologic evaluation of the lung resection candidate. *Clin Chest Med.* 1993; 14:305–320.

Olsen GN, Bolton JWR, Weiman DS, et al. Stair climbing as an exercise test to predict the postoperative complications of lung resection. *Chest.* 1991; 99:587–590.

Peruzzi WT, Smith B. Bronchial hygiene therapy. *Crit Care Clin.* 1995; 11:79–96.

Stiller K, Montarello J, Wallace M, et al. Efficacy of breathing and coughing exercises in the prevention of pulmonary complications after coronary bypass surgery. *Chest.* 1994; 105:741–747.

Sykes LA, Bowe EA. Cardiorespiratory effects of anesthesia. *Clin Chest Med.* 1993; 14: 211–226.

Thomas J, McIntosh J. Are incentive spirometry, intermittent positive pressure breathing, and deep breathing exercises effective in the prevention of postoperative pulmonary complications after upper abdominal surgery? A systemic overview and meta-analysis. *Phys Ther.* 1994; 74:3–16.

Tulla H, Takala J, Alhava E, et al. Respiratory changes after open-heart surgery. *Intensive Care Med.* 1991; 17:365–369.

Zibrak JD, O'Donnell CR. Indications for preoperative pulmonary function testing. *Clin Chest Med.* 1993; 14:227–236.

VII

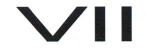

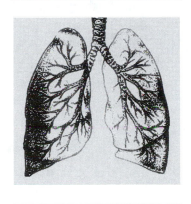

NEOPLASTIC DISEASES
OF THE LUNG

20.

Lung Cancer

Malignant tumors of the lung may be primary, originating in the lung, or metastatic, having their site of origin in other areas of the body. Lung cancer refers to malignant neoplasms that start in the lung tissue. Although any tissue of the lung may undergo malignant change, by far the most common malignant neoplasm in the lung originates from the bronchial mucosa and is called bronchogenic carcinoma. *Lung cancer* and *bronchogenic carcinoma* are used interchangeably in this chapter.

Incidence. At present, primary lung cancer is the most common malignancy in the United States and is one of the leading causes of death. A steady rise in its incidence among males since the early 1940s is recently becoming more evident among females. The alarming yearly increase in its incidence shows no signs of slowing or leveling off, and it is feared that this increase will continue. Presently, one-fourth of Americans dying from cancer die from bronchogenic carcinoma. Although its incidence is lower among females, it is rising much faster than in

males. Since 1986, lung cancer has become the leading cause of death from cancer in women, as has been the case for men for a long time. In 1995, there were 158,700 deaths from lung cancer in the United States.

Etiology and Risk Factors. The exact cause and pathogenesis of cancer in general remains unknown. Certain factors, however, have been incriminated in its causation. In lung cancer, there is an indubitable relationship of prolonged inhalation of air pollutants to its occurrence. Among the pollutants, cigarette smoke has been the most important. Smoking is the cause of lung cancer in 85% of cases. As discussed in Chapter 16, a strong correlation exists between intensity and duration of cigarette smoking and development of lung cancer. Long-time heavy smokers are particularly at high risk. A person who smokes two packs per day for 20 years has a risk almost 70 times higher for developing lung cancer than nonsmokers. Certain histologic types of cancer (ie, small-cell and squamous-cell carcinomas) are almost exclusively observed among smokers. The risk of developing lung cancer diminishes with cessation of smoking. With 15 or more years of abstention after less than 20 years of smoking, the risk of lung cancer approaches that of people who have never smoked.

There seem to be other factors that, when combined with smoking, enhance the carcinogenic effect of the latter. Exposure to asbestos dust and radioactive substances is known to have such an effect. The combined effects of cigarette smoking and asbestos exposure are more multiplicative than additive. This is probably also true in regard to heavy smoking and exposure to naturally occurring radon gas found in certain homes. Moreover, the fact that the incidence of lung cancer is higher in urban populations than in rural dwellers with the same degree of smoking exposure suggests that other pollutants in the atmosphere may play a role in lung cancer. Industrial exposure to certain inorganic and synthetic substances has been implicated in the etiology of lung cancer in some instances (Table 20–1). However, cigarette smoking remains the major offender. The presence of scars and other chronic lung lesions appears to predispose to lung cancer. Cigarette smokers with chronic obstructive pulmonary disease (COPD) have a higher incidence of lung cancer than those without COPD. The Environmental Protection Agency (EPA) has classified environmental tobacco smoke (passive smoking) as a carcinogen.

In addition to environmental causes, there are also genetic and familial factors that predispose to bronchogenic carcinoma. Lung cancer is seen predominantly in persons between the ages of 45 and 75 years, with a peak incidence at age 70. It is

TABLE 20–1. PROVED CAUSES OF LUNG CANCER FROM OCCUPATIONAL EXPOSURE

Asbestos
Ionizing radiation
Chromium
Nickel
Bischloromethyl ether (chemical plants)
Arsenic
Polycyclic aromatic hydrocarbons (coke-oven emission)

a rare occurrence in persons less than the age of 35.

Pathology. Pathologic changes are quite variable and depend on the histologic type, location, duration of disease, tumor size, metastasis, and secondary effects on the surrounding tissues and organs. Except for a small percentage of cases, lung cancer is bronchogenic (ie, it arises from bronchial mucosa). About one-half of the cases are centrally located; that is, their site of origin is in the large bronchi. The other half are peripheral, arising from smaller airways. However, this distinction is often difficult in advanced stages. The upper lobes, particularly the anterior segments, are more commonly involved than the lower lobes, and the right side more commonly than the left.

Although there are several different histologic forms of primary lung cancer, four major types of bronchogenic carcinoma have been recognized that, in addition to their distinctive pathologic characteristics, show different epidemiologic, clinical, radiographic, and prognostic features. They account for 95% of primary lung cancers.

- The *squamous-cell* or epithelial type comprises about one-third of lung cancers and is the most common cell type in men. It is pathologically characterized by keratin formation, bridging between the cells, and the development of large, well-outlined islands of cancer cells. Most of these carcinomas are centrally located, arising from the major bronchi. Because of their exposure to the bronchial lumen, exfoliated tumor cells are often detected in bronchial secretions. Their metastasis is mainly local, involving surrounding structures and regional lymph nodes.

- *Adenocarcinoma* has the same incidence as the squamous-cell type, but is the most common lung cancer in women. It is frequently a peripheral lesion, has a glandular architecture, and may produce mucin. Distant metastasis is common.
- The *large cell undifferentiated* carcinoma is made of large cancer cells that have no resemblance to squamous-cell type or adenocarcinoma. It usually presents as a large peripheral tumor. About 10% to 15% of lung cancers are of this type.
- The three previously described cell types are collectively referred to as non–small-cell lung cancer (NSCLC) to differentiate them from the *small-cell lung cancer* (SCLC), which has distinctive biologic, histologic, and clinical features. The tumors in this group are rapidly growing carcinomas that metastasize to thoracic and extrathoracic sites early and have a very poor prognosis. Most of them originate from central airways, grow submucosally, and involve the mediastinal nodes. Between 15% and 25% of bronchogenic carcinomas are small cell in type. Many of these tumors, by secreting different hormones, have various endocrine functions. Oat-cell carcinoma is the most common

and the best-known category of this highly malignant disease.

Secondary pathologic changes resulting from lung cancer are due to obstruction or compression of structures such as bronchi, blood vessels, and nerves producing various complications. The most common complications—atelectasis, pneumonia, and lung abscess—are due to bronchial obstruction. Metastasis is very common with lung cancer; almost every case ending in autopsy shows metastasis, and more than one-half of the cases at the time of diagnosis have evidence of metastasis. Locally, it usually spreads to the pleura, chest wall, and mediastinal structures. The lymph nodes, liver, bone, brain, and adrenal glands are among common sites for distant metastasis.

Clinical Manifestations. Practically every patient with lung cancer goes through an asymptomatic phase, which comprises the major part of its course. Many patients may even remain symptom-free despite radiographic or bronchoscopic evidence of tumor. Symptoms, when present, are nonspecific and varied depending on the location of the cancer, its size, rapidity of its growth, cell type, and presence of underlying bronchopulmonary disease (Table 20–2). The most common symptom is cough, which unfortunately does not concern most patients because of the frequent concomitance of chronic bronchitis. In these situations, usually a change in the characteristics of cough and expectoration may warn the patients. Bloody sputum, which occurs in about one-half of the patients during their illness, may be the initial symptom prompting the patient to seek medical advice. Severe hemoptysis is much less common. Chest pain with variable inten-

TABLE 20–2. PRESENTING SYMPTOMS OF
LUNG CANCER

Thoracic symptoms
Cough
Dyspnea
Hemoptysis
Chest pain
Wheezing
Dysphagia
Systemic and extrathoracic symptoms
Weight loss
Anorexia
Weakness, fatigue
Bone and joint pain
Swelling of face and arms
Hoarseness
Various neurologic symptoms

sity and other characteristics is fairly common in lung cancer. It may be mild and felt as heaviness or ache, or it may be very severe and unremitting. The presence of pain does not necessarily indicate pleural or chest-wall involvement, although significant steady pain is highly suggestive of this complication. Dyspnea may be due to a tumor causing obstruction of major airways or a large pleural effusion, but often it is due to the presence of significant underlying bronchopulmonary disease. Hoarseness of recent onset usually indicates involvement of the laryngeal nerve, especially the left. Compression of the superior vena cava manifests by vascular congestion and edema of the face, neck, and upper extremities (superior vena cava syndrome).

It is not unusual for bronchogenic carcinoma to manifest as a pulmonary infection such as pneumonia or lung abscess. Systemic symptoms of weight loss, weakness, fatigue, and anorexia, which are common to most advanced malignant diseases, are frequently observed in patients with lung cancer. Other symptoms may be due to distant metastasis to different organs, such as bone, brain, and liver.

The *physical examination* may be entirely normal in the early stage of lung cancer. In advanced cases, the physical findings frequently are due to bronchial obstruction and other complications or metastasis. Localized wheezing, alteration of breath sounds, or other signs of atelectasis, pneumonia, or pleural effusion may be present. Signs of metastasis to extrathoracic structures may be detected on first presentation or may develop later in the course of the disease. In addition to evidence of weight loss and muscle wasting, there are numerous other manifestations of lung cancer that are not related directly to its local or metastatic effects and are known as *paraneoplastic syndromes.* Various endocrine syndromes are due to the secretion by the tumor of certain hormones or hormone-like substances. However, the mechanism in many others such as hematologic, musculoskeletal, neurologic, and cutaneous syndromes are not clearly known. Digital clubbing, a fairly common finding in patients with bronchogenic carcinoma, is another example of paraneoplastic syndromes.

Radiographic Findings. The diagnosis of lung cancer in the majority of patients is strongly suspected by routine chest radiography. Unfortunately, by the time a lung cancer becomes radiographically evident it is already in the invasive stage and is often unresectable. Radiography, therefore, is not an ideal method for diagnosing lung cancer in its early and curable stage. X-ray screening at regular intervals, as carried out in certain centers, has not been demonstrated to add significantly to the overall survival rate from lung cancer. It has been estimated that by the time a lung cancer becomes radiographically detectable it has completed two-thirds to three-quarters of its natural course.

Radiographic changes are quite variable and nonspecific; however, certain manifestations are characteristic. X-ray findings are due to the shadow cast by the tumor itself and secondary pulmonary changes due to bronchial obstruction, infection, or other complications (Fig. 20–1). A peripheral lung lesion may manifest as a small, more or less circumscribed density due to the tumor itself, usually referred to as a *solitary pulmonary nodule* or *coin lesion*. The most common secondary changes are due to bronchial obstruction with development of atelectasis, obstructive pneumonia, and, rarely, hyperinflation. Hilar or mediastinal mass due to direct invasion by tumor or metastasis to the lymph nodes may be observed. Pleural effusion, which may be massive, is sometimes the only radiographic manifestation of lung cancer. The chest x-ray may show evidence of other complications, such as a paralyzed diaphragm or rib lesions.

Different histologic types of lung cancer often have characteristic radiographic features. Most adenocarcinomas manifest as peripheral lesions. Oat-cell carcinoma may present as a large hilar or mediastinal mass (Fig. 20–2). Squamous-cell carcinoma frequently causes bronchial obstruction. Cavitation is common in a peripheral mass due to squamous-cell cancer. The most common radiographic manifestation of large-cell undifferentiated carcinoma is a large peripheral mass.

Special radiologic techniques may be used for further investigation of a suspicious lung lesion. These include fluoroscopy, tomography, bronchography, and pulmonary angiography. Thoracic computed tomography (CT) has proved to be very useful for better delineation of the original lesion and for detection of nodal metastasis. CT scanning of the chest, abdomen, and head is an important part of the staging for lung cancer.

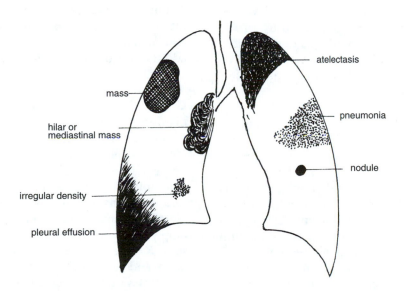

Figure 20–1. Diagrammatic demonstration of various radiographic manifestations of lung cancer.

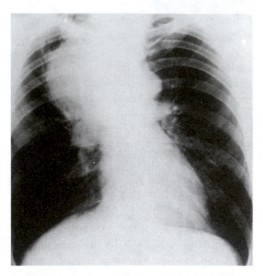

Figure 20–2. Bronchogenic carcinoma. Rapidly growing oat-cell carcinoma involving the right upper lobe and mediastinum.

Diagnosis

Patients who have a suspicious radiographic lesion or present with unexplained symptoms or signs, such as hemoptysis, unremitting cough, or localized wheezing, are subjected to diagnostic procedures that will help in identification, localization, histologic examination, evaluation of extent of the lesion, and detection of metastasis.

Sputum Cytology. One important diagnostic study is the cytologic examination of the sputum. The value of sputum examination in various bronchopulmonary diseases and methods of its proper collection are discussed elsewhere (Chapter 2). Early morning deep-cough technique is most satisfactory if sputum can be produced spontaneously. Otherwise, methods such as heated aerosol therapy or, preferably, ultrasonic nebulization may be used for sputum induc-

tion. Cytologic examination in expert hands has been successful for diagnosis in up to 90% of the cases of bronchogenic carcinoma of squamous-cell type. It is much less useful for detection of small-cell carcinoma because of its frequent submucosal location. Cytologic examination of the pleural fluid, if present, may be helpful for the diagnosis of lung cancer, as well as for confirmation of pleural metastasis.

Bronchoscopy. This procedure is now routinely done on almost every patient suspected to have bronchogenic cancer. The advent of the fiberoptic bronchoscope has significantly increased the usefulness of bronchoscopy in detecting and locating lesions, even when they are situated in the airways as small as subsegmental bronchi. In addition, biopsy, bronchial secretion, and washing can be obtained for histologic and cytologic studies. Transbronchial biopsy in more peripheral lesions and brushing have become much easier with the fiberscope. The transbronchoscopic needle for aspiration of peripheral pulmonary nodules and mediastinal lymph nodes is a useful addition for diagnosing and staging lung cancer.

Other Diagnostic Procedures. Mediastinoscopy has been frequently used for the evaluation of patients with lung cancer for resectability and sometimes for diagnostic purposes. Other biopsy methods include biopsy of peripheral lymph nodes, various forms of percutaneous needle biopsy or aspiration of the lung lesion, and biopsy of the pleura and other metastatic sites. Radioisotope scanning of the liver, brain, and bones is very useful in detecting metastases to these sites. All of these studies, as well as radiologic examination of the chest, are useful not only for diagnosing but also for staging lung cancer. By staging, an accurate assessment of the primary tumor regarding its exact location, size, invasion of neighboring structures as well as involvement of regional lymph nodes, and other metastases is made. Staging is very useful in deciding the most appropriate therapy and in determining the prognosis.

Management. Surgical resection is the most preferred therapeutic approach in the management of patients with NSCLC. Unfortunately, the majority of patients at the time of diagnosis of lung carcinoma are not operable because of advanced disease with evidence of metastasis, location of lesion, or poor general or respiratory state. Of 100 cases of lung cancer, about 25 are usually considered to be operable at the time of diagnosis. Of these 25, some may turn out to be unresectable at the time of thoracotomy. About 25% of resectable cases live 5 years or longer after surgery. Despite significant improvement in diagnostic methods and surgical techniques, the 5-year survival rate of lung cancer patients remains around 10%.

Radiotherapy, alone or combined with surgery, has not significantly changed the survival rate in NSCLC; however, it is a valuable adjunct for palliation such as relieving bronchial obstruction, compression of intrathoracic structures, or pain due to chest-wall metastasis. Various modalities of chemotherapeutic trials for NSCLC are still in progress. Although in rare cases SCLCs are cured by surgery, chemotherapy with or without radiotherapy is the treatment of choice. These tumors are often responsive to appropriate chemotherapeutic agents, which, in many cases, result in an appreciable increase in survival time.

The general care of patients with lung cancer should include pain control, treatment of depression, proper nutrition, and management of other complicating or associated conditions. Lung cancer remains an important health problem and continues to kill more and more people each year. Despite significant progress in diagnostic techniques and therapeutic modalities in lung cancer, the survival rate has not changed much. Prevention by avoidance of known causative factors, particularly cigarette smoking, seems to be the best-known approach to this dreadful health problem at this time.

BIBLIOGRAPHY

Colice GL. Chest CT for known or suspected lung cancer. *Chest.* 1994; 106:1538–1550.

Eddy DM. Screening for lung cancer. *Ann Intern Med.* 1989; 111:232–237.

Gadzar AF, Linnoila RI. The pathology of lung cancer: changing concepts and newer diagnostic techniques. *Semin Oncol.* 1988; 15:215–225.

Goodman GE, Livingston RB. Small cell lung cancer. *Dis Mon.* 1989; 35:779–825.

Harvey JC, Beattie EJ. Lung cancer. *Clin Symp.* 1993; 45(3):1–32.

Haskell CM, Holmes EC. Non–small-cell lung cancer. *Dis Mon.* 1988; 34:61–108.

Hyde L, Hyde CI. Clinical manifestations of lung cancer. *Chest.* 1974; 65:299–306.

Johnson MR. Selecting patients with lung cancer for surgical therapy. *Semin Oncol.* 1988; 15:246–254.

Lillington GA. Management of solitary pulmonary nodules. *Dis Mon.* 1991; 37:271–318.

Little AG, Stitik FP. Clinical staging of patients with non–small-cell lung cancer. *Chest.* 1990; 97:1431–1438.

Martini N. Operable lung cancer. *CA Cancer J Clin.* 1993; 43:201–214.

Parker SL, Tong T, Bolden S, Wingo PA. Cancer statistics, 1996. *CA Cancer J Clin.* 1996; 46:5–27.

Petty TL. Lung cancer and chronic obstructive pulmonary disease. *Med Clin North Am.* 1996; 80(3):645–655.

Sider L. Radiographic manifestations of primary bronchogenic carcinoma. *Radiol Clin North Am.* 1990; 28:583–597.

Silvestri GA, Littenberg B, Colice GL. The clinical evaluation for detecting metastatic lung cancer: a meta-analysis. *Am J Respir Crit Care Med.* 1995; 152:225–230.

Tackman MS. Advances in the early detection of lung cancer. *Semin Respir Crit Care Med.* 1996; 17:335–341.

U.S. Department of Health and Human Services, Office of Smoking and Health. *The Health Consequences of Smoking: Cancer: a report of the Surgeon General.* 1982.

Webb WR, Golden JA. Imaging strategies in the staging of lung cancer. *Clin Chest Med.* 1991; 12:133–150.

Wolpaw DR. Early detection in lung cancer. *Med Clin North Am.* 1996; 80(1):63–82.

VIII

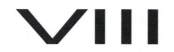

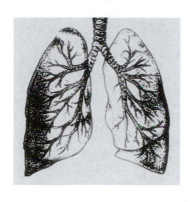

LUNGS IN
CIRCULATORY DISORDERS

21.

Disorders of Pulmonary Circulation

The major components of pulmonary circulation are

1. the right heart chambers, which act as reservoirs and pump mixed venous blood to
2. a system of pulmonary arteries and arterioles that distributes the blood to
3. the capillary bed, which is the gas-exchanging site, and
4. a system of venules and veins that collects the arterialized blood and returns it to the left side of the heart for distribution to the body (Fig. 21–1).

The functional part of pulmonary circulation where gas exchange with alveoli takes place is the capillary bed, which has a surface area of about 70 m^2, or 40 times the body surface area.

The pulmonary vascular bed is a low-resistance system; therefore, the pressure required to circulate blood through it is low. These pulmonary vessels are also very distensible and can adapt to increased blood flow, as occurs with exercise, without a corresponding increase in pressure. The vessels are under control of the autonomic nervous system and are influenced by factors such as vasoactive substances, changes of alveolar oxygen tension, and acidosis. Regional changes in pulmonary blood flow occur as a result of gravity and variation in ventilation. The lowermost parts of the lungs (ie, the bases in upright position) have the highest perfusion per unit lung volume. Under both physiologic and pathologic conditions, poorly ventilated or nonventilated lung regions have reduced blood flow. Conversely, reduction in regional perfusion, such as with occlusion of a branch of the pulmonary artery with an embolus, results in diminished ventilation of that area.

In addition to pulmonary circulation, the lungs receive arterial blood through the bronchial arteries, which are branches of the thoracic aorta. They supply arterial blood to the walls of the tracheobronchial

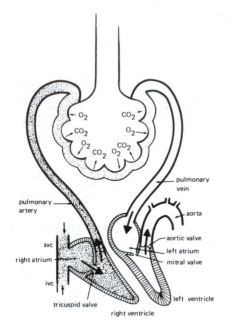

Figure 21–1. Schematic drawing of pulmonary circulation. IVC, inferior vena cava; SVC, superior vena cava.

tree down to and including the terminal bronchioles. The venous return partly enters the pulmonary veins, causing a small amount of shunting.

Disorders of pulmonary circulation may be the result of various abnormalities in the lungs, its blood vessels, or the heart. Vascular changes are an integral part of pulmonary pathology from various causes. These changes may be the result of direct injury by the disease process or indirect effect through the abnormality of blood gases, particularly hypoxemia. Pulmonary blood vessels may be occluded by a local thrombus or, more commonly, by an embolus. They may be obstructed by primary vascular disorders. The close anatomic and physiologic relationship between the heart and the lung is the cause of their mutual effect in pathologic conditions. The function of the right heart chambers is often affected by

lung disorders in which pulmonary vessels are involved. In addition, hypoxemia and disturbance in acid-base balance, which are common in severe lung disease, will have an adverse effect on the function of the myocardium. Conversely, a malfunctioning left side of the heart results in circulatory disturbances in the lung, which may progress to overt heart failure and pulmonary edema.

In this chapter the major disorders of pulmonary circulation, that is, the effect of heart failure on the lung, pulmonary embolism, pulmonary hypertension, and cor pulmonale, are discussed.

■ PULMONARY EDEMA

Pulmonary edema is defined as abnormal accumulation of fluid in the lung tissue and/or alveolar spaces. It is most commonly the result of increased pulmonary microvascular pressure from an abnormal cardiac function (cardiac pulmonary edema). It also may be secondary to causes other than heart disease (noncardiac pulmonary edema). In this chapter, pulmonary edema from heart failure is the main focus of discussion.

Etiology and Pathogenesis. Despite the fact that blood in the pulmonary capillary is separated from the alveolar space by only a very thin membrane that measures no more than 0.5 μ in thickness, the alveoli are normally kept free of excess fluid. This is accomplished by the integrity of permeability characteristics of this membrane and the balance of forces across this membrane, particularly between capillary hydrostatic pressure and plasma oncotic pressure. Although normally the plasma colloid osmotic (oncotic) pressure far exceeds the capillary hydrostatic pressure, the presence of other forces favors the movement of fluid out of the intravascular compartment. These forces are the negative hydrostatic and oncotic pressures of the pericapillary or interstitial space (Fig. 21–2). As demonstrated in the equation in Fig. 21–2, the rate of fluid filtered from the capillary lumen to the interstitial space is determined by these forces, as well as the characteristics of the membrane separating the capillary blood from the interstitial space. Permeability of this membrane to colloids (proteins) affects the plasma-interstitial fluid oncotic gradient.

Variable amounts of fluid that are normally filtered into the interstitial space are readily reabsorbed by the lymphatic channels at this space. However, under pathologic conditions, when the rate of fluid filtration exceeds the absorptive capacity of the lymphatics, pulmonary edema develops. The excess fluid initially accumulates in the interstitial tissue (interstitial edema), and later also floods the alveolar spaces (alveolar edema).

In cardiac failure, pulmonary edema results from an increase in the microvascular hydrostatic pressure that, by increasing the transcapillary pressure, forces the fluid out of the capillary into the interstitial space.

Normally, the outputs of the two sides of the heart are so well adjusted that, despite tremendous changes in circulation with various activities, neither side will be overloaded and, thus, the lungs will not be flooded with blood. This is due to close similarity in the behavior of the two ventricles, which beat at the same rate under various influences and obey *Starling's law of the heart*. This law states that the stretching of the heart muscle, as occurs when more blood returns to the heart, increases the force of its contraction, therefore expelling more blood. Starling's law of the heart is the major mechanism by which the right and left ventricles maintain equal output. A disturbance in balance between the out-

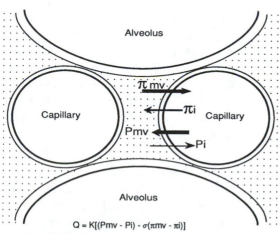

$$Q = K[(Pmv - Pi) - \sigma(\pi mv - \pi i)]$$

Q = filtration rate
K = filtration coefficient
σ = protein reflection coefficient (resistance of membrane to protein leak)
Pmv = microvascular hydrostatic pressure
Pi = interstitial hydrostatic pressure
πmv = plasma oncotic (colloid osmotic) pressure
πi = interstitial fluid oncotic pressure

Figure 21–2. Relationship of forces that determine the rate of fluid filtration from the capillaries to the interstitial spaces of the lungs. Normally these forces result in filtration of a small amount of fluid, which is readily absorbed by the lymphatics.

put of the two sides of the heart will result in overloading of one side of the circulation. In the event of failure of the left ventricle to handle its blood load, the pulmonary capillaries will be congested, and their hydrostatic pressure will rise.

Noncardiac pulmonary edema is most commonly the result of increased permeability of alveolar capillaries to large molecules (leaky capillary). With an influx of proteins in the interstitial space, colloid osmotic gradient between capillary blood and interstitial fluid is decreased, which in turn enhances further the fluid accumulation in the lungs. Acute lung injury from various etiologies is the most frequent cause of noncardiac pulmonary edema. This condition is the underlying mechanism of acute respiratory distress syndrome (ARDS), discussed in Chapter 27. Pulmonary edema that develops as a result of an ascent to high altitude and pulmonary edema that occurs secondary to certain acute disorders of the central nervous system (CNS) (neurogenic pulmonary edema) are two other well-known conditions that are associated with increased permeability of pulmonary capillaries.

Pulmonary edema is also known to result from increased negative intrathoracic and transpulmonary pressures. This may occur when a collapsed lung from a large pneumothorax or pleural effusion is rapidly reexpanded by removing the air or fluid from the pleural cavity too fast (reexpansion pulmonary edema). Pulmonary edema may also develop in upper airway obstruction as a result of forceful inspiratory efforts against the occluded airway. A sudden reduction of the interstitial hydrostatic pressure *and* an increased alveolar-capillary permeability have been implicated in the pathogenesis of pulmonary edema in these two otherwise disparate clinical circumstances.

Increased pulmonary capillary pressure in cardiac pulmonary edema is most commonly due to left-side heart failure from long-standing systemic hypertension, aortic or mitral valve lesion, arteriosclerotic heart disease, and different types of cardiac muscle disorder.

Pathophysiology. As a result of the accumulation of fluid in the interstitial and alveolar spaces, lung compliance diminishes markedly. Lung volumes and capacities are also decreased. The presence of fluid in the airways and edema of the airway walls cause increased airway resistance. These changes result in increased work of breathing, the main cause of breathlessness in heart failure. Reduced blood flow to respiratory muscles and premature lactic acidosis with exertion are other causes of dyspnea in heart failure. The changes in compliance and airway resistance are not uniform throughout the lungs; as a result, the distribution of ventilation is altered. Marked mismatching of ventilation and perfusion and intrapulmonary shunting cause widening of the alveolar-arterial P_{O_2} difference and arterial hypoxemia. Reduced peripheral tissue perfusion from heart failure, as well as arterial hypoxemia, may result in significant tissue hypoxia, lactic acidosis, and dysfunction of other organs.

Clinical Manifestations. Although cardiac pulmonary edema may develop without previous warning or antecedent symptoms of heart disease, most patients have a history of chronic and/or recurrent symptoms of heart failure. Dyspnea is the most common complaint. The mode of onset and characteristics of dyspnea are quite variable, depending on acuteness or chronicity and severity of disease. In mild forms of heart failure, shortness of breath is usually noticed during activity. As heart failure advances, dyspnea occurs with less and less effort until it is present even at rest. **Orthopnea** is a special type of dyspnea that occurs on recumbent position and is relieved by sitting. To avoid this symptom, the patient usually elevates the head of his or her bed or sleeps in a more or less sitting position. Orthopnea is a common manifestation of heart failure, but it also can be associated with severe lung disease. **Paroxysmal nocturnal dyspnea** refers to an attack of severe dyspnea that occurs during the night and awakens the patient from sleep. After sitting upright for a while, dyspnea improves and the patient returns to bed. The attack is due to an episode of acute but transient pulmonary edema, which can be demonstrated by physical examination and radiographic study. Cheyne-Stokes respiration is a fairly common manifestation of heart failure, especially in the elderly.

In fully developed acute pulmonary edema, the patient experiences the sudden onset of dyspnea, which is very severe from the start and reaches the extreme degree within a short time. Cough productive of frothy and blood-tinged sputum is common.

Physical findings in mild heart failure are not striking; a few crackles in the lung bases and, depending on duration of failure, a variable amount of peripheral edema may be present. In patients with acute severe pulmonary edema, the clinical picture is almost diagnostic. The patient is extremely dyspneic, tachypneic, apprehensive, and unable to lie down. The extremities are cool, clammy, and cyanotic. Rales and wheezes are heard throughout the lung fields. There may be evidence of increased peripheral venous pressure manifested by engorged neck veins. The heart rate is rapid and may be irregular. Enlargement of the liver and peripheral edema may or may not be present. There is usually evidence of cardiac enlargement. Auscultation of the heart, although difficult because of a noisy chest, may reveal extra heart sounds and murmurs.

Radiographic Findings. Radiographic examination shows changes of pulmonary venous congestion with interstitial and airspace edema. In full-blown pulmonary edema, there is bilateral, more or less symmetrical, combined interstitial and airspace density involving mostly the lower lung fields and perihilar regions (Fig. 21–3). The vascular markings are prominent in the upper lung fields from pulmonary venous engorgement. A variable amount of pleural effusion, usually bilateral, is commonly observed. The heart shadow is usually enlarged with prominence of the left ventricle. In less severe heart failure, radiographic findings are limited to changes of vascular markings and increased interstitial density.

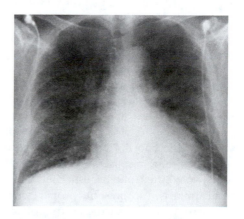

Figure 21–3. Radiograph of cardiac pulmonary edema. Note the enlarged heart and predominantly interstitial edema.

Diagnosis. The diagnosis of pulmonary edema in a setting of known heart disease, characteristic clinical picture, and radiographic findings is usually easy. However, when pulmonary edema develops in critically ill patients, with or without a history of heart disease, in circumstances in which the clinical features are less clear and there are other complicating disorders, the differentiation of cardiac from noncardiac pulmonary edema becomes a difficult diagnostic challenge. The measurement of pulmonary capillary pressure by a flow-directed, balloon-tipped catheter (Swan-Ganz) is most helpful in determining whether pulmonary edema is cardiac or noncardiac in origin. It is also a useful aid in choosing and guiding an appropriate treatment. As expected, pulmonary artery wedge pressure will be high in cardiac pulmonary edema and normal or low in noncardiac cases.

Management. Acute pulmonary edema is a medical emergency requiring prompt and aggressive treatment. Respiratory specialists are frequently involved in the management of patients with this condition. In cardiac pulmonary edema, although therapeutic efforts are mostly directed toward improving the cardiac function and elimination of excess fluid, acuteness and severity of respiratory problems with marked derangement of arterial blood gases necessitate immediate treatment with oxygen administration, maintenance of adequate airways, and sometimes mechanical ventilatory support. The outcome of treatment of these desperately ill patients depends mainly on the coordinated efforts of both the cardiac and respiratory teams. In severely hypoxemic patients, especially when hypercapnia is also present, proper respiratory care is crucial for the efficacy of cardiac measures, because medications intended to improve cardiac function are usually ineffective in the presence of severe hypoxia and acidosis. As morphine is one of the mainstays of management of acute pulmonary edema, its respiratory depressant effect should be closely watched. Mechanical ventilatory support is indicated whenever there is evidence of hypoventilation or severe intractable hypoxemia. Positive end–expiratory pressure (PEEP) has been proved to be of benefit in cardiac pulmonary edema. Medical treatment usually includes the administration of rapid-acting diuretics, vasodilators, and inotropic drugs. Aminophylline is also commonly used.

Prognosis of cardiac pulmonary edema mainly depends on the underlying cause and other associated medical problems. Progressive pump failure and intractable arrhythmia are common causes of death. However, many patients also die from respiratory failure. Aggressive respiratory care and judicious use of mechanical ventilation, together with an appropriate cardiac regimen, have saved the lives of many such patients.

■ PULMONARY EMBOLISM

Pulmonary embolism (PE) is defined as the occlusion of the pulmonary artery or one or more of its branches by matter carried in the blood current. This matter is called *embolus,* which is most commonly a blood clot; however, it may be a fat particle, air, amniotic fluid, tumor or other tissue fragment, parasite, or foreign body. In the practical sense, PE refers to pulmonary arterial occlusion by a blood clot (thromboembolism), unless it is qualified by other causes such as fat embolism, air embolism, and so on.

A blood clot attached to its site of origin in a blood vessel or a heart chamber is called a *thrombus*. A thrombus becomes an embolus once it is detached from its origin and carried by the blood-stream.

PE is one of the most common causes of morbidity and mortality among the adult population. Its true incidence is difficult to ascertain, but autopsy findings indicate that it is much more common than clinical estimates. PE is one of the most common pulmonary pathologic findings at autopsy in large general hospitals.

Etiology and Pathogenesis. Nearly 90% of clinically significant pulmonary emboli result from **deep-vein thrombosis** (DVT) of the lower extremities. Any systemic vein and the right heart chambers, however, may be the site of thrombus formation and a source for PE. Risk of PE from the DVT confined to the calf and from superficial venous thrombosis is much less than when DVT extends to, or occurs at, the thigh.

Three important factors facilitate clot formation in a vessel: abnormal vessel wall, stagnation of blood, and increased coagulability. Although thrombosis may occur in the absence of any detectable predisposing factor, in most cases one or more of such factors is present.

Damage to the vessel wall, particularly to its inner layer, causes adherence of blood platelets and activation of clotting factors. Inflammation of the vein (phlebitis) or its surrounding tissue (periphlebitis) and its traumatic injury are examples in which local intravenous clotting occurs.

Venous stasis seems to be the most important factor in production of a thrombus. Many clinical conditions in which venous thrombosis and PE are observed cause venous stasis. Prolonged bed rest, immobility due to pain of trauma or surgery, presence of orthopedic cast, gen-eral debility, paralysis, pregnancy, varicose veins, heart failure, and many other medical or surgical conditions predispose to stagnation of blood, particularly in the lower extremities.

An increased clotting tendency of blood is known to occur following significant trauma, major surgery, pregnancy and childbirth, and malignant diseases. The role of birth control pills in predisposing to thromboembolic disease is probably due to their effect on blood clotting. Hereditary or acquired quantitative or qualitative abnormalities of certain factors that control or inhibit clotting of circulating blood are uncommon but important causes of recurrent DVT and PE.

Once detached from its source, the blood clot is carried with the blood flow. From the vein, it travels to the right side of the heart and from there to the pulmonary arteries. Depending on its size, it lodges in various parts of the pulmonary artery. A very large embolus may occlude the main pulmonary artery; smaller ones will pass more distally. Because of the large blood flow to the dependent lung regions, they are most commonly involved with PE.

As a result of bronchial arterial blood supply, the occlusion of a pulmonary artery usually does not result in significant pathologic change in the lung parenchyma. A pathologic lesion, known as *pulmonary infarction*, occurs in about 10% of patients with PE, particularly when there is underlying cardiac disease.

Pathophysiology. Mechanical occlusion of a pulmonary artery results in nonperfusion of the part of the lung supplied by that artery. Continuation of ventilation of the nonperfused area will be wasted and, therefore, will add to dead-space ventilation.

Acute occlusion of a regional pulmonary artery results in changes of ventilation and perfusion of other lung regions causing additional ventilation–perfusion ratio ($\dot{V}/\dot{Q}$) mismatching. Diversion of blood to nonoccluded branches of the pulmonary artery causes perfusion to exceed ventilation of the corresponding regions of the lungs, thus resulting in reduction of $\dot{V}/\dot{Q}$. Blood may even be forced to flow through nonventilated regions, causing intrapulmonary shunting. $\dot{V}/\dot{Q}$ mismatching and intrapulmonary shunting are the major causes of an increased alveolar-arterial Po_2 gradient and hypoxemia. Other pathophysiologic changes that contribute to hypoxemia in massive PE are low cardiac output that results in reduced mixed venous oxygen content and right-to-left shunting through incompetent foramen ovale. The latter condition, present in 25% to 30% of the population, results in intracardiac shunting when the right atrial pressure exceeds the left atrial pressure, which may develop as a result of pulmonary hypertension. Hyperventilation, an almost uniform finding in PE, is secondary to the stimulation of lung mechanoreceptors. It occurs with or without hypoxemia.

Elevation of pulmonary artery pressure as a result of PE depends on the size of emboli and the presence or absence of underlying cardiopulmonary disease. As the right ventricle, because of its thin myocardium, is unable to generate high enough pressure, it may fail to maintain an adequate cardiac output if the PE is massive. Reduced cardiac output aggravates hypoxemia, which in turn increases the pulmonary vascular resistance further. Resultant systemic hypotension and circulatory failure are the usual cause of death in severe acute PE. Recurrent unresolved emboli may be the cause of chronic pulmonary hypertension (see later in this chapter).

Clinical Manifestations. Clinical manifestations of PE vary greatly. The presence of significant underlying conditions often obscures or modifies the clinical picture. Many emboli, most often when small, produce little or no symptoms and are hardly suspected. A large embolus may cause sudden death. In most cases, the symptoms are nonspecific and, unless the index of suspicion is high for PE, are often ascribed to other conditions. The symptoms frequently experienced by patients with PE are dyspnea and chest pain. Dyspnea is by far the most common presenting symptom and has certain characteristics, such as sudden onset, severity out of proportion to clinical findings, and associated apprehension. Chest pain may be of the anginal type at the onset, but later becomes pleuritic in nature. Hemoptysis, although a very important symptom, is less common. Other symptoms include cough, faintness, and anxiety.

Physical examination may reveal evidence of DVT, usually of the lower extremities, manifested by pain, tenderness, and swelling. These findings, although very helpful for diagnosis, are lacking in more than one-half of the patients with proved PE. In severe and massive PE, tachypnea, tachycardia, and cyanosis are the usual findings. Local decrease in breath sounds, wheezing, rales, pleural rub, and signs of pleural effusion may be present. Other findings, such as fever, changes in heart sounds, cardiac arrhythmia, and signs of cardiac failure or shock, are sometimes detected. Acute cor pulmonale refers to cardiac changes due to acute obstruction of pulmonary vasculature with embolism.

Radiographic Findings. The chest radiograph may be normal or show only minimal changes. Common findings include loss of lung volume, linear densities of atelectasis, elevation of one side of the diaphragm, evidence of pleural effusion, and parenchymal density of pulmonary infarction. More characteristic changes of local reduction in vascular markings and enlargement of a pulmonary artery in the hilar region are observed uncommonly.

Laboratory Findings and Diagnosis. Arterial blood studies in patients with PE typically show low P_{O_2} and P_{CO_2}. Although arterial hypoxemia is present in most patients, normal arterial P_{O_2} does not exclude the diagnosis. Widening of the alveolar–arterial P_{O_2} gradient, however, is almost always present; a normal gradient makes the diagnosis of PE unlikely.

The *electrocardiogram* (EKG) may show certain abnormalities during PE, suggesting myocardial hypoxia or right ventricular strain.

Radioisotopic lung scanning is one of the most valuable clinical tools for the diagnosis of PE. A normal perfusion lung scan, for all practical purposes, excludes the diagnosis of PE. With multiple large defects on perfusion lung scan in the right clinical setting, the diagnosis of PE is highly probable (Fig. 21–4). Any interpretation of the scan should be made in light of the patient's clinical and laboratory findings, and must never be made without concomitant review of plain chest x-ray films. Combination of ventilation and perfusion lung scanning is very helpful in differentiating PEs from other pulmonary conditions in which the abnormality of perfusion is secondary to a ventilation defect ($\dot{V}/\dot{Q}$ match). In PE, obstruction of a branch of the pulmonary artery results in absent or reduced perfusion of corresponding lung region,

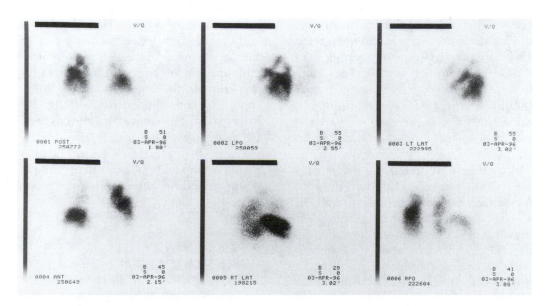

Figure 21–4. Perfusion lung scan in a patient with proved pulmonary embolism. As seen in all six views, there are multiple perfusion defects of various sizes in both lung fields.

whereas ventilation is fairly well preserved ($\dot{V}/\dot{Q}$ mismatch).

Occasionally, *pulmonary angiography* will be necessary for definitive diagnosis of PE when the result of the previously mentioned studies is not conclusive, and the patient has to undergo certain potentially risky therapeutic interventions.

Lower extremity venography is another useful diagnostic study. The presence of a thrombus in a deep vein will support the diagnosis of PE in a proper clinical setting and an abnormal lung scan; a normal venography makes this diagnosis much less likely. Two important noninvasive tests for DVT are impedance plethysmography (IPG) and compression ultrasonography (US). The latter, also known as duplex study, is sometimes combined with venous color Doppler. Because of its higher sensitivity and specificity, compression US is replacing IPG in most medical centers.

Management. As PE results from DVT, every effort should be made to prevent the formation of a clot in the deep veins. The patients at risk of developing DVT should be identified and the conditions that predispose them to venous stasis should be corrected. Proper positioning, active and passive exercises of the lower extremities, early mobilization and ambulation, use of specially designed stockings, and treatment of underlying diseases are some of the measures that can reduce the incidence of venous thrombosis and PE. The use of intermittent pneumatic compression devices is both simple and effective. They should be applied as early as possible *before* the development of venous thrombosis. Therefore, DVT should be excluded before their application. Prophylactic anticoagulation in high-risk patients and early anticoagulant therapy of DVT are effective in preventing pulmonary embolism.

Anticoagulation therapy with heparin remains the therapeutic method of choice for PE. Alleviation of hypoxemia with supplemental oxygen therapy is often indicated. Thrombolytic agents, such as streptokinase and alteplase (tissue plasminogen activator), are known to hasten the lysis of clots in peripheral veins and pulmonary arteries. They are not a substitute for but an addition to anticoagulants. Their therapeutic benefit has been demonstrated in extensive DVT and massive PE associated with significant hemodynamic impairment. Bleeding, especially following recent surgery or from a venous or arterial puncture site, is the main disadvantage of these agents.

Surgical therapy, such as ligation of the inferior vena cava or transvenous insertion of a filtering device, may be necessary in patients who, for some reason, cannot be anticoagulated or have recurrent embolism despite adequate anticoagulation. Currently, the Greenfield filter is the preferred device used as an effective mechanical means for preventing embolization of large-size and medium-size clots to the lungs. Made of stainless steel, this cone-shaped device is usually inserted via the femoral or internal jugular vein and placed inside the inferior vena cava below the renal veins. The filter is able to trap emboli larger than 3 mm in diameter without interrupting the blood flow.

■ PULMONARY FAT EMBOLISM

Inconsequential embolization of a small amount of fat particles to the lung and, possibly, to other organs is a common occurrence in trauma patients and during bone surgery. However, **fat embolism syndrome,** characterized by acute onset of respiratory distress often associated with fever, changes in sensorium, and the appearance of petechiae, is a relatively infrequent but serious complication of severe musculoskeletal trauma.

Etiology   and   Pathogenesis. Although fat embolism has been rarely demonstrated in association with soft-tissue injury, burns, and certain medical conditions, the vast majority of clinically recognizable cases of fat embolism follow multiple fractures, especially of the long bones of the lower extremities and the pelvic bones. Despite continuation of disagreement regarding the mechanism of fat embolism, available data strongly suggest that fat particles from the injured sites, especially bone marrow, enter the blood via disrupted vessels (intravasation). This process is enhanced by movement of the fractured area from manipulation and lack of prompt splinting and immobilization. Embolized fat droplets most often become lodged in the pulmonary microvasculature, whereas only a small fraction of them enter the systemic circulation and are carried to other organs.

The initial mechanical effects are soon followed by a chemical reaction from fatty acids, which are generated by the hydrolysis of the embolized fat. Although mechanical microvascular obstruction contributes to the clinical picture of fat embolism syndrome, it is mainly the local chemical effect of fatty acids that causes diffuse pulmonary injury and disruption of the integrity of the alveolar capillary membrane. Other factors, such as intravascular coagulation and platelet aggregation, also partake in this process. Exudation of fluid into and around the airspaces and reduction of alveolar surfactant complete a pathologic picture of ARDS.

Pathophysiology. As with the other causes of ARDS, the characteristic pathophysiologic changes are reduced lung volumes and compliance with severe gas transport abnormality. Intractable hypoxemia, which is the most significant clinical problem with fat embolism, results from severe $\dot{V}/\dot{Q}$ mismatching and intrapulmonary shunting. Some of the neurologic manifestations of fat embolism are probably due to severe cerebral hypoxia, which aggravates the effect of cerebral fat embolism.

Clinical   Manifestations. The clinical picture is composed of pulmonary and systemic manifestations. Usually 24 to 48 hours after serious injury, the patient presents with progressive respiratory distress with dyspnea, tachypnea, and cyanosis. Pulmonary rales and rhonchi may be heard. Fever and tachycardia are often present. Neurologic manifestations due to fat embolism to the brain include mental confusion, stupor, delirium, and coma. A characteristic sign, which is very helpful for diagnosis of fat embolism, is the occasional appearance of petechiae (small purplish-red spots caused by bleeding into the skin) over the neck, trunk, and conjunctivae.

Radiographic   Findings   and   Diagnosis. Radiographic examination usually reveals diffuse patchy densities due to alveolar edema. Similar changes, however, may be observed following severe trauma and shock without fat embolism. Certain characteristic clinical features, including changes in sensorium, petechiae, and the onset of acute hypoxemic respiratory failure 24 to 48 hours after serious major traumatic injury or surgery of the large bones are important diagnostic features of fat embolism syndrome. These features usually differentiate the syndrome from other causes of posttraumatic respiratory failure.

Management. The principles of management of ARDS are applicable to the treatment of pulmonary fat embolism. Prompt correction of hypoxemia is the key to a successful outcome. Not uncommonly, this may require intubation, mechanical ventilation, and continuous positive pressure breathing. Among several therapeutic modalities used in the management of fat embolism, corticosteroids have the most advocates. Large doses of corticosteroids have been shown to protect against fat embolism syndrome when used early in high-risk patients. Fat embolism, being a self-limited condition, usually has a better prognosis than ARDS from most other causes.

▪ PULMONARY HYPERTENSION

The pulmonary vascular circuit is a low-pressure system due to the low resistance of pulmonary blood vessels. Moreover, because of the adaptability of this vascular bed, increased blood flow, as with exercise, normally does not cause significant elevation of its pressure. Systolic blood pressure in the pulmonary artery in the resting healthy adult averages about 24 mm Hg and diastolic averages about 10 mm Hg. The term *pulmonary hypertension* implies an increase in the pulmonary arterial pressure above the accepted upper limit of normal (ie, 30/16, or mean pressure of 25 mm Hg).

Etiology and Pathogenesis. There are many causes of increased pulmonary artery pressure with various mechanisms for its development. Several factors, singly or in combination, are known to affect pulmonary circulation and its vasculature. Increased pressure in the pulmonary circuit distal to capillaries (ie, left ventricle, left atrium, and pulmonary veins) results in elevated pulmonary artery pressure. Left ventricular failure, mitral valve disease, and occlusion of the pulmonary venous system are among the important causes of "postcapillary" pulmonary hypertension. However, the most common mechanism of elevation of pulmonary artery pressure is reduction in the total cross-sectional area of the pulmonary arterial bed ("precapillary" pulmonary hypertension). Three main processes result in increased pulmonary artery resistance: (1) destruction, (2) obstruction, and (3) constriction. Because of the remarkable distensibility of pulmonary blood vessels, the total area of this vascular bed must be decreased by more than 50% before any elevation of pulmonary arterial pressure develops.

Primary involvement of the pulmonary artery by conditions such as pulmonary vasculitis or its occlusion by PE results in pulmonary hypertension. Chronically increased blood flow to the lungs, as seen in patients with congenital heart disease with left-to-right shunt (eg, atrial or ventricular septal defect), causes increased pulmonary arterial resistance and, hence, pulmonary hypertension.

By far the most common causes of pulmonary hypertension are chronic pulmonary disease and other conditions in which there is sustained hypoxemia. The mechanism involved may be due to significant reduction in pulmonary vasculature as a result of destructive changes in the lung or, more importantly, to the effect of alveolar hypoxia on the pulmonary arteries. Low alveolar P_{O_2}, when acute, causes constriction of pulmonary arteries; whereas when long standing, it causes obstructive changes. Hypercapnia with acidosis enhances the effect of hypoxia. High-altitude residence is known to result in pulmonary hypertension through prolonged hypoxia. In ventilatory insufficiency due to thoracic deformity, neuromuscular disease, sleep apnea syndrome, and primary hypoventilation, pulmonary hypertension may develop as a result of chronic hypoxia. In chronic lung disease, reduced vascular bed and increased pulmonary artery resistance due to hypoxia as well as acidosis contribute to pulmonary hypertension. The mechanism of pulmonary vasoconstriction from hypoxia is not entirely known, but it seems to be from the effect of low oxygen tension on endothelium-derived relaxing factor (nitric oxide).

When there is no identifiable cause for increased pulmonary artery pressure, the diagnosis of primary, or idiopathic, pulmonary hypertension is made. This uncommon but clinically important disorder occurs most commonly in young women.

Clinical Manifestations and Diagnosis. Manifestations of pulmonary hypertension secondary to pulmonary disease are usually overshadowed by the symptoms and signs of the underlying primary condition. It often remains unrecognized until severe right-side heart failure develops (see later in this chapter). When the heart disease or pulmonary vascular disorder is the underlying cause of pulmonary hypertension, clinical manifestations are most often cardiac. Exertional dyspnea, chest pain, weakness, fatigue, and syncope are common presenting symptoms of primary pulmonary hypertension. Although hypoxemia is seen in most cases of pulmonary hypertension, it is much more pronounced when its underlying cause is respiratory.

The diagnosis of pulmonary hypertension is usually suspected on clinical grounds. Radiographic findings of prominent pulmonary artery and its main branches are highly suggestive. Noninvasively, pulmonary artery pressure can be estimated with a reasonable degree of accuracy by Doppler US. Cardiac catheterization for measurement of pulmonary artery and its wedge pressures is considered when postcapillary pulmonary hypertension is suspected. Pulmonary angiography is performed when chronic thromboembolism involving large pulmonary arteries is suggested by radionuclide lung scan, and when surgery is seriously considered for its treatment.

Management. The most important and effective therapeutic measure in pulmonary hypertension is the treatment of the underlying cause, if one can be identified. Almost all cases of pulmonary hypertension in chronic lung disease are associated with significant hypoxemia, which should be adequately but judiciously treated with supplemental oxygen. Despite clinical trials with numerous pharmacologic agents, there has been no truly effective drug against primary pulmonary hypertension, which generally has a poor prognosis. Lung transplantation is the only hope for long-term survival for such patients who are usually considered to be proper candidates for it.

■ CHRONIC COR PULMONALE

Pulmonary hypertension from any cause affects the heart, particularly the right ventricle. Hypertrophy, dilatation, and eventual failure of the right ventricle are the consequences of sustained elevation of pulmonary vascular resistance. *Chronic cor pulmonale* is defined as changes in the right ventricle and its function due to elevation of pulmonary artery pressure resulting from diseases affecting the function or the structure of the lung or its vasculature.

Etiology. Chronic cor pulmonale results from long-standing pulmonary hypertension caused by chronic disease of the lungs and their vasculature. Chronic obstructive pulmonary disease (COPD) leads the long list of such conditions. Chronic diffuse interstitial disease, severe destructive lung diseases following advanced tuberculosis or other chronic inflammatory conditions, cystic fibrosis, extensive resectional surgery, significant chest deformity, and fibrothorax are also common causes of chronic pulmonary hypertension and cor pulmonale.

Recurrent and unresolved pulmonary emboli, primary pulmonary hypertension, and other diseases involving the pulmonary vasculature may manifest by right ventricular hypertrophy and failure. Chronic upper airway obstruction, particularly in infants and children, due to enlarged tonsils and adenoids has been added to the list of disorders leading to chronic cor pulmonale. In chronic hypoventilation syndrome due to obesity, sleep apnea syndrome, neuromuscular disorders, or CNS malfunction, prolonged hypoxemia and perhaps hypercapnia result in pulmonary hypertension and right ventricular failure. As demonstrated schematically in Fig. 21–5, chronic respiratory disease not only results in right ventricular failure, but also may affect the left ventricular function. Hypoxemia and acidosis are known to result in myocardial depression. Moreover, frequent presence of

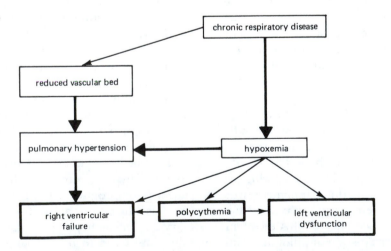

Figure 21–5. Schematic demonstration of the effect of chronic respiratory disease on the heart.

polycythemia, another complication of chronic hypoxemia, may also impair cardiac performance.

Clinical Manifestations and Diagnosis. Because of the presence of significant underlying disease, clinical diagnosis of cor pulmonale is apt to be overlooked. Right ventricular hypertrophy is an early manifestation that is often difficult to prove clinically. Underlying pulmonary disease frequently prevents detection of changes in cardiac impulse or heart sounds. Most often, the diagnosis of cor pulmonale is clinically made when there is evidence of right ventricular failure (ie, increased venous distention, peripheral edema, and enlarged liver).

Radiographic changes of cor pulmonale are usually present in more advanced cases. Signs of underlying pulmonary disease, enlarged pulmonary artery trunk and its main branches with attenuation of distal branches, and right ventricular hypertrophy are characteristic x-ray findings.

Electrocardiographic changes, especially the findings of right ventricular hypertrophy, if present, will be helpful. Cardiac arrhythmias are fairly common with cor pulmonale. By echocardiography and radionuclide ventriculography, the size and contractility of both ventricles can be determined. Cardiac catheterization is rarely indicated in cor pulmonale.

Management. Effective management of cor pulmonale depends on understanding the underlying cause and mechanism of its production. The treatment should be primarily addressed to correction of its cause. The importance of adequate ventilation and oxygenation cannot be overemphasized. If, despite optimal management, the patient remains chronically hypoxemic, continuous oxygen therapy is indicated. The use of a proper cardiac regimen, including rest, digitalis, and diuretics, is usually recommended when heart failure supervenes. It should be emphasized that the successful treatment of cor pulmonale depends much more on improving the underlying respiratory disorder and that right-side heart failure is one of the complications of chronic pulmonary disease that can be prevented or at least delayed by its proper management.

BIBLIOGRAPHY

ACCP Consensus Statement. Primary pulmonary hypertension. *Chest.* 1993; 104: 236–250.

Clagett GP, Anderson FA Jr, Heit J, et al. Prevention of venous thromboembolism. *Chest.* 1995; 108(Suppl):312S–334S.

Cutaia M, Rounds S. Hypoxic pulmonary vasocontriction: physiologic significance, mechanism, and clinical relevance. *Chest.* 1990; 97:706–718.

Fabian TC, Hoots AV, Sanford DS, et al. Fat embolism syndrome. *Crit Care Med.* 1990; 18:42–46.

Fedullo AJ, Swinburne AJ, Wahl GW, Bixby K. Acute cardiogenic pulmonary edema treated with mechanical ventilation. *Chest.* 1991; 99:1220–1226.

Ginsberg JS. Management of venous thromboembolism. *N Eng J Med.* 1996; 335:1816–1828.

Goldhaber SZ. Contemporary pulmonary embolism thrombolysis. *Chest.* 1995; 107 (1Suppl):45S–51S.

Greenfield LJ, Wakefield TW. Prevention of venous thrombosis and pulmonary embolism. *Adv Surg.* 1989; 22:301–324.

Gropper MA, Wiener-Kronish JP, Hashimoto S. Acute cardiogenic pulmonary edema. *Clin Chest Med.* 1994; 15:501–515.

Hanly P, Zuberi N, Gray R. Pathogenesis of Cheyne-Stokes respiration in patients with congestive heart failure: relationship to arterial P_{CO_2}. *Chest.* 1993; 104:1079–1084.

Hull RD, Feldstein W, Stein PD, Pineo GF. Cost-effectiveness of pulmonary embolism diagnosis. *Arch Intern Med.* 1996; 156:68–72.

Hull RD, Hirsh J, Carter CJ, et al. Pulmonary angiography, ventilation lung scanning, and venography for clinically suspected pulmonary embolism with abnormal lung scan. *Ann Intern Med.* 1983; 98:891–899.

Jardin F, Dubourg O, Bourdorias JP. Echocardiographic pattern of acute cor pulmonale. *Chest.* 1997; 111:209–217.

Kelley MA, Carson JL, Palevsky HI, Schwartz JS. Diagnosing pulmonary embolism: new facts and strategies. *Ann Intern Med.* 1991; 114:300–306.

Klinger JR. Right ventricular dysfunction in chronic obstructive pulmonary disease: evaluation and management. *Chest.* 1991; 99:715–723.

Kollef MH, Pluss J. Noncardiogenic pulmonary edema following upper airway obstruction. *Medicine.* 1991; 70:91–98.

Konstantinides S, Geibel A, Kasper W. Role of cardiac ultrasound in the detection of pulmonary embolism. *Semin Respir Crit Care Med.* 1996: 17:39–49.

MacNee W. Pathophysiology of cor pulmonale in chronic obstructive pulmonary disease. *Am J Respir Crit Care Med.* 1994; 150:833-852; 1158–1168.

Moser KM. Venous thromboembolism. *Am Rev Respir Dis.* 1990; 141:235–249.

Peltier LF. Fat embolism: a perspective. *Clin Orthop.* 1988; 232:263–270.

PIOPED Investigators. Value of the ventilation/perfusion scan in acute pulmonary embolism. *JAMA.* 1990; 263:2753–2759.

Salvaterra CG, Rubin LJ. Investigation and management of pulmonary hypertension in chronic obstructive pulmonary disease. *Am Rev Respir Dis.* 1993; 148:1414–1417.

Santolicandro A, Prediletto R, Fornai E, et al. Mechanisms of hypoxemia and hypocapnia in pulmonary embolism. *Am J Respir Crit Care Med.* 1995; 152:336–347.

Sherry S. Thrombolytic therapy for noncoronary diseases. *Ann Emerg Med.* 1991; 20:396–404.

Shure D. Chronic thromboembolic pulmonary hypertension: diagnosis and treatment. *Semin Respir Crit Care Med.* 1996; 17:7–15.

Staub NC. The pathogenesis of pulmonary edema. *Prog Cardiovasc Dis.* 1980; 26:293–315.

Stein PD. Applicability of ventilation/perfusion lung scans in specific populations of patients. *Semin Respir Crit Care Med.* 1996; 17:23–29.

Stein PD, Hull RD, Saltzman HA, Pineo G. Strategy for diagnosis of patients with suspected acute pulmonary embolism. *Chest.* 1993; 103:1553–1559.

Vender RL. Chronic hypoxic pulmonary hypertension. *Chest.* 1994; 106:236–243.

Ward R, Jones D, Haponik, EF. Paradoxical embolism: an underdiagnosed problem. *Chest.* 1995; 108:549–558.

IX

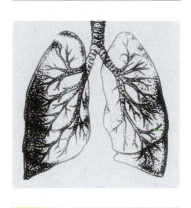

DISEASES OF THE PLEURA AND THE THORACIC WALL: CHEST TRAUMA

22.

Diseases of the Pleura

■ ANATOMIC AND PATHOLOGIC CONSIDERATIONS

The pleura is a serous membrane that lines the inner surface of each side of the thorax, the upper surface of the hemidiaphragm, and the side of the mediastinum where, at the lung root, it deflects to envelop the lung. It invaginates into the interlobar fissures separating the lobes. Thus, a closed space (or potential space) is developed around each lung, with recesses between the lobes (Fig. 22–1). The part of the pleura that envelops the lung is called *visceral* pleura; the part that covers the interior of the thorax, the diaphragm, and the mediastinum is known as *parietal* pleura. Normally, the parietal and visceral pleurae are separated by a thin layer of fluid, which keeps their surfaces moist and smooth, allowing them to slide against one another with minimum friction during respiratory movement.

Because of the close anatomic and physiologic relationship between the lung and pleura, the pathologic condition of one often affects the other. Most diseases of the pleura are secondary to pulmonary lesions that may or may not be apparent. Conversely, significant disease of the pleura impairs the function of the underlying lung. In addition, as a result of proximity of many other organs such as mediastinal structures and subdiaphragmatic viscera, the pleura may be involved in many other disease processes. As part of their manifestations or complications, several systemic diseases are known to affect the pleura. Among them, systemic lupus erythematosus (SLE) and rheumatoid disease are the better known. Primary pleural disease is relatively uncommon.

Being a large interstitial space and because of its anatomic structure as a potential cavity with a subatmospheric pressure, the pleura usually manifests its disorders by the accumulation of fluids in its space. Heart failure, not infrequently, is associated with pleural effusion. Because of the immediate relation of the pleura with the lung and negative intrapleural pressure, the entry and accumulation of

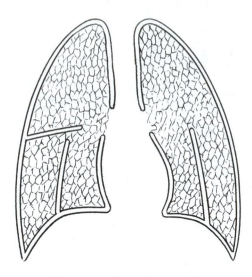

Figure 22–1. Diagram of pleural spaces.

air in the pleural cavity (pneumothorax) occur fairly commonly.

Pleurisy, which is synonymous with *pleuritis*, refers to inflammation of the pleura with or without pleural effusion. It may be mild and transient due to common conditions, such as viral infection, or it may be more severe and indicative of serious illness.

The pleura, like most other tissues, responds to chronic inflammation by proliferation of fibrous tissue. Pleural fibrosis is a common reaction to many prolonged pathologic states, and may result in adhesion of pleural surfaces. Calcium deposition may occur in old pleural fibrosis. Significant fibrous pleural thickening, with or without calcification, results in restriction of respiratory movement.

In view of the importance and the frequency of their occurrence, pleural effusion, empyema, and pneumothorax are discussed in this chapter.

■ PLEURAL EFFUSION

Normally, a very small amount of fluid, which may be occasionally detected only by special radiographic study, is present in the pleural space, serving as a lubricant for pleural surfaces. *Pleural effusion* refers to the accumulation of an easily detectable *abnormal quantity* of fluid in the pleural cavity.

Pathogenesis. Fluid accumulation in the pleural space, as in any part of the body, is the result of an imbalance between its formation and absorption. Continuous exchange of fluid in and out of the pleural cavity in the normal state is so effectively balanced that only a very small amount of fluid is maintained. The difference between the hydrostatic pressure of blood capillaries in the parietal pleura (supplied by systemic circulation) and that of the capillaries of the visceral pleura (supplied mainly by pulmonary circulation) suggests that fluid is formed at the parietal pleura and absorbed by the visceral pleura. Recent studies in experimental animals indicate, however, that normally fluid is formed in the interstitial space of the parietal pleura, enters the pleural cavity, and then is absorbed via the lymphatics in the parietal pleura. The pleural lymphatics have a large reserve capacity, allowing them to absorb varying amounts of fluid, thus maintaining a constant small volume of fluid in the pleural space. Therefore, the pleural cavity normally behaves as an extention of the interstitial space of the parietal pleura.

In disease states, the balance of fluid formation and its absorption is upset, resulting in its accumulation in the pleural space. This occurs because of increased fluid formation, its reduced absorption, or a combination of the two. In pathologic conditions, the source of fluid and mechanism of its absorption may be different from those in a normal state. They also may vary depending on the nature of pathologic processes. For example, pleural effusion in cardiac pulmonary edema results from fluid leak across the visceral pleura from the lung.

When fluid accumulates as the result of a disturbance of the balance between transcapillary pressure and plasma oncotic pressure, it is a **transudate.** Increased capillary pressure in heart failure and reduced plasma oncotic pressure in certain kidney or liver diseases are the known causes of transudative fluid. This kind of fluid has a low specific gravity, a low protein content, and usually a low cell count. When increased fluid formation is due to increased capillary permeability, as in inflammation, it is an **exudate.** The exudative fluid has a higher specific gravity, higher protein content, and often an increased cell count. It may have a significant number of white blood cells, to the point of a purulent appearance.

The accumulation of pleural fluid in association with pneumonia is called *parapneumonic effusion. Pleural empyema* refers to the presence of pus in the pleural cavity; however, in practice, pleural fluid with a large number of polymorphonuclear leukocytes or the presence of pyogenic organisms has been considered to constitute an empyema or *pyothorax.* The accumulation of blood in the pleural cavity is called *hemothorax;* the presence of chyle (milky intestinal lymph fluid) is known as *chylothorax.* Concomitant presence of air with fluid results in *hydropneumothorax;* if the fluid is pus or blood, the terms *pyopneumothorax* or *hemopneumothorax* are applied, respectively.

Causes of Pleural Effusion. Pleural effusion may be associated with many different diseases, the majority of which involve the lung. Sometimes pleural effusion may be the most predominant manifestation of the lung disease. The following list gives the important causes of pleural effusion. The list is not complete, and many other conditions may occasionally or rarely result in pleural effusion:

A. Transudate
1. Congestive heart failure
2. Cirrhosis of the liver
3. Kidney disease

B. Exudate
1. Infections (bacterial, fungal, viral)
2. Neoplasms (primary, metastatic)
3. Pulmonary embolism (PE)
4. Trauma and surgery
5. Systemic diseases (SLE, rheumatoid arthritis)
6. Intra-abdominal diseases (subdiaphragmatic abscess, pancreatitis)
7. Idiopathic (cause cannot be determined)

The most common cause of pleural fluid in clinical practice is congestive heart failure, but various infections, neoplasms, PE, trauma and surgery, and certain systemic diseases are important in causing pleural effusion. Postoperative pleural effusion is a very common occurrence following upper abdominal surgery. The most common cause of massive pleural effusion, which may occupy the entire hemithorax, is metastatic cancer of the pleura. In adult males it is more often from bronchogenic carcinoma, and in adult females, from metastatic breast cancer. Tuberculosis (TB), heart failure, and liver cirrhosis, however, may occasionally result in massive effusion. Sometimes empyema or hemothorax is massive.

Clinical Manifestations. The symptoms of pleural effusion may be absent or overshadowed by the symptoms of the underlying disease. Chest pain of the pleuritic type may be present at the onset when there is pleuritis, but it subsides once the fluid is formed and pleural surfaces are separated. The presence of a significant amount of fluid gives rise to dyspnea, which may be quite severe with massive effusions. The physical findings depend on the quantity of fluid. The typical signs are dullness to percussion, decreased vocal fremitus, and absent breath sounds over the fluid. Small effusions are not usually detectable on physical examination. Sometimes the sound of friction between the pleural surfaces may be heard on auscultation.

When a pleural effusion is large enough to cause significant displacement of the mediastinum to the opposite side, it is referred to as *tension hydrothorax.* In addition to severe dyspnea, patients with tension hydrothorax may be hypotensive from reduced cardiac output and have jugular venous distention.

Radiographic Findings. Radiographic study is the key for diagnosis of pleural effusion. Except for blunting of the costophrenic angle, small effusions may not be easy to identify in routine x-ray films, but they can be demonstrated by the lateral decubitus technique. In more typical cases with moderate amount of pleural fluid, characteristic homogeneous density in the dependent part of the hemithorax will be seen, which obscures the diaphragm and fills the costophrenic angle. This density spreads upward, merging imperceptibly with the rest of the lung field (Fig. 22–2). In massive pleural effusion, the entire hemithorax may be obscured by the fluid. Sometimes, when the fluid is under significant pressure (tension hydrothorax), the mediastinum is pushed to the opposite side. Radiographic study in the lateral decubitus position is important for detecting or verifying small or questionable effusions.

There are various atypical presentations of pleural fluid on chest radiographs, such as loculated fluid in a part of the pleural cavity, particularly in an interlobar fissure, or subpulmonic accumulation of fluid between the lung and diaphragm. In situations in which the diagnosis of pleural effusion remains uncertain after appropriate standard radiographic studies, thoracic ultrasound (US) or computed tomography (CT) scan would be very helpful both for the diagnosis and for the localization of pleural fluid, especially when thoracentesis is being considered.

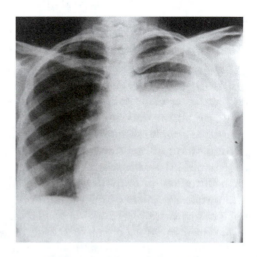

Figure 22–2. Radiograph of pleural effusion.

Examination of Fluid. Although the diagnosis of pleural effusion is often made prior to thoracentesis, sometimes it is necessary to ascertain its presence by diagnostic pleural tap. Frequently, this is done to obtain fluid for examination and occasionally for therapeutic reasons. Etiologic diagnosis may be suspected from the clinical picture; however, examination of fluid is essential for definitive diagnosis in the majority of cases.

The gross appearance of fluid may give a significant clue; grossly bloody fluid following chest trauma or surgery, pus in empyema, or milky appearance in chylothorax are a few examples. Bloody effusion without history of chest trauma suggests malignancy or PE.

Fluid is usually examined for its cell count and differential. Presence of predominantly polymorphonuclear leukocytes is suggestive of pyogenic infection; predominance of lymphocytes may suggest TB or malignancy. In more than 50% of pleural fluids due to malignancy, the cytologic examination will be diagnostic. Determination of biochemical content of the fluid (eg, protein, sugar, certain enzymes) will help in differentiating certain causes of pleural effusion. Determination of pleural fluid pH is also valuable in the differential diagnosis. Bacteriologic examination of the fluid is of special importance in many instances, and probably should be done on all fluids obtained for diagnostic purpose.

Pleural Biopsy. In some cases the etiologic diagnosis of pleural effusion cannot be made despite careful examination of the fluid and other clinical and laboratory studies. Pleural biopsy then becomes necessary; with one of the biopsy needles presently available, small pieces of parietal pleura can be obtained. They are submitted for histologic as well as bacteriologic studies. Biopsy under visual control may be performed with the help of a thoracoscope (pleuroscope). Occasionally, open pleural biopsy is considered when simpler studies remain inconclusive.

Management. The identification and proper treatment of the cause of pleural effusion are the principles of its successful management. Sometimes, when the pleural effusion is large enough to cause symptoms, removal of part or all of the fluid will be helpful for temporary palliation while waiting for the effect of more specific treatment. Tension hydrothorax should be promptly tapped. When the underlying disease is not effectively treatable, such as in malignant pleural effusion, measures to remove the fluid and cause adhesion of pleural surfaces *(pleurodesis)* will be beneficial. For this purpose, tube drainage will be necessary. Tetracycline derivatives (minocycline, doxycycline) are commonly used agents to cause pleurodesis by intrapleural administration. Talc, in the form of poudrage or slurry, is also an effective agent for developing pleural adhesion. A chest tube insertion is necessary for complete evacuation of fluid and administration of agents for pleurodesis. In hemothorax, blood should be evacuated by tube drainage in order to assess the blood loss and prevent the development of fibrothorax.

Pleural Empyema

When the pleural fluid is grossly purulent or contains pyogenic organisms, it is called *empyema.* Pathogenic organisms may enter the pleural space from the underlying infectious focus in the lung, such as pneumonia or lung abscess, following thoracic surgery or penetrating chest wound, and rarely from other sources. The common causative organisms are anaerobic bacteria, pneumococcus, staphylococcus, streptococcus, and certain gram-negative bacteria.

In addition to the symptoms and signs of pleural effusion, the patient with empyema usually has fever and other manifestations of bacterial infection. Thoracentesis with demonstration of characteristic fluid and isolation of causative organisms is diagnostic.

Although in its early stage thoracentesis and proper antibiotic therapy may occasionally suffice, most patients with empyema will need tube drainage for a successful outcome. When the empyema has been present for some time and there is indication of loculation of pus, thoracotomy with rib resection may be necessary. Rarely, with the development of thick pleural peel, decortication will be indicated. The presence of bronchopleural fistula (communication of the pleural space with the bronchial tree), which is fairly common with postpneumonectomy empyema, requires more prolonged tube drainage and suction. Sometimes extensive surgical procedures may be necessary.

■ PNEUMOTHORAX

Pneumothorax, or presence of air in the pleural space, is a relatively common clinical condition. It is classified into the two general categories of *spontaneous* and *traumatic. Artificial pneumothorax,* which is intentional introduction of air into the pleural space, was commonly used for treatment of pulmonary TB before the availability of effective chemotherapeutic agents. It is rarely used currently, and then almost exclusively for special diagnostic purpose (pleuroscopy or thora-

coscopy). Pneumothorax developing in connection with positive pressure ventilation is included in the traumatic category.

Etiology. Pneumothorax is called spontaneous when it develops without accidental or intentional trauma, regardless of the presence or absence of obvious pleuropulmonary disease. When it occurs in apparently healthy individuals, it is called *idiopathic spontaneous pneumothorax.* This type of spontaneous pneumothorax is predominantly a disease of young males. Most patients are tall and thin and have a long and narrow chest. The underlying pathology, which can be demonstrated in most patients undergoing thoracotomy or thoracoscopy, is the presence of apical subpleural air cysts or blebs. It is the rupture of one of these superficial bullous lesions that produces pneumothorax.

In the past, pulmonary TB was considered to be a major cause of spontaneous pneumothorax. It may occur in several diverse pleuropulmonary diseases; however, chronic obstructive lung disease (COLD), especially emphysema, is the most common underlying clinically recognizable disorder. In patients with acquired immunodeficiency syndrome (AIDS), spontaneous pneumothorax may result from *Pneumocystis carinii* pneumonia (PCP). Spontaneous pneumothorax is frequently a repeatedly recurring condition.

Traumatic pneumothorax is a common consequence of chest injury. It is a pneumothorax that is usually due to laceration of the visceral pleura, often with a broken rib, or as the result of a stab wound of the chest. Chest or neck surgery is another traumatic cause of air entry into the pleural cavity. It may occur following tracheostomy. Several diagnostic and therapeutic procedures may induce pneumothorax by inadvertent or unavoidable perforation or laceration of visceral pleura. Thoracentesis, pleural biopsy, percutaneous or transbronchial lung biopsy, subclavian vein puncture, and some other procedures may be complicated by pneumothorax.

The use of positive pressure breathing, either intermittently or continuously, particularly when higher pressures are required, may result in pneumothorax (barotrauma). This potential complication of positive pressure respiration should be emphasized to the healthcare professionals involved with such therapeutic interventions.

Pathophysiology. When there is free communication between the pleural space and atmospheric air, the "negative" pressure in the pleural cavity will become atmospheric and, because of its recoil, the lung will collapse. The ventilation of the collapsed lung will be markedly reduced; as a result, that of the opposite lung will increase. Reduced O_2 and increased CO_2 tension, and perhaps other factors, cause diminution of blood flow to the collapsed lung; thus, the contralateral lung will receive a larger share of blood supply. Although this regulatory mechanism is not complete, it will greatly improve the ventilation–perfusion relationship, and thus will prevent severe hypoxemia.

When the communication between the pleural space and the atmosphere is sealed, the trapped air will undergo absorption, resulting in gradual reestablishment of subatmospheric pressure and reexpansion of the lung. As oxygen content of the pneumothorax is absorbed faster, the air in a pneumothorax has higher nitrogen and CO_2 tensions than atmospheric air.

In some instances, the communication behaves as a one-way valve, allowing the air to enter the pleural cavity during elevation of intrathoracic pressure with cough or other expiratory efforts but preventing its exit. Under this circumstance the pressure in the pneumothorax will become higher than atmospheric. This increased pressure may cause significant shift of the heart and other mediastinal structures to the opposite side, thus impairing the function of the other lung also (Fig. 22–3). Moreover, elevated intrathoracic pressure may impede cardiac function by reducing venous return. This condition is called *tension pneumothorax.* Severe respiratory distress with profound hypoxemia and circulatory collapse are the consequences of this life-threatening event, which necessitates immediate treatment. Tension pneumothorax is more commonly seen when pneumothorax occurs following chest trauma or as a result of ventilator-induced barotrauma.

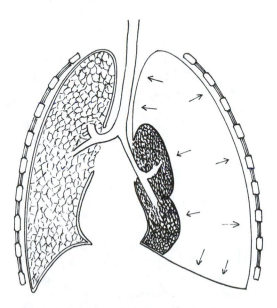

Figure 22–3. Diagrammatic demonstration of tension pneumothorax on the left side. There is a shift of the heart and mediastinum to the right.

Clinical Manifestation. The most common presenting symptom of pneumothorax is dyspnea. The severity of dyspnea and its progression depend on the extent of the pneumothorax, presence or absence of underlying pulmonary condition, and tension. In many cases it is more severe at the beginning than several hours later, despite lack of change in the amount of pneumothorax. The combination of sudden onset of sharp chest pain and dyspnea in an otherwise healthy young adult male is highly suggestive of spontaneous pneumothorax. The initial severe sharp pain is usually followed soon by a dull ache. Sudden aggravation of dyspnea in patients with COLD, spontaneously or with certain diagnostic or therapeutic interventions mentioned earlier, should arouse suspicion of pneumothorax. Severe dyspnea immediately after an accident frequently is due to pneumothorax, which may be a tension pneumothorax.

Physical examination may show evidence of respiratory distress and cyanosis if the pneumothorax is significant. Reduced to absent breath sounds with resonant percussion note over one hemithorax are the most common physical findings when the pneumothorax is large. In a small pneumothorax, physical examination may be entirely normal. Development of pneumothorax in a patient on a ventilator manifests by an acute deterioration of respiratory mechanics and arterial blood gases. If unrecognized, it may rapidly progress to severe hemodynamic impairment, difficulty with mechanical ventilation, and eventual death.

Radiographic Findings and Diagnosis. Radiographic examination is the key to the diagnosis of pneumothorax, assessment of its amount, and evaluation of underlying and associated conditions. X-ray films taken at full expiration accentuate the pneumothorax and, therefore, help in demonstration of a small amount of air in the pleural cavity. With significant pneumothorax, the entire lung seems to have detached from the chest wall, maintaining its connection with the lower half of the mediastinum and medial portion of the diaphragm (Fig. 22–4). Because of reduction of its blood and presence of air around the lung, the density of moderately collapsed lung usually will not be increased. It is the difference between the lung with its markings and air in the pleural space without such markings that helps in the detection of pneumothorax. When the lung is completely collapsed, its volume is markedly diminished and its density is increased. Tension pneumothorax results in total collapse of the underlying lung and significant deviation of the heart and mediastinum to the opposite side (see Fig. 22–3).

Management. Small to moderate asymptomatic pneumothorax, except in association with advanced lung disease or in patients on mechanical ventilation, will

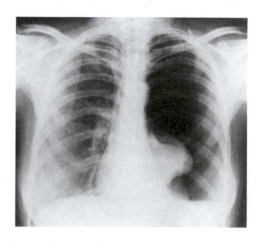

Figure 22–4. Left pneumothorax resulting in complete collapse of the left lung.

require no special treatment, but only adequate follow-up until the lung is totally expanded. Once the pleural tear is sealed, which often happens spontaneously, the air in the pleural space will be absorbed, but it may require several days to weeks for completion. Symptomatic patients, those with underlying respiratory insufficiency, and those on mechanical ventilation, will need a chest tube for more rapid evacuation of the air. Tension pneumothorax is an emergency and should be immediately relieved by any available means, such as insertion of a needle into the pleural space, which will allow the air under positive pressure to escape. This should be followed by tube thoracostomy or insertion of a Heimlich catheter. The application of excessive negative pressure for evacuation of air from the pleural cavity should be avoided; otherwise, pulmonary edema may develop.

Spontaneous pneumothorax, being a recurrent problem, requires a well-planned follow-up. Most thoracic surgeons recommend thoracotomy in suitable patients when more than one episode of pneumothorax develops spontaneously, at the same or the opposite side, or when there is persistent air leak with a chest tube, preventing the expansion of the lung. The commonly recommended surgical procedures are excision of lung blebs, pleural abrasion, or both. Pleural abrasion results in the adhesion of pleural surfaces. It appears that the simpler methods of pleurodesis with intrapleural sclerosing agents, such as a tetracycline derivative and talc, is increasingly replacing surgical methods for prevention of recurrent spontaneous pneumothorax, especially in patients who are poor surgical risks.

BIBLIOGRAPHY

Bartter T, Santarelli R, Akers SM, Pratter MR. The evaluation of pleural effusion. *Chest.* 1994; 106:1209–1214.

Broaddus VC. Infections in the pleural space: an update on pathogenesis and management. *Semin Respir Crit Care Med.* 1995; 16:303–314.

Hott JW. Malignant pleural effusion. *Semin Respir Crit Care Med.* 1995; 16:333–339.

Jantz MA, Pierson DJ. Pneumothorax and barotrauma. *Clin Chest Med.* 1994; 15(1): 75–91.

Joseph J, Sahn SA. Connective tissue diseases and the pleura. *Chest.* 1993; 104:262–270.

Kennedy L, Sahn SA. Talc pleurodesis for the treatment of pneumothorax and pleural effusion. *Chest.* 1994; 106:1215–1222.

Kinsasewitz GT. Pneumothorax. *Semin Respir Crit Care Med.* 1995; 16:293–302.

LeMense GP, Strange C, Sahn SA. Empyema thoracis: therapeutic management and outcome. *Chest.* 1995; 107:1532–1537.

Light RW. Management of spontaneous pneumothorax. *Am Rev Respir Dis.* 1993; 148: 245–248.

Light RW. Pleural diseases. *Dis Mon.* 1992; 38:263–331.

Quigley RL. Thoracentesis and chest tube drainage. *Crit Care Clin.* 1995; 11:111–126.

Sahn SA. The diagnostic value of pleural fluid analysis. *Semin Respir Crit Care Med.* 1995; 16:269–278.

Sahn SA. The pathophysiology of pleural effusion. *Annu Rev Med.* 1990; 41:7–13.

Sepkowitz KA, Telzak EE, Gold JWM, et al. Pneumothorax in AIDS. *Ann Intern Med.* 1991; 114:455–459.

Strange C. Hemothorax. *Semin Respir Crit Care Med.* 1995; 16:324–332.

Walker-Renard PB, Vaughan LM, Sahn SA. Chemical pleurodesis for malignant pleural effusions. *Ann Intern Med.* 1994; 120: 56–64.

Diseases of the Thoracic Wall and Chest Trauma

The thoracic wall and diaphragm, which enclose and protect vitally important organs, are essential structures for the production of necessary forces and their effective utilization for respiratory movements (respiratory pump). A proper interaction between the chest wall and respiratory muscles determines the forces necessary to change the geometry of the thorax, which in turn changes the lung volume for effective ventilation. Therefore, disorders of the chest wall, either congenital or from trauma and surgery, may result in ventilatory impairment more or less similar to one caused by respiratory neuromuscular diseases (see Chapter 24).

■ DISEASES OF THE CHEST WALL

By far the most important pathologic condition of the bony thorax is traumatic injury. Among the various thoracic defor-mities, *funnel chest (pectus excavatum)* and *pigeon breast (pectus carinatum)* are quite common. In funnel chest, the sternum is depressed and the ribs on each side protrude more anteriorly. In pigeon breast, there is abnormal prominence of the sternum due to its forward projection. These deformities, which may be quite remarkable in their physical and radiographic appearances, rarely result in significant respiratory disturbance.

Kyphoscoliosis

Because of the insertion of the ribs to the vertebrae, significant deformity of the thoracic cage may result from abnormal curvature of the dorsal spine. *Kyphosis* is the increased posterior convexity of the thoracic spine; *scoliosis* is the sideways deviation of the spine (Figs. 23–1 and 23–2). For some unknown reason, the convexity of the curvature in scoliosis is toward the right in most cases. Angles of curvature in both scoliosis and kyphosis are inscribed

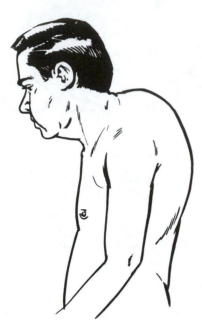

Figure 23–1. Kyphosis of the dorsal spine.

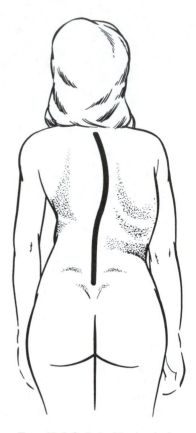

Figure 23–2. Scoliosis of the dorsal spine.

by the straight lines parallel to the upper and lower limbs of the curvature. The combination of these two deformities is referred to as *kyphoscoliosis*.

In scoliosis and kyphoscoliosis, in addition to its abnormal curvature, the spine is usually rotated around its longitudinal axis so that the spinous processes of the vertebrae are directed toward the lateral concavity of the curve (Fig. 23–3). The ribs on the convexity protrude posteriorly; the ribs on the concave side, which are crowded together, are more prominent anteriorly. In severe kyphoscoliosis, the deformity of the chest is, therefore, quite extensive.

Abnormal curvature of the thoracic spine has various causes, such as congenital, traumatic, paralytic, and infectious. Tuberculosis (TB) of the spine used to be a very common cause of this deformity. Among neuromuscular disorders, poliomyelitis and syringomyelia are fre-

quently associated with spinal deformity. However, the vast majority of patients with scoliosis or kyphoscoliosis have no known underlying disease. This condition, which is four times more common in females than in males, is called *idiopathic kyphoscoliosis*. This deformity may become apparent in childhood or adolescence, and progresses with the patient's growth.

Children and young adults with kyphoscoliosis usually are asymptomatic. In severe cases, the symptoms and signs of cardiorespiratory embarrassment do not ordinarily appear until the fourth or fifth decade of life. Dyspnea, frequent pulmonary infection, progressive respiratory

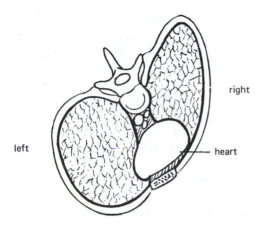

Figure 23–3. A transaxial diagrammatic view of the chest in kyphoscoliosis. There is a rotation of the spine along its longitudinal axis contributing to the deformity of the rib cage.

insufficiency, hypoxemia, hypercapnia, and eventual cardiac failure are the common cardiorespiratory manifestations of severe kyphoscoliosis.

Pulmonary function tests (PFTs) show reduced vital capacity and other changes of restrictive ventilatory impairment; however, the residual volume is usually increased. Low vital capacity is secondary to reduced chest-wall expansion and abnormal geometry of the diaphragm. Increased residual volume is mainly from limitation of the thoracic cage in reducing its volume with maximum expiration. There is uneven ventilation in relation to the blood flow, causing increased dead-space ventilation and hypoxemia. In more advanced disease, alveolar hypoventilation further aggravates the hypoxemia when cor pulmonale also occurs. Severe arterial blood desaturation during sleep is a common problem in advanced kyphoscoliosis. When combined with hypercapnia, nocturnal mechanical ventilation may be necessary.

Alveolar hypoventilation results from the progressive diminution of tidal volume associated with increased physiologic dead-space volume. Both mechanical factors and reduction in the efficiency of respiratory muscles contribute to ventilatory failure. As in other causes of chronic respiratory insufficiency, respiratory infections are major causes of frequent exacerbations. Early detection of spinal deformity, especially idiopathic kyphoscoliosis, is the key for its successful treatment and prevention of its progression. Various orthopedic procedures, such as spinal bracing, casting, and surgery may be considered dependent on the patient's age and stage and severity of the condition. Advanced cases in adult and middle-age patients are usually not amenable to corrective procedures. Therapeutic measures in such cases should be centered around prevention and early treatment of respiratory tract infection and proper supportive care.

■ CHEST TRAUMA

Chest trauma continues to be one of the most common causes of morbidity and mortality among casualties of military conflicts and victims of peacetime accidents and violent crimes. Respiratory care providers will be involved in the management of patients with thoracic trauma and surgery, which almost invariably affect respiration. Mechanisms through which respiration is affected in such patients vary and depend on the severity and extent of injury and the structures involved.

Disruption of integrity of the thoracic wall and diaphragm, tear of the pleura with resultant accumulation of air and/or blood in the pleural cavity, and injury to the lung parenchyma and tracheobronchial tree are among the lesions resulting from chest trauma that directly impair respiration. However, because of the presence of other structures in the thorax, such as the heart, pericardium, aorta and other major blood vessels, and the esophagus, chest trauma may involve these organs as well. Moreover, injury to the chest is frequently accompanied by trauma to other areas of the body, such as the abdomen, head, neck, spine, and extremities. Respiration, therefore, not only is affected by direct trauma to the chest, but also may be impaired indirectly by injury elsewhere. Severe trauma to the head and the neck may result in upper airway obstruction. Head injury, in addition, may cause respiratory difficulty as a result of loss of consciousness. Spinal cord injury, particularly in the cervical region, affects respiration through respiratory muscle paralysis. Shock due to blood loss, severe trauma, or infection may cause diffuse pulmonary lesion ("shock lung"). Fat embolism is another possible complication of traumatic injury, especially following fractures of large bones. Patients with such injuries are also prone to develop thromboembolic disorders.

Because of the scope of this book, the remainder of this chapter is limited to a brief discussion of traumatic injuries to various structures of the chest.

Simple Rib Fracture

Mild chest-wall injury from blunt trauma usually results in no more than transient pain or tenderness of no significant consequence. Associated rib fracture, however, which is a very common occurrence, may be accompanied or followed by other more significant lesions. Splinting of the chest movement because of severe pain and inability to cough may result in atelectasis or pneumonia, especially

in the elderly. Patients with underlying chronic respiratory impairment are particularly susceptible to these complications. Associated pneumothorax or hemothorax should be looked for.

Rib fracture may occur at the point of impact or may result from its excessive bending by indirect forces (Fig. 23–4). Uncomplicated rib fracture is usually treated symptomatically with analgesics. Sometimes injection of a local anesthetic at the fracture site or an intercostal nerve block may be necessary to

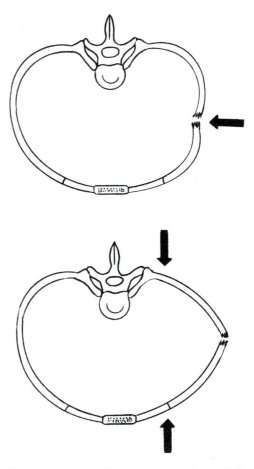

Figure 23–4. Diagrams of rib fractures due to direct and indirect forces.

control the pain and allow the patient to take deep breaths and cough. Multiple broken ribs often indicate the presence of other intrathoracic injuries, especially when the first rib is also fractured.

Flail Chest

Single fracture of a few ribs at one point of their length without separating from their cartilage does not result in mechanical impairment of the chest wall. However, when there are double fractures of three or more adjacent ribs, or fracture of several ribs with separation from their cartilage or fracture of the sternum, a portion of the rib cage will lose its continuity with the rest of the bony thorax (Figs. 23–5 and 23–6). This condition is commonly known as *flail chest.*

Flail chest is usually the result of severe chest trauma and, therefore, is frequently accompanied by evidence of pleural lesion, pulmonary contusion, and injury to other structures. Steering wheel injury is a common cause of this condition.

The mechanical effect of flail chest and the resultant ventilatory disturbance are due to paradoxical movement of the unsupported portion of the chest wall (Fig. 23–7). During inspiration, while the rest of the chest is expanding, the unstable portion moves inward due to more negative intrathoracic pressure. On expiration, particularly during forced expiration, it bulges outward. If the flail segment is large, the mediastinum swings in the same direction as the unsupported portion. The amplitude of paradoxical movements will depend on the size of the flail segment and pressure changes inside the thorax. As the pressure changes in the chest during the respiratory cycle

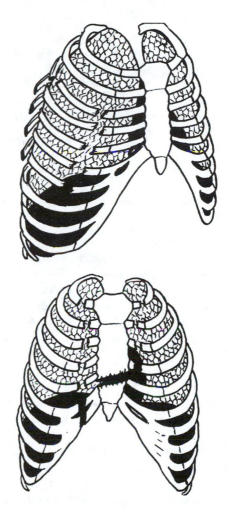

Figures 23–5 and 23–6. Drawings of the rib cage showing flail chest by two mechanisms. The upper diagram shows double fractures of several ribs. The lower drawing shows fractures of cartilages of ribs and the sternum.

vary with the compliance of the lungs and thoracic wall, as well as with airway resistance, conditions that result in reduced compliance or increased airway resistance will augment the amplitude of the paradoxical movements. Associated pleuropulmonary lesions due to direct or

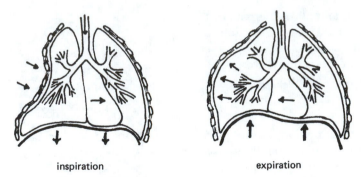

inspiration   expiration

Figure 23–7. Paradoxical movement in flail chest. During inspiration, the flailed segment is sucked in, whereas during expiration, it bulges out.

indirect effects of injury makes the presence of flail chest more evident and its ventilatory effects more manifest. Inefficient ventilation results in increased work of breathing. Ineffective cough and accumulation of secretions result in further ventilatory impairment and eventual respiratory failure.

In the management of patients with flail chest, every effort should be made to correct the conditions that increase airway resistance and/or reduce the compliance. Restoration and maintenance of adequate airway, tracheobronchial toilet, control of infection, treatment of pulmonary congestion, restriction of fluid, and evacuation of air or fluid from the pleural cavity are measures that minimize the deleterious effect of flail chest. Supplemental oxygen is necessary in most patients. Multiple intercostal nerve blocks or epidural block are often used for pain relief. Strapping the chest, especially circumferential adhesive taping, should be avoided as it further compromises ventilation and promotes retention of secretions and atelectasis. Therapeutic success in management of flail chest will depend more on these measures than preoccupation with stabilization of the flail seg-

ment. Many of these patients can be successfully managed without mechanical ventilation or other measures intended to stabilize the chest wall.

The old methods of external chest-wall stabilization, such as traction of the loose segment by various devices, are rarely, if ever, used currently. Surgical fixation, however, is occasionally performed when concomitant intrathoracic injury requires open thoracotomy or when, with a large flail segment, more conventional methods fail to improve paradoxical movement in a reasonable amount of time. A simple and quick way in emergency situations is gentle but firm pressure with the palm of the hand against the flail segment, the placement of sandbags or even turning the patient onto the injured side while being transported to the hospital or waiting for more definitive therapy.

Internal stabilization by mechanical positive pressure ventilation has been much more effective and practical in most situations in need of stabilization. Moreover, associated pulmonary and extrathoracic injury may necessitate assisted ventilation, regardless of the presence or absence of flail chest. For the purpose of internal fixation, intubation or tracheostomy with a large tube is usually required. It is often necessary, at least initially, to sedate the patient or even paralyze the respiratory muscles for effective ventilation (controlled ventilation) and prevention of excessive movement of the flail segment. In recent years an increasing number of patients with flail chest have been successfully managed by nonventilatory means. With proper respiratory care and prevention of complications that impair the mechanical properties of the lung, the need for prolonged ventilatory support can be lessened. The patients who initially require ventilatory assistance may be weaned off the respirator successfully, even before the chest wall regains stability, provided that other complications are brought under control.

Diaphragmatic Injury

Diaphragmatic injury may result from a perforating wound but, in civilian practice, it is more commonly due to blunt trauma to the chest and/or abdomen. As with chest-wall injury, automobile accidents are the most frequent causes of diaphragmatic injury. Falls from heights may also result in rupture of the diaphragm. Although diaphragmatic injury is usually indicative of severe trauma, sometimes rupture of the diaphragm may follow a blow to the chest or abdomen that appears to be insignificant. Diaphragmatic rupture from blunt trauma occurs on the left side more frequently than on the right side.

Usually, the manifestations of diaphragmatic lesion are overshadowed by those of more obvious injuries to the chest or other organs. It may, therefore, remain unrecognized. Many such lesions are identified during abdominal exploration for treatment of other traumatic injuries, especially laceration of the spleen or the liver. *Herniation* of the abdominal viscera through the diaphragmatic rent may take place immediately or some variable time after the trauma. The symptoms and signs of diaphragmatic injury, which are usually due to herniation, are cardiorespiratory and/or gastrointestinal (GI) in nature. Dyspnea, cough, and palpitation are common cardiorespiratory symptoms due to significant herniation. Diminished thoracic excursion, impairment of percussion note, reduction of breath sounds, and presence of bowel sounds in the chest may be detected on physical examination of the thorax. Respiratory embarrassment may be severe in large diaphragmatic ruptures. GI manifestations are usually due to compression and obstruction of the stomach and bowels. Nausea, vomiting, and abdominal distension may indicate such complications.

Radiographic studies are essential for diagnosis of diaphragmatic injury. Plain x-ray films may be highly suggestive of diaphragmatic hernia, but examination with contrast material is necessary for definitive diagnosis.

The diaphragmatic rupture is treated surgically when noted during abdominal exploration or after the diagnosis is established by appropriate radiographic studies.

Pleural Injury

Penetrating chest wounds often result in pleural laceration, but blunt chest trauma, which is much more common in civilian medicine, may also cause injury to both the parietal and visceral pleurae, especially when accompanied by rib fractures.

Traumatic pleural injury results in accumulation of air and/or blood in the pleural cavity. It is only rarely that air gains access to the pleural space from a chest-wall wound, producing *open pneumothorax* (sucking chest wound). By far the most common mechanism of production of traumatic pneumothorax is the entrance of air through a visceral pleural rent. (Pneumothorax is discussed on page 322.) It should be emphasized that tension pneumothorax is more frequent with traumatic pneumothorax. Moreover, traumatic pneumothorax is commonly associated with the accumulation of blood in the pleural space, which is then called *hemopneumothorax*. The accumulation of air in subcutaneous tissue (*subcutaneous emphysema*), which may be quite extensive, is common with traumatic pneumothorax.

Hemothorax, with or without pneumothorax, is a common complication of thoracic injury, either penetrating or blunt. Bleeding into the pleural space is mostly due to laceration of the parietal pleura along with a thoracic wall vessel, usually an intercostal artery and sometimes the internal mammary artery. The amount of blood varies from minimal to massive. The immediate problems with hemothorax are related to acute blood loss as well as respiratory embarrassment. Shock and tension hemothorax may result.

Minimal hemothorax requires no treatment except for close observation. When small, blood usually is resolved within a couple of weeks without residue. Moderate hemothorax may be managed by thoracentesis; however, if blood reaccumulates, it should be drained by a chest tube. Accurate measurement of blood loss is important for its replacement by transfusion. The patient's own blood from the pleural cavity may be used (autotransfusion), provided that it is not contaminated and is collected aseptically.

Massive hemothorax, which usually indicates rapid and continuous bleeding from a large vessel, is an emergency and should be treated promptly by pleural drainage and restoration of circulating blood volume. Continuation of significant bleeding is an indication for exploratory surgery.

Rarely, as a result of injury to the thoracic duct (the major lymph vessel in the chest), milky effusion, or *chylothorax*, may develop.

Pulmonary Parenchymal Injury

Lung contusion, or pulmonary bruise, is the most common parenchymal pulmonary injury due to direct chest trauma. It results from the accumulation of edema fluid and blood inside the alveoli, as well as interstitial tissue. The mechanism of its development is thought to be sudden compression and decompression of lung tissue, causing severe pressure changes in the distal airways, alveolar spaces, and interstitium. Pulmonary contusion may be associated with injuries to the chest wall and other parts of the thoracic structures. It is almost always present when chest-wall injury is severe enough to cause flail chest. A small area of lung contusion does not result in significant symptoms referable to the lesion. However, when the contusion is more extensive, respiratory symptoms and signs of dyspnea, cough, hemoptysis, rales, and cyanosis may be present. In more severe cases the clinical picture of acute respiratory distress syndrome (ARDS) will develop. Radiographic examination will show airspace consolidation of patchy or homogeneous pattern, which has no segmental distribution. The changes become apparent within a few hours following trauma and start to resolve in 24 to 48 hours.

Laceration and hematoma of the lung often result from a penetrating injury, but it may be secondary to blunt chest trauma. Several alveolar spaces are disrupted, resulting in the formation of a cavitary space filled with blood. Sometimes an air-filled cystic lesion may develop. Thoracic computed tomography (CT) has shown that lung laceration, often missed by standard chest radiography, is very common in association with pulmonary contusion.

The trachea or bronchi may uncommonly be the site of traumatic injury, which may range from mild laceration of the mucosa to partial or complete fracture, with or without separation of the fragments. These injuries are frequently overlooked because of other associated injuries. Hemoptysis, surprisingly, is not common. Pneumothorax, pneumomediastinum, and subcutaneous emphysema are commonly present. Persistent and progressive pneumothorax, despite a chest tube, is highly suggestive of tracheobronchial injury. Complete atelectasis may be the result of separation of fractured bronchial fragments. Bronchoscopy is the key to accurate diagnosis in most cases.

ACUTE TRAUMATIC RESPIRATORY FAILURE

From the foregoing discussion it is evident that acute respiratory failure in patients with severe chest trauma may have various causes that, singly or in combination and by different mechanisms, impair respiratory function. Furthermore, the common association of extrathoracic injury may contribute significantly to respiratory complications. Figure 23–8 schematically demonstrates the various factors involved in causing respiratory failure in patients with severe traumatic injury to the chest and extrathoracic structures. Mechanical effects of flail chest, pneumothorax, hemothorax, diaphragmatic tear, and airway laceration

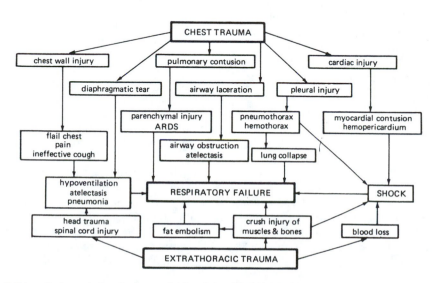

Figure 23–8. Schematic demonstration of pathogenesis of respiratory failure in thoracic and extrathoracic trauma. Note the multiplicity of factors that cause or contribute to respiratory failure.

with resultant hypoventilation and atelectasis are usually combined with and intensified by pulmonary parenchymal injury from direct trauma as well as indirect causes. Shock may result from both intrathoracic and extrathoracic injuries including hemothorax, cardiac tamponade from bleeding inside the pericardial sac, other severe internal hemorrhage, myocardial contusion, and crush injury. As one of the important causes of ARDS, shock is a major factor in the pathogenesis of acute traumatic respiratory failure (Chapter 27). Pulmonary fat embolism from multiple bone fractures is also known to result in ARDS.

In the management of patients with traumatic respiratory failure, all of the previously mentioned factors should be identified and properly treated. Restoration and maintenance of an adequate airway, optimal oxygenation, and ventilatory support whenever needed are the most important steps in their successful management. The obvious mechanical problems, such as significant pneumothorax or hemothorax, should be corrected immediately. Hypovolemic and cardiogenic shock should be promptly treated, avoiding overhydration. Every effort should be made to prevent avoidable complications, such as atelectasis, aspiration, or infection.

BIBLIOGRAPHY

Bollinger CT, Van Eeden SF. Treatment of multiple rib fractures: randomized controlled trial comparing ventilatory with nonventilatory management. *Chest.* 1990; 97: 943–948.

Campbell DB. Trauma to chest wall, lung, and major airways. *Semin Thorac Cardiovasc Surg.* 1992; 4:234–240.

Ciraulo DL, Elliott D, Mitchell KA, Rodriguez A. Flail chest as a marker for significant injuries. *J Am College Surg.* 1994; 178:466–470.

Jackinczyk K. Blunt chest trauma. *Emerg Med Clin North Am.* 1993; 11:81–96.

Keim HA, Hensinger RN. Spinal deformities: scoliosis and kyphosis. *Clin Symp.* 1989; 41(4):3–32.

Kshettry VR, Bolman RM III. Chest trauma: assessment, diagnosis, and management. *Clin Chest Med.* 1994; 15(1):137–146.

McRitchie DI, Matthews JG, Fink MP. Pneumonia in patients with multiple trauma. *Clin Chest Med.* 1995; 16:135–146.

Pate JW. Chest wall injuries. *Surg Clin North Am.* 1989; 69:59–70.

Pehrsson K, Larsson S, Oden A, Nachemson A. Long-term follow-up of patients with untreated scoliosis. *Spine.* 1992; 17:1091–1096.

Pepe PE. Acute post-traumatic respiratory physiology and insufficiency. *Surg Clin North Am.* 1989; 69:157–173.

Pinilla JC. Acute respiratory failure in severe blunt chest trauma. *J Trauma.* 1982; 22:221–226.

Richardson JD, Adams L, Flint LM. Selective management of flail chest and pulmonary contusion. *Ann Surg.* 1982; 196:481–487.

Rinsky LA. Advances in management of idiopathic scoliosis. *Hosp Pract.* 1992; 27(4): 47–53.

Shamberger RC. Congenital chest wall deformities. *Curr Probl Surg.* 1996; 33:474–542.

Symbas PN, Gott JP. Delayed sequelae of thoracic trauma. *Surg Clin North Am.* 1989; 69:135–142.

van der Werken C, Lubbers EJC, Goris RJA. Rupture of the diaphragm by blunt trauma as a marker of injury severity. *Injury.* 1983; 15:149–152.

Wardle EN. Shock lungs: the post-traumatic respiratory distress syndrome. *Q J Med.* 1984; 53:317–329.

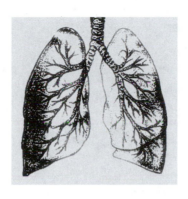

DISORDERS OF
RESPIRATORY CONTROL

24.

Neuromuscular and Central Nervous System Disorders Affecting Respiration

■ RESPIRATORY MUSCLES

Numerous muscles under various circumstances contribute to mechanical respiratory function. They include the diaphragm, muscles of the rib cage, abdominals, scalenes, and accessory muscles (Figs. 24–1 and 24–2).

The main respiratory muscles of the rib cage are the *external* and *internal intercostal muscles,* which are arranged in two layers—an outer layer and an inner layer—between the ribs and differ in their position and the direction of their fibers. It is generally accepted that the external intercostal muscles and interchondral portion of the internal intercostals (parasternals) are inspiratory, whereas the remaining internal intercostal muscles are expiratory. In addition, the contraction of these muscles serves to stabilize the intercostal spaces, preventing them

from being pulled in or pushed out during the respiratory cycle. The innervation of these muscles is by the intercostal nerves, which originate from the spinal cord at corresponding levels of the dorsal spine.

The diaphragm is the principal muscle of inspiration. It is a musculotendinous partition between the abdomen and thorax, anchored all around the circumference of the lower border of the thoracic cage. In its relaxed position it is dome shaped, but on contraction its central part will move downward, increasing the vertical dimension of the thorax. It also raises the lower ribs, thus enlarging the chest cavity further. In quiet breathing, the diaphragm appears to be the only active inspiratory muscle, but the external intercostal, interchondral, and scalene muscles are also active during inspiration. The diaphragm is not dispensable

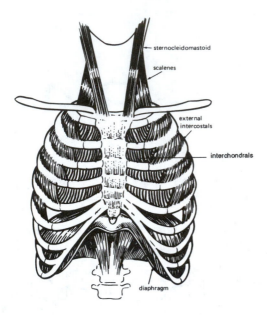

Figure 24–1. Inspiratory muscles. The diaphragm and external intercostals are used with normal breathing. Sternocleidomastoids, scalenes, and other accessory inspiratory muscles are also used when the work of breathing is markedly increased. Note that the interchondral parts of the internal intercostals are also inspiratory muscles.

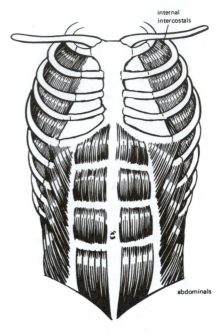

Figure 24–2. Expiratory muscles. The major expiratory muscles are abdominals and internal intercostals except for their interchondral portion.

for breathing as long as the thorax and its muscles are normal; respiration can be maintained without the diaphragm participating, as in bilateral diaphragmatic paralysis. With general anesthesia, as the other inspiratory muscles become inactive, the diaphragm remains the only muscle to sustain spontaneous ventilation. The diaphragm is also essential when the intercostal muscles are paralyzed or when the bony thorax becomes rigid and immobile. Each half of the diaphragm is innervated by the phrenic nerve, which originates chiefly from the fourth cervical nerve, but is augmented by fibers from the third and fifth nerves.

In addition to the diaphragm and the intercostal and scalene muscles, other muscles are called into play when there is special need during increased inspiratory effort. Among these, the sternocleidomastoids are the most important. Serratus, trapezius, pectoralis, and other muscles may participate under certain situations.

Expiration is passive with quiet breathing. During the active contraction of the inspiratory muscles, the elastic tissues of the lung and chest wall are stretched, storing potential energy. It is the release of this stored energy by recoil of stretched tissues that engenders expiratory movement. Expiratory muscles, however, actively participate when there is increased ventiliation and under certain situations in which high expiratory pressures are required, such as with airway obstruction, coughing, sneezing, blowing, straining, and talking. The most important expiratory muscles are the abdominals.

Contraction of these muscles reduces the volume of the thoracic cavity by forcing the diaphragm upward with increased abdominal pressure and by depressing the lower ribs. As mentioned previously, the internal intercostal muscles, except for the interchondral portion, are also expiratory muscles.

■ DISEASES OF THE MUSCLES

The diaphragmatic muscle may be the site of certain congenital or acquired defects that may impair its function. *Herniation* through congenital or acquired defects in the diaphragm is common, but rarely causes significant respiratory difficulty. The most common diaphragmatic hernia is that which occurs through an abnormality of the opening in the diaphragm through which the esophagus passes *(hiatus hernia)*. Congenital defects in other parts of the diaphragm may result in the entrance of abdominal viscera into the thoracic cavity, sometimes resulting in respiratory symptoms. A rare cause of respiratory distress in newborns is a large diaphragmatic hernia through one of these defects.

Penetrating or blunt trauma to the chest or abdomen may result in a diaphragmatic tear. Herniation through such a rupture may be immediate or may take place some time after the injury. The respiratory difficulty resulting from such a traumatic hernia may be overshadowed or complicated by associated injuries to the chest wall, lungs, and other organs. This is discussed in Chapter 23.

Respiratory muscles may be involved in various generalized muscular disorders of diverse causes. Deficiencies of certain enzymes essential for muscle metabolism are known to cause respiratory difficulty,

most commonly in infants and children, but these may also affect the ventilatory function later in life. *Acid maltase deficiency* is an especially important metabolic cause of myopathy in which ventilatory failure may be its predominant manifestation. In its adult form, acid maltase deficiency may manifest as bilateral diaphragmatic paralysis.

The major primary muscular diseases that often involve respiratory function are muscular dystrophies and inflammatory myopathies.

Muscular Dystrophies

Muscular dystrophies are a group of hereditary conditions characterized by progressive degeneration of the striated muscles, resulting in increasingly severe weakness. They have been classified according to certain clinical and genetic features. The most common form is *Duchenne dystrophy*, which because of its genetic characteristics (X-linked recessive) is essentially a disease of males. Becker dystrophy has the genetic and clinical features similar to Duchenne dystrophy, but Becker dystrophy manifests later and evolves more slowly. Other forms of muscular dystrophy, with an autosomal type of inheritance, are seen equally in both sexes.

The onset of muscular weakness, which is the only presenting symptom in most cases, is quite variable. In Duchenne dystrophy, the weakness starts early in life in the proximal muscles of the extremities. Once the child starts to walk, certain abnormalities can be detected, which become more evident as he grows older. Movements such as getting up from a sitting position or climbing stairs, which require proximal muscle strength, become more and more difficult. In early adolescence, the victim is usually unable to walk. Respiratory muscle weakness can be detected in the early teens, but the diaphragm is usually spared until later. Ventilation, which may be maintained during daytime, becomes impaired during sleep. Progressive increase in the severity of respiratory difficulty is aggravated further with each episode of frequently occurring respiratory tract infection. Rarely do patients with Duchenne dystrophy live beyond the age of 20 years. In other forms of muscular dystrophy, the onset is later and the type of dystrophy is usually designated according to the group of muscles that are primarily involved.

In *myotonic* muscular dystrophy, in addition to progressive muscular weakness, there are certain distinctive features. Difficulty in relaxing the contracted muscles, as in a hand grip, is quite characteristic (myotonia). Early development of cataracts, testicular atrophy, and frontal baldness are other associated features. Pulmonary complications are much more common in myotonic dystrophy than in other forms.

In muscular dystrophies, in addition to respiratory muscle involvement, there are frequent problems with swallowing and aspiration. Pulmonary function studies in most cases of muscular dystrophy demonstrate some abnormalities. Reduced vital capacity, maximum voluntary ventilation, and maximum expiratory and inspiratory forces are quite common. The severity of these abnormalities depends on the degree of respiratory muscle involvement.

As respiratory failure is the usual cause of death in these unfortunate young patients, their comprehensive management should include a well-planned respiratory care program.

Inflammatory Myopathies

Polymyositis, which is the major inflammatory muscle disease, is discussed in Chapter 14.

■ DISORDERS OF THE NEUROMUSCULAR JUNCTION

The junction of the motor nerve endings with the striated muscle (muscle end plate) is the area through which the nerve impulses are transmitted to the muscle (Fig. 24–3). This transmission is accomplished by liberation of acetylcholine from the nerve endings and its reaction with the special receptors at the muscle cell membrane. This interaction results in increased permeability of this membrane to such cations as sodium, potassium, and calcium. The crossing of these ions through the membrane results in the depolarization of muscle and the initiation of its action potential and contraction. An enzyme called *acetylcholinesterase* inactivates acetylcholine by hydrolysis; thus the muscle is repolarized and becomes ready for reception of another nerve impulse and initiation of another contraction. The proper function of this junctional region is, therefore, essential for orderly muscle activity.

Certain agents are known to disrupt the normal function of the neuromuscular junction. Drugs that interfere with the action of acetylcholinesterase (eg, neostigmine) result in the accumulation of acetylcholine in this region, thus facilitating the transmission of impulses through the myoneural junction; however, large doses of these drugs will result in muscle weakness. Neuromuscular blocking agents paralyze the muscles by blocking the access of acetylcholine to the motor end plate. Tubocurarine and other curariform drugs,

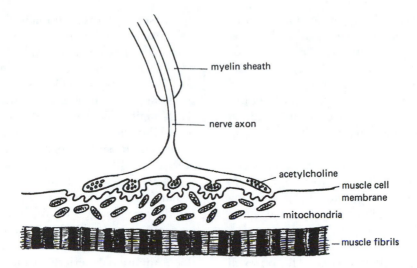

Figure 24–3. Neuromuscular junction.

such as pancuronium (Pavulon), act through this mechanism. Succinylcholine (Anectine), another type of paralyzing agent, causes depolarization of muscles, as does acetylcholine, but succinylcholine is inactivated much more slowly. Repolarization, which is essential for transmission of impulses from the nerve endings, is therefore prevented. These paralyzing agents are used as an adjunct in general anesthesia and for facilitation of management of patients undergoing intubation and mechanical ventilation.

In *botulism,* which is a form of food poisoning from absorption of the toxin produced by the bacterium *Clostridium botulinum,* paralysis is due to the effect of the toxin on the nerve endings, preventing them from releasing acetylcholine. Rapid ventilatory failure due to respiratory muscle paralysis is the usual cause of death in botulism.

A certain group of antibiotics, known as aminoglycosides (eg, gentamicin, tobramycin), may on rare occasion result in neuromuscular blockade by interference with the release of acetylcholine.

Myasthenia Gravis

Myasthenia gravis is a disease of the neuromuscular junction manifested by muscular weakness and fatigability. It is an acquired autoimmune disorder in which autoantibodies against the acetylcholine receptors are produced. These receptors are located in the muscle-cell membrane, where motor nerve endings meet the muscle fibers. The antibodies cause quantitative and qualitative deficiency of these receptors. The relationship of the thymus gland and myasthenia gravis has long been demonstrated, but its pathogenetic role remains undetermined; 70% of patients have hyperplasia of this gland and another 10% have thymoma (neoplasm of the thymus). The relationship of the thymus gland to myasthenia gravis is probably through its putative role in the production of antiacetylcholine-receptor antibodies.

Most frequently involved in myasthenia gravis are the muscles of the face, eyes, pharynx, and larynx. Every skeletal muscle, however, may be affected. Involvement of the respiratory muscles may result in abrupt development of ventilatory failure. This grave complication is the most common cause of death from this disease.

Myasthenia gravis occurs at all ages; females are affected more often than males. The highest incidence is during the third decade of life in females and sixth decade in males.

Clinical Manifestations. The onset of myasthenia gravis is usually slow and insidious, but occasionally it may be abrupt. Weakness of the eye muscles, which is the most common manifestation, may result in drooping of the eyelids and double vision. In about 15% of patients, weakness remains limited to extraocular and palpebral muscles. In the remining 85%, other different muscles are also involved. Characteristic facial appearance results from the involvement of the facial muscles. Abnormal speech may be due to weakness of facial, tongue, or laryngeal muscles. These symptoms are more apparent at the end of the day or following repetitive movements of the involved muscles, and they improve with rest. Difficulty with chewing, swallowing, and choking upon eating causes problems with nutrition. Excessive fatigability of the muscles of the trunk and extremities can be demonstrated with exercise. Sometimes the weakness may be extreme, and the patient may seem to be totally paralyzed.

Myasthenia crisis refers to the rapid development of weakness to the extent of impairment of respiration. It is usually provoked by infections, especially those involving the respiratory tract. Emotional upset, surgery, discontinuation of medications, or the intake of certain drugs known to increase neuromuscular blockade (such as aminoglycoside antibiotics and institution of high-dose corticosteroids) are other causes of myasthenia crisis. A similar picture may develop in patients who have taken an excessive amount of anticholinesterase drugs (cholinergic crisis).

The course of myasthenia gravis is usually unpredictable; it may progress rapidly or slowly, remain unchanged, or remit spontaneously. Certain factors, such as infection, general fatigue, lack of sleep, menstrual period, or other causes of physical or mental stress, may aggravate its course. Respiratory complications as a result of impairment of respiratory muscle function, difficulty with clearing the secretions, aspiration, and frequent respiratory tract infections are continuous threats to these patients.

Diagnosis. A diagnosis of myasthenia gravis is strongly suspected from the characteristic history and usually made by demonstration of muscular weakness and fatigue on repetitive or sustained contraction of certain muscles, particularly the eye muscles. Regaining strength after a period of rest further supports the diagnosis. With the administration of anticholinesterase drugs such as neostigmine or, preferably, edrophonium chloride (Tensilon), regaining strength can be demonstrated in dramatic fashion. This test is also useful in differentiating the weakness of myasthenia from that of excessive anticholinesterase therapy. The characteristic muscle fatigability can also be demonstrated by electric stimulation of muscles and recording their response (electromyography). Determination of circulating antibodies against acetylcholine receptors, present in 80% to 90% of patients with myasthenia gravis, is helpful in establishing the diagnosis. Appropriate imaging of the thymus gland, preferably with a computed tomography (CT) scanner, is important for detecting thymomas. It is also useful when thymectomy is being considered.

Management. With a better understanding of myasthenia gravis, the treatment of patients with this disease has undergone significant changes in recent years; however, the principles of management remain essentially the same. These are proper and adequate treatment of acute episodes of severe muscle weakness, including myasthenia crisis, and measures directed to alter the basic pathophysiologic process and to prevent the recurrence of symptoms.

Initially, most patients with myasthenia gravis are hospitalized for further studies, observation of the course of the disease, and evaluation of response to treatment. More severely involved patients are usually put in an intensive care unit. Diligent respiratory care is the most important part of management of these patients during the acute phase of their illness. Unpredictability of the progress of disease requires frequent and regular monitoring of the patients' respiratory functions, such as measuring and recording their vital capacities and maximum inspiratory and expiratory pressures. They should be closely watched for problems such as difficulty with swallowing, aspiration, and effective cough. Infection and other factors known to precipitate myasthenia crisis should be prevented and/or promptly eliminated. Ventilatory failure in myasthenia is the result of increasing weakness of the respiratory pump, usually aggravated by difficulty in handling secretions and aspiration. Repeated measurements of pulmonary

mechanics are important in determining the necessity for and proper timing of assisted ventilation. The choice of intubation for mechanical ventilation has been influenced by the advent of endotracheal tubes with low-pressure, high-compliance cuffs. Early tracheostomy is no longer necessary or advisable. However, as some patients may require prolonged ventilatory support, tracheostomy may be indicated later in the course of such patients.

The main pharmacologic agents in the treatment of acute attacks are anticholinesterase drugs, especially pyridostigmine (Mestinon) or sometimes neostigmine, which result in significant improvement in most cases. Difficulty with arriving at a proper maintenance dosage, variability in response, and occasional development of refractoriness make these agents less than ideal for continuous long-term therapy. Less severe cases, however, can be managed safely with these agents. Mild forms may require no treatment except during relapse. Corticosteroids, particularly prednisone, given in a large single dose every other day, have been demonstrated to result in remission of cases that responded poorly to other forms of therapy. Therapy with large doses of corticosteroids should be instituted in the hospital while the patient is being closely monitored, as initial worsening before eventual improvement may occur. Other immunosuppressive drugs, especially azathioprine and cyclosporine, have also been effective for maintaining remission in myasthenia gravis.

Removal of the thymus gland (thymectomy) is frequently performed, particularly in patients with generalized or rapidly progressive myasthenia gravis. Although the result of surgery for thymus tumor (thymoma) is less than satisfactory, the majority of patients with thymic hyperplasia show long-term benefit from a thymectomy. Because of the seriousness of postoperative complications in myasthenia patients, the necessity for adequate preoperative preparation and proper postoperative care should be emphasized.

Plasma exchange (plasmapheresis) has shown to result in significant, albeit temporary, improvement of some patients with refractory disease. The purpose of this treatment is to remove the circulating acetylcholine-receptor antibodies. It is useful in preparing patients for thymectomy. Intravenous immune globulin seems to have an efficacy comparable to plasmapheresis. It has the advantage of not requiring special equipment. Its effect is also temporary.

With the improvement of therapeutic measures, the prognosis of myasthenia gravis has markedly improved. With proper care, a great majority of patients will lead a fairly normal life. Many patients, however, must continue immunosuppressive treatment indefinitely.

■ DISEASES OF PERIPHERAL MOTOR NERVES

Peripheral nerves may be affected by various toxic agents, metabolic disorders, inflammatory states, vascular disease, trauma, and some unknown causes. Despite the frequency of peripheral nerve disease in clinical practice, involvement of the respiratory motor nerves is uncommon. Many critically ill patients with sepsis and multiple organ failure requiring prolonged mechanical ventilatory support have been recognized who show evidence of polyneuropathy. Involvement of the respiratory muscle nerves is implicated as one of the causes of difficulty in weaning these patients off the respirator.

Unilateral paralysis of the diaphragm is a relatively common occurrence and is often due to invasion or compression of one of the phrenic nerves along its long intrathoracic course by a tumor mass; however, there are other causes of this condition. It may even occur without any apparent cause (idiopathic). Unilateral paralysis of the diaphragm by itself causes no significant symptoms. The physiologic effect, as measured by pulmonary function tests, includes reduction of total lung capacity, particularly when the subject is supine. Radiologic changes are quite characteristic. They include elevation of one hemidiaphragm and its absent or paradoxical movement with respiration. The latter can be more precisely demonstrated fluoroscopically with a rapid inspiratory maneuver, such as sniffing.

Bilateral paralysis of the diaphragm, as an isolated disease, is a rare condition and, as mentioned earlier, is compatible with maintenance of adequate ventilation at rest, and even with a moderate amount of physical activity, provided that other respiratory muscles function normally. Respiration at night does not seem to be affected. Exertional dyspnea and orthopnea, as well as the characteristic physical finding of paradoxical abdominal–thoracic, movement, are the usual manifestations. The chest x-ray film shows marked bilateral elevation of the diaphragm. On fluoroscopy, paradoxical upward movement of the diaphragm on inspiration will be observed. In this condition, there is a significant reduction of vital capacity to less than one-half of the normal.

Guillain-Barré Syndrome

Guillain-Barré syndrome is the acute form of inflammatory polyneuritis of unknown cause that predominantly affects the peripheral motor nerves and may involve the respiratory muscles. About 20% to 25% of patients require respiratory assistance.

Guillain-Barré syndrome is a relatively common condition, which has its highest incidence in young and middle-age persons. Since the virtual elimination of poliomyelitis, this syndrome has become the most common cause of acute generalized paralysis. There is frequently a history of preceding upper respiratory tract infection, although the etiology remains unknown. Its association with certain viral diseases, including infectious mononucleosis, influenza, infectious hepatitis, and infection with human immunodeficiency virus (HIV) and cytomegalovirus (CMV), has been demonstated in some cases. Pathologically, there is segmental loss of the myelin sheath of the peripheral nerves and mononuclear cell infiltration. Delayed hypersensitivity against the myelin sheath has been implicated in its pathogenesis. There is also evidence for humoral mechanism with production of antibodies against the peripheral nerve myelin.

Clinical Manifestations. Typically, the onset is rapid with progressive and more or less symmetrical weakness that starts in the legs and spreads upward to affect the trunk, arms, and face. It may, however, start in the face or the upper extremities. Respiratory muscles are involved in more severe cases. The paralyzed muscles are flaccid, with loss of deep-tendon reflexes. Mild sensory changes may also be present. After the establishment of maximum weakness, which is quite variable in individual cases, spontaneous recovery begins. Weakness progresses for 1 to 3 weeks before a plateau state. Recovery is

expected within 2 to 4 weeks after cessation of its progression. There are other atypical presentations of Guillain-Barré syndrome. It may have a chronic and relapsing course.

Involvement of the muscles of the pharynx and larynx may result in swallowing difficulty and aspiration. Weakness of the abdominal and chest muscles impairs the cough mechanism and, thus, airway clearance, predisposing to respiratory infection and atelectasis. Other respiratory muscles, including the diaphragm, may be affected. Ventilatory failure is expected under these circumstances. As a result of autonomic dysfunction, the hemodynamic state may be unstable. Both hypertension and hypotension, especially postural, may occur.

Diagnosis. Although early in its course the diagnosis of Guillain-Barré syndrome may be difficult and mistaken for other neuromuscular disorders, its fully evolved pattern in typical cases is easily recognized by its characteristic clinical features. Abnormal nerve conduction and analysis of cerebrospinal fluid are helpful for diagnosis of more difficult cases.

Management. The management of patients with Guillain-Barré syndrome is primarily *respiratory*. These patients should be hospitalized. Patients with advanced paralysis and reduced vital capacity, or when there is evidence of cardiovascular instability, should be admitted to a critical care unit and closely monitored. Proper respiratory care includes regular monitoring of the respiratory function, with frequent measurement of vital capacity and maximum inspiratory and expiratory pressures, careful bronchopulmonary toilet, and ventilatory assistance. Recovery will depend on adequate maintenance of the patient's respiratory status; therefore, the importance of respiratory care in patient management cannot be over-stressed. With the proved benefit from plasmapheresis in the early stage of the disease, the importance of early and accurate diagnosis should be emphasized. It has been demonstrated that plasmapheresis, when administered within the first 2 weeks, results in shortening the course of the disease and in reducing its complications. Intravenous administration of immunoglobulin has also been shown to be equally effective during the early stage of the disease. Because of the increased incidence of venous thromboembolic disease in Guillain-Barré syndrome, prophylaxis against deep-vein thrombosis (DVT) should be undertaken.

When there is evidence of respiratory difficulty, as judged by significant reduction in vital capacity and respiratory forces and other signs of ventilatory failure, mechanical ventilatory support should be instituted. Although tracheostomy has been the preferred mode of intubation for ventilatory support in the past, availability of soft cuffs has made endotracheal intubation an acceptable, even preferable, alternative. As the vast majority of patients will eventually recover despite marked impairment of their muscle function, every effort should be made to support their lives until remission takes place. The respiratory therapists and nurses play crucial roles in this rewarding endeavor. An occasional patient may require prolonged mechanical ventilation before any sign of improvement can be demonstrated. Corticosteroids have no proven benefit in Guillain-Barré syndrome; they may even be detrimental.

■ DISORDERS OF THE SPINAL CORD

Acute anterior poliomyelitis, commonly known as *polio,* used to be the most important cause of ventilatory failure of neuromuscular origin. Fortunately, it is now almost totally eradicated, and its importance has become mostly historic. A catastrophic epidemic of poliomyelitis, which occurred in 1952 in Copenhagen, was an important impetus in the improvement of mechanical ventilators. Some victims of polio, many years after a severe paralytic form of the disease, show evidence of progressive weakness in their already involved muscles. This condition is recognized as *postpolio syndrome.* Ventilatory difficulty from this syndrome occurs in patients in whom the respiratory muscles were affected at the time of their acute polio.

Many other diseases of the spinal cord may occasionally result in respiratory difficulty. Diseases such as **amyotrophic lateral sclerosis,** multiple sclerosis, and various forms of inflammatory or neoplastic diseases of the spinal cord may result in respiratory muscle weakness and ventilatory failure. As the origin of the phrenic nerves is from the high cervical cord, diseases that involve only the lower regions spare the diaphragm, and adequate ventilation is maintained. However, significant weakness of other respiratory muscles, especially the abdominals, may result in impairment of effective cough and, thus, cause respiratory problems.

Respiratory involvement and complications from spinal cord injury depend on the level of the cord lesion (Fig. 24–4). Traumatic injury to the cervical spinal cord below the fourth cervical vertebra results in *quadriplegia* (also known as

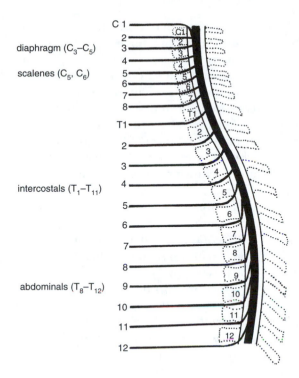

diaphragm (C_3–C_5)

scalenes (C_5, C_6)

intercostals (T_1–T_{11})

abdominals (T_8–T_{12})

Figure 24–4. A diagram showing cervical and thoracic spines and their motor nerve roots. Levels of the spinal cord and vertebral column corresponding to the nerve supply to the major respiratory muscles are indicated.

tetraplegia) with maintenance of respiration by the unaffected diaphragm. Injury above this level, however, will result in paralysis of all respiratory muscles except for the accessory inspiratory muscle, sternocleidomastoid, which is unable to maintain adequate ventilation. Permanent mechanical ventilatory support is necessary for victims of such an injury. Even with intact diaphragmatic function, quadriplegics are predisposed to respiratory difficulties from frequent bouts of pneumonia and atelectasis as a result of impairment of cough and clearing of the airways, as well as lack of mobility. In addition, these patients are prone to develop thrombophlebitis and repeated pulmonary embolism. Pulmonary functional impairment in the early acute stage following cervical spinal

cord injury is more severe than it is during the chronic stage. Most early deaths following acute traumatic quadriplegia are due to pulmonary complications; therefore, the importance of adequate respiratory care in the management of such patients should be stressed. Some of the early complications following acute spinal cord injury are reduced by kinetic therapy, using a rotating bed. Continuous respiratory care should be included in overall chronic management and rehabilitation of these unfortunate patients. Although cough in quadriplegics is generally considered to be a passive process that results from the elastic recoil of the lungs and abdomen, it has been demonstrated that part of the pectoralis major muscles contribute actively to cough by compressing the upper rib cage.

Therefore, appropriate training and strengthening of these muscles should be part of the rehabilitation program of quadriplegics.

■ RESPIRATION IN DISORDERS OF THE CENTRAL NERVOUS SYSTEM (BRAIN)

Respiration is frequently affected by disorders of the central nervous system (CNS). This is understandable considering the particular function of the "respiratory center" and the importance of various reflexes in pulmonary defense, which may be impaired by many diseases involving the brain.

The term "respiratory center" should not impart the notion that it is a compact mass of nerve cells confined to a closely restricted area. It is rather a physiologic center that is concerned with the integration of the activity of muscles of respiration. Although most of the nervous elements for this purpose are collected in the brainstem, especially the medulla, other parts of the CNS have influence over this neurologic function.

The center receives impulses not only from various peripheral and central chemoreceptors, stretch lung receptors, and other mechanical receptors, but also from higher cerebral centers. Normally, respiration is readily effected by voluntary control and influenced by such factors as wakefulness or sleep, emotional change, and mental or physical stress. In many diseases of the CNS, despite lack of involvement of the brainstem, there is alteration of the respiratory pattern, commonly in the form of hyperventilation, periodic breathing (Cheyne-Stokes respiration) or other abnormal respiratory patterns.

Depression of ventilation in CNS disorders generally implies reduced activity of the respiratory center. Although there are several causes of respiratory depression of central origin, the most common cause in clinical practice is overdose with CNS-depressant drugs, including general anesthetics. Except for rare cases in which the respiratory center is primarily and exclusively depressed, there is always a certain degree of impairment of the other functions of the CNS with central hypoventilation. Indeed, in a majority of such conditions, depression of respiration occurs *after* most other CNS functions are suppressed.

In CNS disorders, respiration is not only affected through the influence of the respiratory center, but also altered by derangement of normal mechanisms that ensure airway patency. Impairment or loss of consciousness from any cause may result in respiratory difficulty, even when the respiratory center is not involved. Obstruction of the hypopharynx from relaxation of the pharyngeal walls and tongue, with its backward fall; impairment of reflexes that prevent the entry of secretions, vomitus, and foreign matter to and/or help with their removal from the air passages; and absence or inadequacy of certain respiratory maneuvers that normally help to prevent small airway closure and pulmonary atelectasis are some of the problems facing patients with CNS malfunction. Reflexes that are normally operative to close the laryngeal entrance by the epiglottis and vocal cords (glottis) are usually absent. The respiratory maneuvers that result in periodic deep breathing, such as coughing, sighing, yawning, sneezing, talking, crying, laughing, sniffing, blowing, and straining, are abolished in unconscious patients. Any patient with impaired consciousness is, therefore, highly predisposed to respiratory complications resulting from inadequate protection of airways and diminished lung expansion, even though there may be no evidence of ventilatory depression. Lack of mobility and positional change contributes further to these complications. Among them, pulmonary atelectasis, aspiration pneumonitis, bacterial pneumonia, and thromboembolism are quite common. Neurogenic pulmonary edema may develop following acute CNS events. Severe head trauma is known to cause acute hypoxemia immediately after injury without evidence of pulmonary pathology. Patients with underlying chronic pulmonary disease are, obviously, at much higher risk if they develop impaired consciousness.

Acute and transient disturbance of consciousness, such as seen during and for a short time following epileptic seizure, may result in profound respiratory impairment. Marked hypoxemia and respiratory and metabolic acidosis are common during such episodes. In *status epilepticus* (frequent epileptic seizures without restoration of consciousness between them), the most feared fatal complication is respiratory, which may be due to seizures as well as the large amount of sedatives necessary for their control.

In the management of patients with impairment of CNS function, especially when the patient is unconscious, respiratory care plays a major role. Pulmonary complication is the most common cause of death in most such situations.

■ DRUG OVERDOSE

The subject of drug overdose is selected for discussion with more detail because of its common occurrence and the frequency of respiratory complications. Drug overdose is a leading cause of unconsciousness among patients admitted to critical care units. The principles of respiratory management of this condition are applicable equally well to any comatose or stuporous patient from other causes. Although overdose from any drug may have deleterious and even fatal effects, the more frequently encountered drug overdose in clinical practice is due to accidental or, more commonly, suicidal intake of large amounts of CNS-depressant drugs. These include sedatives, hypnotics, tranquilizers, narcotics, alcohol, and numerous other drugs used in the treatment of psychiatric disorders. Discussion of common clinical features and principles of management of overdoses by CNS-depressant drugs is followed by a brief outline of individual characteristics of commonly occurring specific drug overdoses that affect respiration.

Clinical Manifestations. The most common clinical manifestation of overdose by drugs is depression of CNS function. Variable degrees of impairment of consciousness, from sleepiness to deep coma, may be observed depending on the nature and the amount of drug and the time that it has been ingested. Various classifications, including the Glasgow Coma Scale, are used for staging the level of responsiveness. However, for descriptive purposes, the following classification is widely used for staging the severity of intoxication from CNS-depressant drugs.

- *Stage 0.* Sleepy state from which the patient can be aroused and can answer questions.
- *Stage I.* Comatose state, but the patient responds to painful stimuli by

withdrawal. Respiration and blood pressure are normal and the deep-tendon reflexes are intact.

- *Stage II.* Comatose and no response to pain. Most reflexes are intact and there is no respiratory or circulatory depression.
- *Stage III.* Comatose, most or all reflexes are absent; there is no response to pain, but respiration and blood pressure are maintained.
- *Stage IV.* Comatose, most reflexes are absent, and there is depression of respiration and/or decreased blood pressure.

This classification is not intended for narcotic overdose in which respiration may be markedly depressed *before* total loss of consciousness or changes in reflexes. Indeed, respiratory depression out of proportion to the severity of coma is strongly suggestive of narcotic drug overdose.

In addition to ventilatory depression, unconscious patients with drug overdose, like other comatose patients, are prone to respiratory complications from multiple causes. *Aspiration* is a common complication in drug overdose. It may be spontaneous or secondary to therapeutic procedures such as induced vomiting, gastric lavage, or tracheal intubation. Pulmonary *atelectasis* and maldistribution of ventilation are frequent and result from retained secretions, lack of intermittent deep breaths, and immobility. Widening of the alveolar–arterial Po_2 difference and even clinically significant hypoxemia may be observed without hypoventilation.

Many overdosed patients will have some fever with or without transient infiltration on the chest radiograph, probably as a result of pulmonary aspiration or in-fection. Some patients may develop frank pneumonia, lung abscess, or empyema. Aspiration of contaminated upper airway secretions is often the cause of these infectious complications. Sometimes contaminated respiratory therapy equipment may be the culprit.

Circulatory impairment is common in severe overdose from many centrally acting drugs. Reduction in effective circulatory volume from decreased vascular tone and myocardial depression are usual causes. Hypotension and reduced tissue perfusion may complicate the direct toxic effects of drugs on many organs, including the brain. Anoxic brain damage may result from hypoxemia and reduced cerebral perfusion.

Patients with shock or severe hypoxemia may develop pulmonary edema from alveolar capillary damage, which would be enhanced by cardiac failure and made worse by overzealous fluid infusion. Pulmonary edema is more common in narcotic drug overdose.

Diagnosis. Diagnosis of drug overdose is considered from history and clinical presentation and confirmed by appropriate toxicologic studies of blood, urine, or gastric content. Sometimes response to a specific antidote supports the clinical suspicion, such as naloxone in narcotic drug overdose and flumazenil in benzodiazepine overdose (see later).

Management. Patients with mild intoxication are usually managed by close observation and monitoring of the vital signs, level of consciousness, reflexes, and urinary output. The removal of unabsorbed drug from the GI tract by such measures as gastric lavage and the use of cathartics is usually tried. However, if the patient is poorly responsive or comatose, attempt at gastric lavage should only be made after an adequate airway with cuffed endotracheal tube has been established.

The most important aspect of management of patients with drug overdose is supportive therapy, particularly the maintenance of cardiovascular and respiratory functions. Respiratory care includes establishment and maintenance of adequate airway, tracheobronchial toilet, adequate oxygenation, and ventilatory assistance. The establishment of adequate airway is the first priority in any comatose patient. The assurance of an adequate intravenous (IV) access is mandatory, and the status of urine output should be monitored by an indwelling bladder catheter. Blood, urine, and gastric lavage samples should be obtained for toxicologic analysis. When there is deep coma (Stage II and higher), signs of respiratory depression, risk of vomiting and aspiration, or evidence of significant hypoxemia, an endotracheal tube should be inserted. Patients with drug overdose will need proper bronchial toilet by adequate humidification, frequent change of position, postural drainage, and tracheobronchial suctioning. A variable degree of hypoxemia is common in these patients due to atelectasis or aspiration. Severe hypoxemia is strongly suggestive of pulmonary edema or aspiration pneumonitis. An adequate amount of oxygen should be administered to combat hypoxemia. Change of position, bronchial toilet, and intermittent positive pressure breathing or periodic bagging will help to prevent atelectasis.

Mechanical ventilation should be instituted when there is any indication of inadequate ventilation, severe hypox-

emia, or risk of the respiratory state worsening. Most clinicians prefer to put deeply comatose patients on a respirator regardless of their ventilatory states, as they may change quite unpredictably. Large tidal volumes (10–12 mL/kg) at a respiratory rate necessary to maintain adequate alveolar ventilation are recommended. In patients with pulmonary edema, as may occur with narcotic overdose or severe aspiration pneumonitis, addition of positive end-expiratory pressure will assure more satisfactory oxygenation, and will obviate the necessity for administration of a toxic concentration of oxygen.

Hemodynamic status should be closely monitored by frequent examination of blood pressure, pulse, and peripheral perfusion. Determination of hourly urinary output is important as an indicator of adequacy of tissue perfusion. In certain situations, especially when there is evidence of myocardial depression, poor tissue perfusion, unstable blood pressure, or pulmonary edema, direct hemodynamic monitoring with a Swan-Ganz catheter may be helpful as a guide for proper fluid therapy and administration of inotropic and vasoactive drugs.

Except for overdose with narcotics and benzodiazepines, there is no effective antidote for CNS depressant drugs. If narcotic drug intoxication is suspected, a narcotic antagonist such as naloxone hydrochloride (Narcan) is administered. Response to the proper dose of this agent in the case of narcotic overdose is rapid and often dramatic.

The measures to prevent the absorption of the drug after its ingestion are effective when they are employed within a few hours of the time of its intake. They include induction of vomiting, gastric lavage, and the administration of activated charcoal and cathartics. Protection of airways should always be carried out whenever there is a chance of aspiration resulting from any of these therapeutic measures. Activated charcoal is considered to be the most effective for the purpose of prevention of absorption in most common drug overdoses. Removal of the drug after its absorption may be enhanced by various methods, depending on the pharmacokinetics of the drug and the necessity and usefulness of its faster removal. In most situations of overdose by CNS-depressant drugs, it is neither effective nor significantly beneficial toward eventual clinical outcome. Forced diuresis, hemodialysis, hemoperfusion, and multiple-dose activated charcoal administration are some of the methods used for enhancing drug elimination.

The emphasis in management of CNS-depressant drug overdose should be placed on *supportive measures,* especially proper and diligent respiratory care and maintenance of an adequate circulatory state. With such measures, patients with drug overdose are expected to survive. The rare fatal cases in the hospital are seen among patients with severe cardiac depression unresponsive to optimal therapeutic measures, advanced anoxic brain damage, or severe infectious complications.

■ SPECIFIC DRUG OVERDOSE

Narcotics

Narcotic drugs with a significant overdose potential include heroin, methadone, codeine, meperidine (Demerol), pentazocine (Talwin), and propoxyphene (Darvon). With a few exceptions, the clinical picture of acute poisoning and its man-

agement are similar for overdose from any of these drugs. They are notorious for their ventilatory-depressant action through their direct effect on the respiratory center. Both the rate and volume of ventilation are depressed, and Cheyne-Stokes respiration is common. Except for meperidine, narcotics result in constriction of pupils, unless there is extreme hypoxemia. The well-known triad of coma, respiratory depression, and pinpoint pupils is highly suggestive of narcotic drug overdose. Noncardiac pulmonary edema, especially with heroin and codeine poisoning, is another fairly common feature of narcotic overdose. Most of the fatal cases of narcotic overdose are caused by or associated with pulmonary edema with or without concomitant aspiration. Pulmonary edema may develop even after the CNS effect has improved. The exact mechanism of pulmonary edema in narcotic intoxication is not clear, although increased alveolar capillary permeability resulting from severe hypoxia and hypotension seems likely. Other possible causes are aspiration of acid gastric content, neurogenic effect on pulmonary vessels, and hypersensitivity reaction.

Other complications of overdose from narcotics include hypotension and hypothermia. Convulsive seizures may also occur, especially in overdose with meperidine and propoxyphene. Poisoning from the latter drug is also known to cause cardiac arrhythmias.

Principles of management of poisoning from CNS-depressant drugs in general are applicable to narcotic overdose. In addition, the highly specific narcotic antagonist naloxone (Narcan) is very effective in reversing the CNS effect of narcotic drugs, including respiratory depression. Because of its shorter half-life than that of many narcotics, especially methadone, repeated administration or continuous infusion of Narcan may be necessary. This drug has both a diagnostic and a therapeutic use for coma of unknown cause. A rapid response is diagnostic of narcotic drug poisoning. Naloxone has no effect on pulmonary edema from narcotic overdose.

Sedative–Hypnotic Drugs

Overdose from sedative–hypnotic drugs—which include barbiturates, benzodiazepines such as diazepam (Valium) and alprazolam (Xanax), meprobamates, and other "tranquilizers" and "sleeping pills"—results primarily in CNS depression ranging from mild sedation to deep coma. In combination with alcohol and other CNS depressants, the toxic effect of these drugs is markedly enhanced. With severe toxicity, respiratory depression and hypotension may develop. The management principles outlined earlier are best applicable to overdose from these drugs. Rarely are measures such as dialysis for the drugs' increased elimination necessary or advisable. Because of a significant difference in the metabolism and excretion of these drugs, the duration of coma from their overdose varies. With proper supportive care, barring rare fatal complications, survival from sedative–hypnotic drug overdose is the rule. In overdose with a benzodiazepine, IV administration of flumazenil results in rapid improvement of the level of consciousness. Patients treated with this agent should be observed for agitation and seizure.

Antidepressant Drugs

Tricyclics, the most commonly used antidepressants, are the leading cause of serious and potentially lethal drug overdose. The early manifestations of toxicity from these drugs are the result of their anticholinergic effects, which include tachycardia, dry mucous membranes, blurred vision, and dilated pupils. The early CNS symptoms of agitation, restlessness, confusion, and hallucination may be rapidly followed by coma with or without convulsions. The cardiovascular toxic effects include sinus tachycardia, various forms of arrhythmia and other electrocardiographic abnormalities, and hypotension. Pulmonary edema may occur in some patients, especially when there is hypotension. Among other pulmonary complications of tricyclic antidepressant overdose, respiratory center depression, pulmonary aspiration, atelectasis, and pneumonia are fairly common. Hypoxemia and marked increase in alveolar-arterial oxygen tension gradient occur in most patients, even in those without clinical or radiographic evidence of pulmonary involvement. Acidosis from various causes, including hypotension and convulsive seizures, increases the toxicity of these drugs. Lower blood pH increases the proportion of free (not bound to proteins) drug concentration. Most of the toxic effects on the cardiovascular system are especially enhanced with acidosis.

In the management of patients with tricyclic antidepressant overdose, in addition to proper respiratory care and other supportive measures for coma, cardiovascular abnormalities should be adequately evaluated and treated. Acidosis should be appropriately corrected by adequate ventilation, control of seizures, treatment of hypotension, and the administration of sodium bicarbonate. Most of the toxic effects of tricyclics, especially cardiac arrhythmias and hypotension, are ameliorated by the correction of acidosis and alkalinization of blood. Hypotension often responds to fluid administration and correction of acidosis, but may also require vasopressor drugs. Seizures and arrhythmias should be controlled with specific drugs as needed. Although physostigmine has been used as an "antidote" for tricyclic drug toxicity, it is rarely recommended because of its unpredictable side effects.

Aspirin

An important cause of accidental drug overdose in children is aspirin. In adults, in addition to suicidal ingestion, aspirin overdose may occur as a result of cumulative effects of its regular chronic use, especially in the elderly. As there is significant individual variation in its pharmacodynamics, a toxic effect may develop even with a usual daily "therapeutic" dose if taken for a long period. In very high blood levels, aspirin has CNS-depressant effects, including respiratory suppression. However, with moderate toxicity and early in the course of severe toxicity, it is a strong respiratory center stimulant, resulting in hyperventilation and respiratory alkalosis. Metabolic acidosis, especially in children, further complicates the acid-base status. With acute aspirin poisoning, vomiting is very common. CNS effects of aspirin poisoning include confusion, delirium, convulsion, and coma. Aspirin at normal blood pH is mostly ionized and, thus, difficult to penetrate the cells of various tissues, including the CNS. However, in acidemia, the nonionized portion is increased, which enhances its toxicity. A serious complication of aspirin poisoning is the development of pulmonary edema, which occurs mostly in elderly patients. Some patients with chronic aspirin poisoning may present with clinical features of sepsis ("pseudosepsis syndrome"). A high index of suspicion is necessary for the diagnosis of aspirin poisoning, which is readily confirmed by the determination of blood aspirin levels.

In treatment of aspirin poisoning, measures to inhibit its further absorption and increase its elimination should be combined with the correction of fluid, electrolytes, and acid-base abnormalities. Activated charcoal not only inhibits the absorption of aspirin, but also, when given in repeated doses, reduces its plasma half-life (increases its removal). Sodium bicarbonate is given to correct metabolic acidosis and, by so doing, to reduce the toxic effect of aspirin. By alkalinizing the urine, bicarbonate also increases its renal excretion. Mechanical ventilation may be necessary in unconscious patients, when pulmonary edema develops, or when there is evidence of respiratory depression. Peritoneal dialysis or hemodialysis may be necessary in severe aspirin intoxication.

Cocaine

With the widespread use of cocaine, especially since the introduction of its free alkaloid form (free-base, "crack") in the illicit drug market in the United States, the number of cases of toxicity and complications from this agent continues to increase. Because of its use as a smoking substance, "crack" cocaine not only results in various CNS and cardiovascular effects, but also causes several pulmonary complications. They include noncardiogenic pulmonary edema, alveolar hemorrhage, hypersensitivity pneumonitis, pneumothorax, pneumomediastinum, and exacerbation of asthma. "Crack lung" is a generic term, usually referred to as a syndrome, manifested by chest pain, hemoptysis, and diffuse alveolar infiltrates. Although most of these complications resulting from smoking cocaine are self-limited, some may have a serious and even fatal outcome if not properly managed. As a significant number of "crack" cocaine users also are injection-drug abusers or may have other risk factors for HIV infection, cocaine-related lung lesions should be differentiated from HIV-related pulmonary complications.

BIBLIOGRAPHY

Baydur A. Respiratory muscle function in systemic disorders. *Sem Respir Med.* 1988; 9:223–238.

Bennett DA, Bleck TP. Diagnosis and treatment of neuromuscular causes of acute respiratory failure. *Clin Neuropharmacol.* 1988; 11:303–347.

Braun SR, Giovannoni R, O'Connor M. Improving the cough in patients with spinal cord injury. *Am J Phys Med.* 1984; 63(1): 1–10.

Celli BR. Clinical and physiologic evaluation of respiratory muscle function. *Clin Chest Med.* 1989; 10:199–214.

Colice GL, Bernat JL. Neurologic disorders and respiration. *Clin Chest Med.* 1989; 10: 521–543.

Coronel B, Mercatello A, Couturier JC, et al. Polyneuropathy: potential cause of difficult weaning. *Crit Care Med.* 1990; 18:486–489.

Dec GW, Stern TA. Tricyclic antidepressants in the intensive care unit. *J Intensive Care Med.* 1990; 5:69–81.

DeVivo MJ, Ivie CS III. Life expectancy of ventilator-dependent persons with spinal cord injuries. *Chest.* 1995; 108:226–232.

Drachman DB. Myasthenia gravis. *N Engl J Med.* 1994; 330:1797–1810.

Estenne M, DeTroyer A. Cough in tetraplegic subjects: an active process. *Ann Intern Med.* 1990; 112:22–28.

Forrester JM, Steele AW, Waldron JA, Flint A. Crack lung: an acute pulmonary syndrome with a spectrum of clinical and histopathologic findings. *Am Rev Respir Dis.* 1990; 142:462–467.

Gibson GJ. Diaphragmatic paresis: pathophysiology, clinical features, and investigation. *Thorax.* 1989; 44:960–970.

Gracey DR, Howland FM Jr, Divertie MB. Plasmapheresis in the treatment of ventilator-dependent myasthenia gravis patients. *Chest.* 1984; 85:739–743.

Haim DY, Lippmann ML, Goldberg SK, Walkenstein MD. The pulmonary complications of crack cocaine: a comprehensive review. *Chest.* 1995; 107:233–240.

Heffner JE, Sahn SA. Salicylate-induced pulmonary edema. *Ann Intern Med.* 1981; 95:405–409.

Hughes RAC. The management of Guillain-Barré syndrome. *Hosp Pract.* 1992; 27(3A): 107–125.

Juan G, Calverley P, Talamo C, et al. Effect of carbon dioxide on diaphragmatic function in human beings. *N Engl J Med.* 1984; 310:874–879.

Laroche CM, Carroll N, Moxham J, Green M. Clinical significance of severe isolated diaphragm weakness. *Am Rev Respir Dis.* 1988; 138:862–866.

Lynn DJ, Woda RP, Mendell JR. Respiratory dysfunction in muscular dystrophy and other myopathies. *Clin Chest Med.* 1994; 15:661–674.

Mansel JK, Norman JR. Respiratory complications and management of spinal cord injuries. *Chest.* 1990; 97:1446–1452.

McGuigan MA. Treatment of poisoning. *Clin Symp.* 1984; 36(5):3–32.

Mier A. Respiratory muscle weakness. *Respir Med.* 1990; 84:351–359.

Mulder DG, Graves M, Herrmann C. Thymectomy for myasthenia gravis: recent observation and comparison with past experience. *Ann Thorac Surg.* 1989; 48:551–555.

NHLBI. Workshop summary. Respiratory muscle fatigue. *Am Rev Respir Dis.* 1990; 142: 474–480.

Parsons PE. Respiratory failure as a result of drugs, overdoses, and poisonings. *Clin Chest Med.* 1994; 15(1):93–102.

Reines HD, Harris RC. Pulmonary complications of acute spinal cord injuries. *Neurosurgery.* 1987; 21:193–196.

Rochester DF, Esau SA. Assessment of ventilatory function in patients with neuromuscular disease. *Clin Chest Med.* 1994; 15: 751–763.

Ropper AH. The Guillain-Barré syndrome. *N Engl J Med.* 1992; 326:1130–1136.

Roussos C. Respiratory muscle fatigue and ventilatory failure. *Chest.* 1990; 97(suppl): 89S–96S.

Roy TM, Ossorio MA, Cipolla LM, et al. Pulmonary complications after tricyclic antidepressant overdose. *Chest.* 1989; 96: 852–856.

Scanlon PD, Loring SH, Pichurko BM, et al. Respiratory mechanics in acute quadriplegia. *Am Rev Respir Dis.* 1989; 139:615–620.

Sherman MS, Paz HL. Review of respiratory care of the patient with ALS. *Respiration.* 1994; 61:61–67.

Slack RS, Shucart W. Respiratory dysfunction associated with traumatic injury to the central nervous system. *Clin Chest Med.* 1994; 15:739–749.

Smith PEM, Edwards RHT, Calverley PMA. Ventilation and breathing pattern during sleep in Duchenne muscular dystrophy. *Chest.* 1989; 96:1346–1351.

Spinelli A, Marconi G, Gorini M, et al. Control of breathing in patients with myasthenia gravis. *Am Rev Respir Dis.* 1992; 145: 1359–1366.

Steinhart CM, Pearson-Shaver AL. Poisoning. *Crit Care Clin.* 1988; 4:845–872.

Steljes DG, Kryger MH, Kirk BW, Millar TW. Sleep in postpolio syndrome. *Chest.* 1990; 98:133–140.

Strumpf DA, Millman RP, Hill NS. The management of chronic hypoventilation. *Chest.* 1990; 98:474–480.

Teitelbaum JS, Borel CO. Respiratory dysfunction in Guillain-Barré syndrome. *Clin Chest Med.* 1994; 15:705–714.

Zulueta JJ, Fanburg BL. Respiratory dysfunction in myasthenia gravis. *Clin Chest Med.* 1994; 15:683–691.

Sleep-Related Breathing Disorders

The effect of sleep on breathing and its role in various respiratory disorders have been extensively studied in recent years. Both basic research and clinical investigation have resulted in significant advances in knowledge and understanding of this important but hitherto neglected area of pulmonary medicine. It has been realized that sleep-related disorders of respiration are quite common and may be the cause of significant mortality and morbidity. The clinical entity known as *Pickwickian* or *obesity–hypoventilation syndrome* is recognized to be only part of the wide spectrum of these disorders.

■ RESPIRATION DURING SLEEP

The effects of sleep on respiration vary according to the state and the stage of sleep. There are two entirely different states of sleep: non–rapid eye movement (NREM) and rapid eye movement (REM). They occur cyclically at about 90-minute intervals. NREM sleep, with its four successive stages, is referred to as *quiet sleep* and is characterized by progressive deepening of sleep and slowing of brain waves as shown on an electroencephalogram (EEG). With the onset of sleep, there is gradual reduction of sympathetic activity during NREM sleep; unopposed parasympathetic activity causes slowing of the heart rate. Systemic blood pressure also diminishes with the progression of NREM sleep. During drowsiness and early stages of NREM sleep, the pattern of breathing may be periodic, with cyclic waxing and waning of respiratory rate and tidal volume. In older individuals, true Cheyne-Stokes respiration may occur. With deeper NREM sleep, breathing becomes regular and steady. In healthy persons, minute ventilation at the later stages of NREM sleep is somewhat less than during resting but wakeful state; as a result, the arterial Pco_2 rises and Po_2 decreases by about 5 mm Hg.

359

REM sleep is characterized by bursts of rapid eye movements and changes in the EEG, indicative of increased neuronal activity. Dreaming occurs in this sleeping period and, if awakened, the subject recalls vividly the content of his or her dream. Changes in autonomic nervous system activity result in fluctuation of the heart rate and blood pressure. Skeletal muscle tone is markedly diminished during REM sleep. Intercostal muscle activity is also decreased, resulting in paradoxical motion of the rib cage with breathing. During REM sleep, respiration is characteristically irregular and may even be interrupted by short periods of apnea. Up to 30 apneic episodes in a 7-hour sleep period is considered to be normal. Alteration in rate, rhythm, and depth of breathing causes fluctuation in the state of alveolar ventilation during REM sleep.

In addition to changes characteristic of each sleep period, there are certain alterations in pulmonary defense and ventilatory control mechanisms with sleep. Mucociliary clearance, protective reflexes of the airways, and arousal responses to noxious stimuli are decreased during REM and late stages of NREM sleep. As a result, small amounts of upper airway secretions may be aspirated during sleep. Ventilatory and arousal responses to both hypercapnia and hypoxemia are also diminished to variable degrees depending on the sleep state. Activity of the upper airway muscles is important in maintaining the patency of its muscular portion (pharynx). Active pharyngeal muscle contraction with each inspiration plays a significant role in preventing the airway from collapsing, which otherwise would occur as a result of negative pressure of inspiration. It has been demonstrated that pharyngeal muscle activity is reduced during sleep.

■ SLEEP APNEA SYNDROME

Sleep apnea syndrome refers to a pathologic condition in which repeated episodes of apnea and/or hypopnea during sleep results in clinically significant hypoxemia, sleep fragmentation, and daytime somnolence. Apnea is defined as a cessation of airflow (at the level of both the nostrils and mouth) lasting for at least 10 seconds. Hypopnea is generally defined as a 30% or more decline in airflow associated with a reduction of arterial oxygen saturation of at least 4%. Usually 5 or more apneic episodes per hour of sleep (apnea index), 15 or more hypopneic episodes per hour of sleep, or an equivalent combination characterize sleep apnea syndrome. The presence of symptoms and signs resulting from sleep disruption and hypoxemia and their resolution by elimination of apneic–hypopneic episodes are necessary for its diagnosis.

Classification and Mechanism. Conventionally, sleep apnea is classified into three types:

1. The **central** type is an apnea in which cessation of airflow is the result of absence of ventilatory effort.
2. The **obstructive** or occlusive type is characterized by cessation of airflow despite the presence of chest and abdominal movements.
3. The **mixed** type is a combination of central and obstructive apnea in which the initial cessation of ventilatory effort is followed by its resumption without airflow because of upper airway obstruction.

This classification is also applied to hypopnea, which is different from apnea simply by having reduced rather than absent airflow. To simplify the discussion, the term apnea is used in the remainder of this chapter to include both apneic and hypopneic events.

In the majority of patients, apneic episodes are a variable combination of central, obstructive, or mixed apneas suggesting that a functional defect in the central respiratory drive during sleep affects both inspiratory muscle contraction and upper airway muscle activity. Central apnea without an obstructive component is very uncommon, except for brief and infrequent episodes during REM sleep. Diminished respiratory center output may on rare occasions occur in patients with central nervous system (CNS) lesions involving the respiratory control system. In central apnea, the inspiratory drive ceases, as manifested by the lack of diaphragmatic and intercostal muscle activity.

In the obstructive type, intermittent closure of the upper airway at the level of the oropharynx prevents the airflow despite inspiratory muscle contractions. Several structural abnormalities predispose to obstructive apnea, such as hypertrophic tonsils and adenoids, large tongue, and recessed jaw. In most patients, however, no clinically apparent anatomic abnormality of the upper airway can be identified.

As most patients with obstructive sleep apnea are overweight, it appears that obesity contributes to pharyngeal obstruction during sleep. Studies of the upper airways by various means, including computed tomography (CT), have shown that in these patients the upper airway at the level of the oropharynx has smaller than normal dimensions and is more collapsible. The soft palate (including the uvula), base of the tongue, and loose pha-

ryngeal wall contribute to airway narrowing. It is readily apparent (Fig. 25–1) that lack of muscle tone in this region would result in further narrowing of the oropharynx.

The genioglossus is the most important muscle of the tongue, and its active contraction with inspiration prevents the closure of the airway at this level. Whenever the negative pressure during inspiration, which tends to collapse the pharynx, cannot be overcome by dilating muscular force, airway occlusion occurs. As mentioned earlier, the inspiratory activity of the pharyngeal muscles is normally diminished during sleep. In obstructive sleep apnea, the inspiratory activity of these muscles, particularly the genioglossus, has been shown to be absent during apnea; as a result, the base of the tongue touches

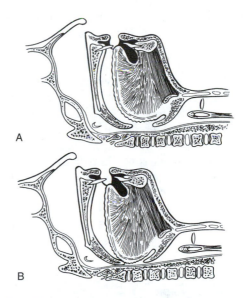

Figure 25–1. Upper airway in obstructive sleep apnea: (A) During wakefulness, (B) during sleep. Note that during sleep the relaxation of the genioglossus muscle results in backward displacement of the base of the tongue, which touches the soft palate, uvula, and posterior pharyngeal wall, causing upper airway obstruction.

the soft palate and the uvula, pushing them against the posterior pharyngeal wall. With the inspiratory effort, the intraluminal negative pressure of the upper airway completes its obstruction. Thus in obstructive apnea, both anatomic abnormality of the upper airway and functional impairment of its musculature from lack of inspiratory neural drive are involved in airway obstruction during sleep. Progressive increase in hypoxemia, hypercapnia, and inspiratory muscle effort results in arousal and subsequent reactivation of upper airway dilating muscles and resumption of ventilation. The cycle repeats throughout the sleeping hours with varying frequency and duration, depending on the stage of sleep and arousability.

REM sleep, in which arousability is reduced, is associated with more frequent and more severe apneic episodes. It should be noted that loud snoring, an invariable feature of this disorder, is the result of vibration of the soft palate and the uvula between the tongue and the pharyngeal wall when the air passage is incompletely obstructed. Habitual snoring is considered to be an important risk factor for the development of obstructive sleep apnea. It has been demonstrated that the upper airway in snorers is narrower and flabbier than in nonsnorers. It seems that from both temporal and pathophysiologic standpoints, snoring represents an intermediate stage between a normal upper airway function and airway obstruction of sleep apnea.

Pathophysiology. The major physiologic consequence of sleep apnea is the development of hypoxemia, which depends not only on the frequency and duration of apneic episodes, but also on the baseline arterial oxygen content and lung volume. Cessation of ventilation, as expected, results in both hypoxemia and hypercapnia; however, the severity of hypoxemia during apneic episodes is out of proportion to the degree of alveolar hypoventilation indicated by the rising $Paco_2$. Reduced functional residual capacity (FRC), which may be less than closing volume, results in a significant abnormality of gas transport and, therefore, contributes to hypoxemia. Oxygen desaturation is usually more pronounced with obstructive apnea than with central apnea.

Repeated interruption of sleep during the night results from frequent arousals when hypoxemia and hypercapnia are severe enough at the end of apneic episodes. The resumption of respiration signifies arousal or change in the state of sleep from a deeper to a lighter stage. Fragmented and restless sleep is the major cause of daytime somnolence, which is one of the characteristic features of sleep apnea syndrome. Severe hypoxemia in association with altered autonomic nervous system function causes cardiac arrhythmia and elevation of blood pressure. In the advanced stage of the syndrome, repeated episodes of nocturnal hypoxemia and hypercapnia over several years may result in pulmonary hypertension, polycythemia, and eventual heart failure. It seems that with progression of this syndrome, there is further impairment of ventilatory control due to changes in blood gases as well as sleep deprivation; thus, a vicious circle develops (Fig. 25–2). Sleep apnea syndrome in association with severe obesity, if untreated, often advances to a state of persistent hypoventilation throughout the day, and the characteristic picture of Pickwickian syndrome develops. Ventilation–perfusion $(\dot{V}/\dot{Q})$ mismatch contributes significantly

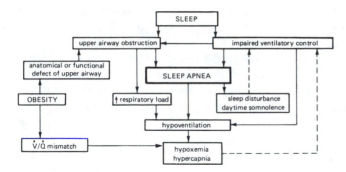

Figure 25–2. Schematic demonstration of pathogenesis of sleep apnea syndrome. Note that the abnormalities of both the upper airway and ventilatory control mechanisms are involved.

to the gas transport abnormality in morbidly obese patients.

Clinical Manifestations. Although people with infrequent and short apneic episodes have no significant symptoms, patients with sleep apnea syndrome have readily recognizable clinical manifestations resulting from disturbance of both sleep and respiration. Most patients with sleep apnea syndrome are middle-age males. Excessive daytime sleepiness and nocturnal insomnia are the most common complaints. In the most prevalent obstructive type, loud snoring, silence of cessation of breathing, and its resumption with a blasting snort are invariably present and reported by the distraught spouse. Restlessness and abnormal motor activities, such as flinging the arms and the legs around, are common. Patients usually wake up in the morning tired and often with a headache. Alcohol intake and sleeping medications make the matter worse. Daytime somnolence may occur at any time, even during physical activity. Personality changes and decreased intellectual function have been reported. Systemic hypertension is a frequently associated condition.

The findings on the physical examination may be normal, but most patients with this disorder are obese. In severe cases, patients may fall asleep during the interview or the physical examination. In a minority of patients, gross abnormalities of the upper airway (such as nasal obstruction, large tonsils and adenoids, enlarged tongue, or recessed lower jaw) may be detected. Pickwickian syndrome is characterized by extreme obesity, cyanosis, and signs of right-side heart failure.

Diagnosis. A diagnosis of sleep apnea syndrome should be suspected in patients presenting with the previously mentioned symptoms and physical findings. Although careful observation of the patient during sleep gives important clues to the diagnosis, study in a sleep laboratory is necessary not only to establish the diagnosis, but also to assess its severity and the mechanism of its production. Polysomnography is the simultaneous recordings of CNS, respiratory, and cardiac functions during sleep. Recording of the airflow at the mouth and the nostrils, and of thoracic and abdominal movement shows the number and the duration of apneas and identifies their type. Pulse oximetry is important in assessing the clinical significance of apneic episodes. The state and the stage of sleep are determined by EEG and electrooculogram (EOG). The electrocardiographic tracing shows changes in the heart rate and rhythm in association with apnea. Cardiac arrhythmia is a frequent finding with severe sleep apnea and is the cause of significant morbidity and even mortality. The presence of more than 30 apneic episodes during a night's sleep, especially when they occur during the NREM sleep, is abnormal. Most patients with sleep apnea syndrome will have up to 300 such episodes during a 7-hour sleep period. They may spend more than one-half the sleeping time without ventilation. Oxygen desaturation to critically low levels is not unusual. Figure 25–3 represents some polysomnographic tracings of one episode of obstructive apnea and one episode of central apnea.

Functional and anatomic studies of the upper airways by different methods may demonstrate abnormalities. The maximum flow-volume loop and the CT scan are most informative in this regard.

Management. The proper management of patients with sleep apnea syndrome necessitates an accurate diagnosis of its presence, severity, and cause. In all cases, factors that are known to increase the frequency and duration of apneic episodes, such as sleep deprivation, alcohol use, and intake of CNS depressant drugs, should be avoided. Such measures may suffice in less severe cases that should, however, be followed closely as they may progress to more severe stages of the disease. Medications for treatment of sleep apnea have been disappointing. Administration of oxygen during sleep should be considered for patients who have significant hypoxemic episodes and

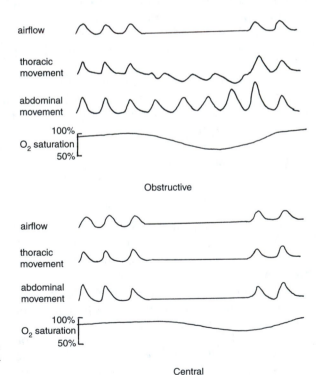

Figure 25–3. Patterns of some of the polysomnographic tracings in obstructive and central sleep apneas. In the obstructive type, despite the activity of respiratory muscles (thoracic and abdominal movement), there is no airflow. In the central type, cessation of airflow is the result of lack of respiratory muscle activity (no thoracic or abdominal movement).

who are intolerant or unwilling to use more effective treatment.

No uniformly effective therapy exists for predominantly central sleep apnea; respiratory stimulants, a rocking bed, a negative pressure ventilator such as the chest cuirass, and, occasionally, a positive pressure ventilator may be used. Electrical pacing of the diaphragm has been used in a few patients with some success.

In predominantly obstructive or mixed apneas, bypassing the obstructing site with a tracheostomy is considered to be the most effective therapeutic measure. However, technical difficulty in some patients, the potential complications, and lack of its acceptability by most patients are its main drawbacks. Methods that can maintain upper airway patency have proved successful in numerous instances. One such method is the application of continuous positive airway pressure (CPAP) through the nose. Acting as an internal pneumatic splint, nasal CPAP prevents upper airway collapse during inspiration. Its beneficial effect is almost as dramatic as the tracheostomy. With the restoration of a consolidated sleep pattern, daytime somnolence improves rapidly. The level of CPAP needed to maintain patency of the upper airway during sleep is usually determined by the sleep study. Some patients may be intolerant of an adequate level of positive pressure. A system with a ramp that allows a gradual increase of CPAP to optimal level within several minutes may be more acceptable to the patient. After nightly application of nasal CPAP for several weeks, most patients will not need it every night. Its periodic use, however, will be necessary for prevention of relapse.

Reconstructive surgery of the pharynx and the palate and the application of various prosthetic devices in selected patients appear to be effective in relieving the obstruction, but more studies and longer follow-up are necessary before their role in treatment of this disorder is established. The benefit of surgery in patients with well-defined anatomic lesions is obvious.

■ EFFECT OF SLEEP ON CHRONIC RESPIRATORY DISORDERS

Sleep apnea syndrome may also occur in a setting of chronic respiratory disorders. Because of the presence of an already recognized underlying condition, sleep apnea syndrome in patients with these disorders is usually not suspected. Many patients with chronic obstructive pulmonary disease (COPD), kyphoscoliosis, and various neuromuscular disorders are identified by sleep study to also have obstructive sleep apnea.

Other sleep-related respiratory dysfunctions, discussed at the beginning of this chapter, are known to contribute to the symptoms and the complications in patients with chronic pulmonary or ventilatory disorders. The worsening of arterial oxygen desaturation during sleep, especially in the REM state, is commonly observed. The severity of the disturbance of blood gases during sleep cannot reliably be predicted from the abnormality of pulmonary function tests or arterial blood studies during wakefulness. However, it has been demonstrated that in COPD, blue bloaters tend to have more severe nocturnal oxygen desaturation than pink puffers.

Certain features should alert the respiratory care provider to the possibility of sleep-related disturbances in patients with chronic respiratory disease. These include insomnia, sudden awakening with a choking sensation, and severe morning headaches. Pulmonary hypertension and cor pulmonale out of proportion to the degree of pulmonary functional impairment and awake blood gas values are other manifestations. When sleep-related disorders are suspected, the monitoring of oxygen saturation by pulse oximetry and electrocardiography during a night's sleep are indicated. Selected patients may require polysomnography. Patients with chest-wall deformity and chronic neuromuscular disorders who demonstrate evidence of chronic hypoventilation, polycythemia, pulmonary hypertension, and daytime somnolence and fatigue should be considered for sleep studies. It is important to identify the subjects who will benefit from nocturnal oxygen therapy.

Patients with other chronic respiratory problems may likewise have sleep-related worsening of their conditions. In congestive heart failure, in addition to well-known Cheyne-Stokes respiration, recurrent apneas may occur during sleep. Some of these patients may benefit from nasal CPAP. Many asthmatics are known to have nocturnal exacerbation of their asthma (see Chapter 9).

BIBLIOGRAPHY

American Thoracic Society. Indications and standards for cardiopulmonary sleep studies. *Am Rev Respir Dis.* 1989; 139:559–568.

American Thoracic Society. Indications and standards for use of nasal positive airway pressure (CPAP) in sleep apnea syndrome. *Am J Respir Crit Care Med.* 1994; 150: 1738–1745.

Block AJ, Faulkner JA, Hughes RL, et al. Factors influencing upper airway closure. *Chest.* 1984; 86:114–122.

Collop NA, Block AJ, Hellard D. The effect of nightly nasal CPAP treatment on underlying obstructive sleep apnea and pharyngeal size. *Chest.* 1991; 99:85–860.

Culver BH. Pulmonary responses to sleep. *Respir Care.* 1989; 34:510–515.

Douglas NJ, Flenley DC. Breathing during sleep in patients with obstructive lung disease. *Am Rev Respir Dis.* 1990; 141:1055–1070.

Funsten AW, Suratt PM. Evaluation of respiratory disorders during sleep. *Clin Chest Med.* 1989; 10:265–276.

Hoffstein V. Snoring. *Chest.* 1996; 109:201–222.

Hudgel DW. Treatment of obstructive sleep apnea: a review. *Chest.* 1996; 109:1346–1358.

Kuna ST, Bedi DG, Ryckman C. Effect of nasal airway positive pressure on upper airway size and configuration. *Am Rev Respir Dis.* 1988; 138:969–975.

Laks L, Lehrhaft B, Grunstein RR, Sullivan CE. Pulmonary artery pressure response to hypoxia in sleep apnea. *Am J Respir Crit Care Med.* 1997; 155:193–198.

Midgren B. Oxygen desaturation during sleep as a function of the underlying respiratory disease. *Am Rev Respir Dis.* 1990; 141:43–46.

Pack AI. Obstructive sleep apnea. *Adv Intern Med.* 1994; 39:517–567.

Parish JM, Shepard JW Jr. Cardiovascular effects of sleep disorders. *Chest.* 1990; 97: 1220–1226.

Peter JH, Koehler U, Grote L, Podszus T. Manifestations and consequences of obstructive sleep apnea. *Eur Respir J.* 1995; 8:1572–1583.

Phillips B. Sleep apnea: underdiagnosed and undertreated. *Hosp Pract.* 1996; 31(3): 193–205.

Remmers JE. Sleeping and breathing. *Chest.* 1990; 93(3 Suppl):77S–80S.

Sanders MH, Kern N. Obstructive sleep apnea treated by independently adjusted inspiratory and expiratory positive airway pressure via nasal mask: physiologic and clinical implications. *Chest.* 1990; 98:317–324.

Shepard JW Jr. Cardiopulmonary consequences of obstructive sleep apnea. *Mayo Clin Proc.* 1990; 65:1250–1259.

Strohl KP, Redline S. Recognition of obstructive sleep apnea. *Am J Respir Crit Care Med.* 1996; 154:279–289.

Strollo PJ Jr, Rogers RM. Obstructive sleep apnea. *N Engl J Med.* 1996; 334:99–104.

Sullivan CE, Issa FG, Berthon-Jones M, Eves L. Reversal of obstructive sleep apnea by continuous positive airway pressure applied through the nares. *Lancet.* 1981; 1:862–865.

Ten Brock E, Shucard DW. Sleep apnea. *Am Fam Phys.* 1994; 549:385–394.

Waldhorn RE, Herrick TW, Nguyen MC, et al. Long-term compliance with nasal continuous positive airway pressure therapy of obstructive sleep apnea. *Chest.* 1990; 97: 33–38.

Wiegand L, Zwillich CW. Obstructive sleep apnea. *Dis Mon.* 1994; 40:197–252.

XI

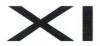

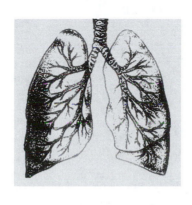

RESPIRATORY FAILURE

26.

Respiratory Failure

Impairment of respiratory function may be minimal and only detectable by very sensitive laboratory tests, or it may be severe enough to result in symptoms and easily detectable abnormalities on physical examination and routine laboratory studies. As the respiratory system fails to maintain its principal functions, that is, adequate oxygenation of arterial blood and/or proper elimination of carbon dioxide (CO_2) with normal activities, it is no more *sufficient*. This state of functional impairment is, thus, termed *respiratory insufficiency* or *failure*.

Respiratory insufficiency may be acute, chronic, or both. In *chronic respiratory insufficiency*, slow development and long duration of disturbances of lung function will allow for intervention of various *compensatory mechanisms*, which prevent, or at least diminish, the harmful effect on the body homeostasis. These compensatory mechanisms include changes in respiratory pattern and utilization of accessory respiratory muscles to overcome the increased airway resistance and reduced compliance; hyperventilation to increase CO_2 elimina-

tion and alveolar oxygen tension; circulatory adjustment to improve oxygen transport, particularly to more vital organs; alteration in blood to facilitate oxygen delivery to tissues; and renal compensation to ameliorate acid-base derangement. Reduction in physical activity, which is a major mechanism to cope with respiratory insufficiency, determines the degree of disability that results.

In *acute respiratory insufficiency* or *failure,* because of rapidity of development of respiratory impairment, the compensatory mechanisms will be inadequate for prevention of serious consequences. Inadequate tissue oxygenation and/or severe acid-base disturbance will become life threatening unless appropriate measures are taken. Acute respiratory failure is somewhat arbitrarily defined as acute reduction of arterial blood P_{O_2} below 60 mm Hg (at sea level) and/or acute elevation of arterial blood P_{CO_2} above 50 mm Hg as a consequence of impaired respiratory function.

It should be emphasized that the previous definition is valid only in cases in which baseline arterial blood gases (ABGs) are known or assumed to be normal. In patients with established chronic hypoxemia and/or hypercapnia, it is the *acute deterioration* of blood gases, rather than their absolute values, that characterizes acute respiratory failure. In other situations, although the acuteness of hypercapnia can be inferred from the expected reduction in arterial blood pH, the acuteness of hypoxemia can only be ascertained retrospectively by its clinical course.

Classification. In addition to its division into acute and chronic forms, respiratory failure is classified according to the predominance of its pathogenetic mechanism:

- Ventilatory failure, or hypercapnic respiratory failure, is the result of inadequate alveolar ventilation. It may develop with or without significant lung disease. Hypoxemia is secondary to reduced alveolar Po_2 and proportional to hypercapnia. Alveolar-arterial oxygen gradient, or $P(A\text{-}a)o_2$, therefore should not be increased.
- Hypoxemic respiratory failure, or oxygenation failure, is the result of abnormal oxygen transport secondary to pulmonary parenchymal disease. Alveolar ventilation is often increased (low arterial Pco_2). $P(A\text{-}a)o_2$ is always increased in this type of respiratory failure. Acute respiratory distress syndrome (ARDS) is the prototype of hypoxemic respiratory failure.
- Hypoxemic-hypercapnic respiratory failure develops as a result of a combination of inadequate alveolar ventilation and abnormal gas transport. The severity of hypoxemia is out of

proportion to hypercapnia; therefore, $P(A\text{-}a)o_2$ is also increased in this type of respiratory failure. It is usually indicative of a markedly deranged ventilation–perfusion relationship, as in severe obstructive airway disease.

Pathogenesis and Etiology. To understand the pathogenesis of respiratory failure under diverse pathologic conditions, it is important to know how ABGs are regulated and maintained within physiologic range despite continuous changes in metabolic activities. Although oxygenation of arterial blood and elimination of CO_2 are interrelated, the mechanisms of their regulations are quite different.

The *control of carbon dioxide,* being part of a delicate hydrogen ion regulation, is much more precise. It is accomplished by ventilatory response through various sensitive receptors. The level of alveolar ventilation is so well adjusted to the metabolic rate that, under normal conditions, the arterial blood pH is maintained within a remarkably narrow range (7.4 ± 0.04) by elimination of CO_2, the byproduct of tissue metabolism. Thus the arterial blood CO_2 tension is also held within normal range. Central chemoreceptors are primarily sensitive to the hydrogen ion concentration, and their apparent sensitivity to CO_2 is probably mediated through local production of H^+.

The stimuli from chemoreceptors as well as from other sources are integrated in the *respiratory center,* which sends nerve impulses to the *respiratory muscles.* The orderly contraction of these muscles performs the work necessary for rhythmic expansion of thoracic cavity, which results in ventilation. Normally, in young adults, about 70% of ventilation is effective in gas exchange, which is known as *alveolar ventilation*. It is the alveolar ventilation that eliminates the CO_2 accumulated in alveoli, thus maintaining its tension at normal range. Because of its ready diffusibility, CO_2 tension in the alveoli is practically the same as in the blood leaving them (ie, arterial blood). The integrity of this sensitive ventilatory control system ensures the elimination of the exact amount of CO_2 produced with the body metabolism, and thus maintains the arterial blood pH and P_{CO_2} within the normal range.

The mechanism of *regulation of oxygen intake* is not that precise, and the ventilatory response to O_2 lack is less sensitive and less effective. In health, the control of oxygen uptake is operative, at least partly, through CO_2 and H^+ regulation. There is only a small ventilatory response to low arterial blood P_{O_2} per se until it has fallen to less than 50 mm Hg. The increased tissue requirement of O_2 most often is met by circulatory response to various stimuli. The ventilatory response to CO_2 and H^+ regulation along with increased blood flow provides the necessary supply of oxygen. Other factors, including change of affinity of hemoglobin, also facilitate oxygen delivery.

In respiratory failure there is derangement of these regulatory mechanisms at various parts of the ventilatory system and/or marked abnormality of pulmonary gas transport. Respiratory failure may, therefore, result from malfunction of the respiratory center, abnormal respiratory neuromuscular system, diseases of the chest wall, airway obstruction, or parenchymal lung disorders. The important disorders leading to respiratory failure, classified according to the major areas of involvement of respiratory control system, are as follows:

I. Intrinsic lung and airway diseases
  A. Large airway obstruction
    1. Congenital deformities
    2. Acute laryngitis, epiglottitis
    3. Foreign bodies
    4. Intrinsic tumors
    5. Extrinsic pressure
    6. Traumatic injury
    7. Enlarged tonsils and adenoids
    8. Obstructive sleep apnea
  B. Bronchial diseases
    1. Chronic bronchitis
    2. Asthma
    3. Acute bronchiolitis
  C. Parenchymal diseases
    1. Pulmonary emphysema
    2. Pulmonary fibrosis and other chronic diffuse infiltrative diseases
    3. Severe pneumonia
    4. Acute lung injury from various causes (ARDS)
  D. Cardiovascular disease
    1. Cardiac pulmonary edema
    2. Massive or recurrent pulmonary embolism
    3. Pulmonary vasculitis

II. Extrapulmonary disorders
  A. Diseases of the pleura and the chest wall
    1. Pneumothorax
    2. Pleural effusion
    3. Fibrothorax
    4. Thoracic wall deformity
    5. Traumatic injury to the chest wall: flail chest
    6. Obesity
  B. Disorders of the respiratory muscles and the neuromuscular junction
    1. Myasthenia gravis and myasthenia-like disorders

2. Muscular dystrophies
3. Polymyositis
4. Botulism
5. Muscle-paralyzing drugs
6. Severe hypokalemia and hypophosphatemia

C. Disorders of the peripheral nerves and spinal cord
1. Poliomyelitis
2. Guillain-Barré syndrome
3. Spinal cord trauma (quadriplegia)
4. Amyotrophic lateral sclerosis
5. Tetanus
6. Multiple sclerosis

D. Disorders of the central nervous system (CNS)
1. Sedative and narcotic drug overdose
2. Head trauma
3. Cerebral hypoxia
4. Cerebrovascular accident
5. CNS infection
6. Epileptic seizure: status epilepticus
7. Metabolic and endocrine disorders
8. Bulbar poliomyelitis
9. Primary alveolar hypoventilation
10. Sleep apnea syndrome

Many of these disorders are discussed in appropriate chapters of this book.

In addition to the basic disease leading to respiratory failure, certain precipitating or exacerbating factors are operative, such as the following:

1. Changes of tracheobronchial secretions
2. Infection: viral or bacterial
3. Disturbance of tracheobronchial clearance

4. Drugs: sedatives, narcotics, anesthesia, oxygen
5. Inhalation or aspiration of irritants, vomitus, foreign body
6. Cardiovascular disorders: heart failure, pulmonary embolism, shock
7. Mechanical factors: pneumothorax, pleural effusion, abdominal distension
8. Trauma, including surgery
9. Neuromuscular abnormalities
10. Allergic disorders: bronchospasm
11. Increased oxygen demand: fever, infection
12. Inspiratory muscle fatigue

These precipitating factors play a very important role in exacerbation of preexisting respiratory insufficiency. In practically every case of acute respiratory failure superimposed on chronic pulmonary disease, one or more of these factors can be identified. Because of their reversibility, their early detection and prompt treatment are essential in the proper management of acute respiratory failure. Respiratory muscle fatigue is considered to be an important factor in precipitating as well as in perpetuating respiratory failure.

Certain factors associated with respiratory failure are considered both among leading causes and precipitating causes. For example, pulmonary infection may be the major or even the only cause of acute respiratory failure in widespread pneumonia, whereas it is a frequent precipitating factor in chronic obstructive lung disease (COLD).

Pathophysiologic Mechanisms. Abnormal gas exchange is the dominating physiologic alteration in respiratory failure. Hypoxemia, common to all forms of respiratory failure, may be caused by any of the following basic mechanisms, singly or in various combinations:

1. **Alveolar hypoventilation** results in an increase in the alveolar P_{CO_2}, which in turn is the cause of low alveolar P_{O_2}. Even with a normal alveolar-arterial P_{O_2} gradient, low alveolar P_{O_2} results in arterial hypoxemia. Hypoxemia in ventilatory failure is due to this mechanism.

2. **Impairment of diffusion,** although present in emphysema and other diffuse lung injury, has only an insignificant role in the hypoxemia of acute respiratory failure. The alveolar-arterial oxygen tension gradient solely from a diffusion defect is usually small and readily compensated by even a small increase in the fractional concentration of inspired oxygen (FIO_2).

3. **Ventilation–perfusion mismatching** is the most common cause of hypoxemia in clinical situations. Disorders involving the airways result in uneven ventilation of various lung regions and units whose perfusion frequently fails to match the changes of ventilation (Fig. 26–1). Both chronic lung diseases and

most acute leading or precipitating causes of respiratory failure are known to be associated with ventilation–perfusion inequality.

4. **Right-to-left shunt** as a cause of hypoxemia in acute respiratory failure is the result of continuous perfusion of nonventilated regions of the lung (Fig. 26–2). It almost always indicates the closure of the air passages, especially the distal airways and alveoli, by various causes so common in acute respiratory failure.

5. **Reduced oxygen in mixed venous blood.** In addition to the previously mentioned basic mechanisms, extrapulmonary factors such as cardiac output and metabolic rate are known to affect arterial P_{O_2} tension, particularly in association with abnormal pulmonary gas exchange. Increased oxygen extraction from the arterial blood in these clinical situations results in reduced mixed venous blood P_{O_2}. Any degree of hypoxemia from pulmonary causes, especially with a right-to-left shunt and ventilation–perfusion mismatching, is aggravated by this extrapulmonary mechanism, which is almost invariably present in critically ill patients (Fig. 26–3).

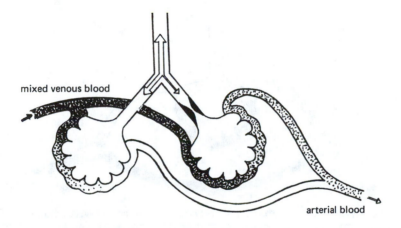

mixed venous blood

arterial blood

Figure 26–1. Mismatching of ventilation with perfusion. Perfusion in excess of ventilation resulting in arterial hypoxemia.

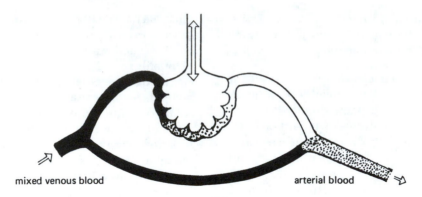

Figure 26–2. Hypoxemia resulting from intrapulmonary shunting.

Unless hypoxemia is solely from low alveolar P_{O_2} (as in alveolar hypoventilation), it is always associated with increased $P(A-a)_{O_2}$. (For calculation of alveolar-arterial O_2 gradient, see Appendix D.)

Hypercapnia, the hallmark of ventilatory failure, is indicative of an alveolar ventilation that is inadequate for the proper elimination of CO_2. Ventilation–perfusion mismatching, when not compensated by increased ventilation of well-perfused regions, is a significant cause of hypercapnia in chronic obstructive pulmonary disease (COPD). The clinical type of hypercapnic-hypoxemic respiratory failure most characteristically occurs in this setting.

In acute hypercapnia, as expected, arterial blood pH will be reduced, indicating acute respiratory acidosis. It should, however, be mentioned that the

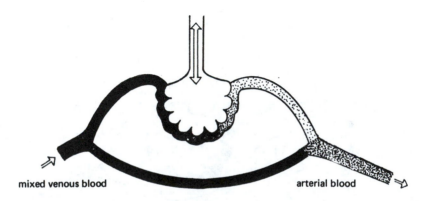

Figure 26–3. Effect of very low venous oxygen content on arterial hypoxemia. Hypoxemia resulting from shunting or $\dot{V}/\dot{Q}$ mismatch becomes more severe when venous blood oxygen is decreased as a result of increased peripheral extraction (low cardiac output and/or high metabolic rate).

superimposition of metabolic acidosis on preexistent chronic respiratory alkalosis produces an ABG picture indistinguishable from that of acute respiratory acidosis. With chronic hypercapnia, as seen in advanced cases of COPD, the onset of acute respiratory failure is indicated by a further increase of arterial P_{CO_2} to a very high level and a reduction of blood pH. Serum bicarbonate levels will be significantly increased.

In hypoxemic respiratory failure, arterial blood pH is usually alkalotic as a result of hyperventilation, unless it is offset by concomitant metabolic acidosis of tissue hypoxia. The combination of acute hypercapnia in ventilatory failure and metabolic acidosis causes a more severe reduction in pH (mixed respiratory and metabolic acidosis).

The major impact of respiratory failure on various organs is through hypoxemia and disturbance in acid-base balance, mainly from hypercapnia. However, it should be emphasized that hypoxemia usually has more disastrous consequences and its effect on vital organs is more damaging than hypercapnia. Practically every organ and tissue may suffer from hypoxemia, and acidosis is known to impair many cellular functions. As a result of low O_2 in poorly ventilated regions, pulmonary vascular resistance increases. Hypercapnia (acidosis) enhances this effect of hypoxia further. Therefore, preexistent cor pulmonale in patients with chronic lung disease is aggravated by acute respiratory failure. The effect of hypoxemia on the myocardium not only is an additional cause of right-side heart failure, but left ventricular function is also impaired. Reduced cardiac output and cardiogenic pulmonary edema exacerbate hypoxemia. Respiratory muscles are also known to be affected by both hypoxemia and hypercapnia. Diaphragmatic fatigue, which can occur as a result of increased workload, may be precipitated by hypoxemia, reduced perfusion, and hypercapnia. It appears, therefore, that acute respiratory failure may reach a point when a positive feedback mechanism is established. This vicious circle results in the precipitous deterioration of respiratory failure and death unless appropriate treatment is instituted.

Clinical Manifestations. The clinical presentation of acute respiratory failure is a combination of clinical features of underlying disease and precipitating factor(s) and manifestations of hypoxemia and/or hypercapnia. As numerous pulmonary and extrapulmonary disorders may lead to acute respiratory failure and various factors may precipitate it, the clinical picture will be quite variable. Moreover, the presence or absence of preceding chronic respiratory insufficiency and predominance of hypoxemia or hypercapnia will further change the clinical manifestations.

The commonly mentioned symptom of dyspnea, which is the hallmark of hypoxemic respiratory failure, may be entirely absent in ventilatory failure resulting from depression of the respiratory center. The rate of respiration, likewise, will be quite variable; it is generally increased in hypoxemic respiratory failure and decreased in ventilatory failure due to respiratory center depression. Although inadequacy of alveolar ventilation is pathognomonic for ventilatory failure, its bedside detection is often difficult if not impossible in most instances. It is not uncommon to make an assumption of ad equacy of alveolar ventilation from the respiratory rate and apparent depth of breathing that turns out to be quite inaccurate by ABG analysis. Use of accessory muscles of respiration and intercostal or supraclavicular retraction are indicative of significant mechanical impediment to respiration and increased ventilatory effort. As with dyspnea, these signs may be totally absent in central hypoventilation. In diaphragmatic weakness or fatigue, paradoxical abdominal movement is a characteristic finding.

Cyanosis, although not very sensitive, is a common feature of hypoxemic respiratory failure. Lack of improvement of cyanosis after breathing oxygen usually signifies severe gas transport abnormality, shunting, or poor tissue perfusion.

Other respiratory symptoms and physical findings on examination of the chest will depend on underlying chronic or acute pulmonary disease leading to or aggravating respiratory failure. These have been discussed in appropriate chapters dealing with specific disease states. Signs of right-side heart failure (cor pulmonale), including peripheral edema, engorged neck veins, and enlarged liver, are usually indicative of chronic underlying pulmonary condition.

Clinical manifestations of hypoxemia and hypercapnia are discussed in Chapter 1. It should be emphasized that most of these manifestations are common for both hypoxemia and acidosis from hypercapnia. They include change in mental state, headaches, weakness, lassitude, and muscle tremor or twitching. Drowsiness, confusion, somnolence, irritability, agitation, and coma are some of the usual mental changes due to severe hypoxemia with or without hypercapnia. Increased intracranial pressure, sometimes manifested by changes in the eyeground, is

fairly common in both of these conditions. Cardiac arrhythmias are common manifestations of acute respiratory failure. Bronchodilators, including aminophylline and beta-adrenergics, are known to cause or aggravate cardiac arrhythmias, especially in patients with hypoxemia and/or acidosis. (See also clinical manifestations of ARDS in Chapter 27.)

Radiographic Findings. Radiographic examination of the chest is essential for the diagnosis of underlying, as well as precipitating, causes of respiratory failure. As with symptoms and physical findings, chest x-ray changes in respiratory failure will vary with underlying disease. It may be entirely normal in ventilatory failure due to extrapulmonary disorders. Changes of COPD or diffuse fibrosis, with or without superimposed acute changes due to infection or other complicating and precipitating pulmonary events, are common radiographic findings in chronic cases. Most cases of acute hypoxemic respiratory failure without underlying chronic lung disease manifest with bilateral diffuse interstitial and airspace densities suggesting pulmonary edema as discussed in Chapter 27.

Radiographic studies are important for the proper follow-up of patients with acute respiratory failure and for the early detection of complications such as superinfection, atelectasis, pneumothorax, and other mishaps of intubation and mechanical ventilation.

Diagnosis. Although the history, physical examination, and radiographic findings are very important for the diagnosis of respiratory failure, it can be conclusively established only by determination of the blood gases and pH. These tests are essential not only for the diagnosis, classi-fication, and assessment of the severity of respiratory failure, but are also indispens-able for the evaluation of its progress and response to therapeutic measures. With a diagnosis of respiratory failure, the iden-tification of its underlying cause and the recognition of the precipitating event(s) are crucial for an appropriate manage-ment plan.

The presence and the extent of parenchymal lung disease, particularly acute lung injury and inflammation, are best assessed by radiographic examina-tion. Infection, being one of the most common causes of respiratory failure, should always be suspected and properly evaluated. Examination of the sputum, among other bacteriologic studies, is es-sential for its detection. Airway obstruc-tion should be confirmed and its severity gauged by flow studies such as measure-ment of peak expiratory flow. Other vari-ables of respiratory mechanics are evalu-ated by determining tidal volume, minute ventilation, vital capacity, and maximum inspiratory and expiratory pressures. De-termination of the latter is essential for the diagnosis of disorders of the respira-tory pump resulting in ventilatory failure or contributing to other forms of respira-tory failure.

As is discussed in Chapter 27, one of the important differentiations in respira-tory failure is between cardiogenic pul-monary edema and acute respiratory dis-tress syndrome (ARDS). Pulmonary artery catheterization with a balloon-flotation catheter is useful for this purpose. It may also give valuable information for the proper management of patients with acute respiratory failure in whom con-comitant cardiac impairment and fluid imbalance are quite common.

■ MANAGEMENT OF RESPIRATORY FAILURE

General Principles

Principles of management are applicable to all forms of acute respiratory failure, although the therapeutic approach will vary according to the particular underly-ing disease, predisposing factor(s), and pathophysiologic abnormalities. In every patient with respiratory failure, the fol-lowing measures should be undertaken:

- Establishment and maintenance of an adequate airway
- Oxygenation
- Correction of acid-base disturbance
- Restoration of fluid and electrolyte balance
- Optimizing cardiac function
- Identification and treatment of un-derlying correctable conditions and precipitating causes
- Prevention of potential complica-tions and their early detection
- Nutritional support
- Periodic assessment of the course, progress, and response to therapy
- Determination of a need for me-chanical ventilatory support

Management of patients with acute respiratory failure superimposed on chronic pulmonary disease is somewhat different from management of patients whose respiratory failure is due to acute pulmonary injury or extrapulmonary conditions. This distinction is especially important in deciding for tracheal intu-bation and mechanical ventilation (see Chapter 28).

Although the following steps in the management of respiratory failure are discussed separately, in most clinical set-tings they are carried out more or less concurrently. Moreover, certain measures are effective in correcting more than one abnormality.

Establishment and Maintenance of an Adequate Airway. It is essential that an adequate airway be provided at all times for a patient with respiratory failure. In patients with upper airway obstruction as the cause of respiratory failure, the establishment of a patent airway will immediately restore ventilation. This is discussed in Chapter 7. Use of simple devices, such as oropharyngeal or nasopharyngeal tubes, will suffice in certain situations (eg, during transient loss of consciousness). In many instances, particularly when there is a need for ventilatory support, tracheal intubation is necessary (page 399). In addition to providing an appropriate airway for mechanical ventilation, tracheal intubation may be indicated for protecting the lungs from aspiration, for maintenance of airway patency, and for effective suctioning.

As secretions and other materials in the airways are frequent causes of airway obstruction, the importance of adequate tracheobronchial toilet, with or without tracheal intubation, cannot be overstressed. Deep breathing, coughing, and other physiotherapeutic maneuvers, as well as tracheobronchial suctioning should be considered in every patient with respiratory failure. Many times, the success or failure of therapy will depend on the adequacy and proper application of these measures. The presence of a tracheal tube makes its care, as well as tracheobronchial hygiene, even more important.

Oxygenation. The proper supply of oxygen to the tissues is the major concern in the management of patients with respiratory failure, as the lack of adequate tissue oxygenation is the most important deleterious consequence of this condition.

In addition to the arterial blood oxygen content, tissue oxygenation depends on its blood supply. For an adequate tissue oxygen delivery, cardiac output and tissue perfusion are at least as important as the arterial blood oxygen level.

Chronic hypoxemia, sometimes to a severe degree, is usually well tolerated. Certain adaptive mechanisms, including changes in blood perfusion, shift of the oxyhemoglobin dissociation curve, reduced metabolic activities, and perhaps more efficient oxygen extraction by the tissues, are operative in chronic hypoxemia. However *acute* hypoxemia usually results in significant tissue hypoxia because of the lack of or inadequacy of adaptive mechanisms. Obviously, the easiest way to improve the arterial oxygen tension is to increase the inspired oxygen concentration. It should be emphasized, however, that the maneuvers that improve alveolar ventilation and gas distribution will also result in enhancement of arterial blood oxygenation.

In acute respiratory failure, oxygen may be administered by various means to increase the arterial oxygen tension to a satisfactory level, which varies according to the duration of hypoxemia and other circumstances of respiratory failure. Increasing FIO_2 is expected to improve arterial Po_2 in all conditions except when there is significant ($>30\%$) right-to-left shunting (Fig. 26–4). Administration of oxygen in hypoxemia with adequate ventilation, unless the FIO_2 exceeds 0.5 for a prolonged period of time, is quite safe.

In hypercapnic states, oxygen should be given more judiciously. As many patients with hypercapnia have decreased

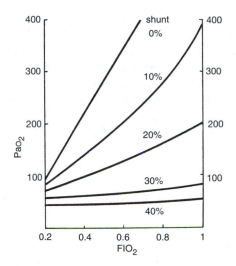

Figure 26–4. The relationship between FIO_2 and Pao_2 with varying percentage of shunt. With a shunt over 30% of cardiac output, hypoxemia cannot be corrected with high FIO_2s.

ventilatory response to Pco_2 and H^+, hypoxemia is their major remaining respiratory stimulus. In addition, by eliminating hypoxic pulmonary vasoconstriction, oxygen administration may enhance ventilation–perfusion mismatching. This mechanism may be even more important than inhibition of hypoxic ventilatory drive. Regardless of the mechanism involved, inappropriate oxygen administration in hypercapnic patients may result in further CO_2 retention and respiratory acidosis. Fortunately, in most instances of hypoxemia with ventilatory impairment, a small increment in concentration of inspired oxygen is sufficient for a clinically significant improvement in oxygenation. Because of the steepness of the oxyhemoglobin dissociation curve in hypoxemic range, a modest increase in the arterial oxygen tension results in a significant improvement of the oxygen content.

For example, raising the arterial oxygen tension from 30 to 50 mm Hg results in an increase in its saturation from 57% to 83.5% (Fig. 26–5). This is the rationale for controlled oxygen therapy in patients with acute respiratory failure due to COPD. It is conveniently accomplished by the administration of oxygen via a Venturi mask or judicious use of nasal O_2, which, along with monitoring arterial blood gases, will allow one to manage the acute and critical reduction of the arterial Po_2 in these patients without aggravating their respiratory acidosis. In practice, there is no significant advantage in increasing the arterial Po_2 to more than 60 mm Hg; and in many cases, Po_2 levels in the low 50s are acceptable. Continuous monitoring of arterial oxygen saturation with pulse oximetry is an important addition to a safer way of oxygen therapy.

As reduced mixed venous oxygen content aggravates arterial hypoxemia resulting from abnormal pulmonary gas transport, measures that reduce the difference between arterial and venous oxygen content should increase arterial Po_2 in hypoxemic states. Such measures in-

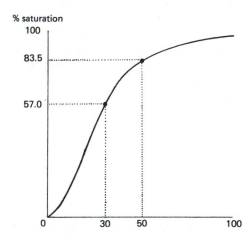

Figure 26–5. Oxygen-hemoglobin dissociation curve. At hypoxemic level, a small rise in arterial Po_2 results in significant improvement of its oxygen content.

clude improving cardiac output (see later in this chapter), correcting anemia, and reducing metabolic rates (as by controlling fever). These therapeutic interventions, in addition, will improve tissue oxygenation.

As mentioned earlier, in oxygenation failure when there is significant intrapulmonary shunting, such as in ARDS, it is difficult to adequately oxygenate patients by simply increasing their FIO_2 (see Fig. 26–4). In certain selected patients, especially when they are alert and cooperative, the addition of continuous positive airway pressure (CPAP) or expiratory positive airway pressure (EPAP) by a nasal or facial mask with a soft, tight seal helps oxygenation and may obviate the necessity for intubation and mechanical ventilation. In more severe cases with refractory and progressive hypoxemia, mechanical ventilatory support will be necessary (Chapter 28).

Correction of Acid-Base Disturbance. As discussed earlier, respiratory failure is almost always accompanied by certain degrees of acid-base abnormalities. In *ventilatory* failure and hypoxic-hypercapnic respiratory failure, an increase in PCO_2 results in reduction of pH (acidemia) until renal compensation increases the serum bicarbonate level. Renal compensation at very high PCO_2 levels is usually not complete, and the resultant pH will remain somewhat acidotic. In acute ventilatory failure, renal compensation, which requires a certain amount of time to take place, will be lacking; therefore, acidemia is always present. Furthermore, superimposition of metabolic acidosis, which is a fairly common occurrence, results in further reduction of the pH. In hypoxemic respiratory failure,

however, hyperventilation and, thus, respiratory alkalosis may be evident. Severe tissue hypoxia may result in anaerobic metabolism, production of lactic acid, and, hence, metabolic acidosis.

Because in acute respiratory failure pH abnormality is more deleterious to the proper functions of vital organs than are changes of PCO_2, emphasis should be placed on correction of pH and its maintenance rather than that of PCO_2. Metabolic acidosis is usually treated by administration of bicarbonate; however, correction of causes of metabolic derangement, such as severe hypoxemia, is essential for successful outcome. In acute hypercapnia with significant acidosis, improving the alveolar ventilation is the most logical approach. This can be accomplished by various means. In addition to mechanical ventilatory support (see Chapter 28), simpler measures intended for improvement of alveolar ventilation, such as establishment and maintenance of an adequate airway, treating bronchospasm, controlling heart failure, and eliminating other precipitating factors should be undertaken. Controlling fever, sepsis, and other hypermetabolic states results in reduced CO_2 production and improvement of hypercapnia. Dietary adjustment (see later in this chapter) is known to alter the respiratory exchange ratio and thus may also be helpful in reducing CO_2 production. Often such measures will obviate the necessity for mechanical ventilation. The use of "respiratory center stimulants," except for aminophylline and occasionally other drugs, has not shown significant therapeutic benefit. The use of depressant drugs, including indiscriminate oxygen administration, should be avoided. The use of bicarbonate in acute respiratory acidosis is controversial but may be considered in certain unusual circumstances, as in permissive hypercapnia.

Restoration of Fluid and Electrolyte Balance. Proper attention to fluid and electrolyte status is an important part of management of patients with respiratory failure. The lungs are easily affected by excess fluid from various causes. In addition to heart failure, certain renal and hepatic disorders may result in fluid overload and alteration of plasma oncotic (colloid osmotic) pressure. Excessive intravenous fluid administration is known to increase the water content of injured lungs and worsen respiratory failure. Conversely, poor fluid intake and other causes of dehydration by reducing cardiac output adversely affect oxygen transport. Monitoring of fluid intake and output and periodic measurement of body weight will be helpful in assessment of fluid balance. Among electrolyte abnormalities affecting respiratory function are hypokalemia and hypophosphatemia, which should be prevented and treated promptly if present.

Optimizing Cardiac Function. Cardiac malfunction is common in pulmonary disease, particularly in acute respiratory failure. Injured lungs, by being sensitive to changes in cardiac function, tend to retain fluid easily because of loss of integrity of the alveolar-capillary membrane. Adequate cardiac output is essential for oxygen delivery to body organs and tissues. At a time when arterial oxygen content is reduced as a result of respiratory failure, adequate tissue oxygenation becomes dependent on increased perfusion. Respiratory muscles, because of their increased workload, need addi-

tional blood flow for their metabolic needs. Reduced cardiac output, therefore, may impair the ventilatory function of these muscles resulting in their fatigue. Conversely, hypoxemia and acidosis of respiratory failure adversely affect myocardial function. Thus, in treatment of respiratory failure, optimizing cardiac function may be crucial for a successful outcome. For proper management of combined respiratory and cardiac failure, hemodynamic monitoring, preferably with a pulmonary artery catheter, is advisable.

Identification and Treatment of Underlying Correctable Conditions and Precipitating Causes. While patients with acute respiratory failure are being managed for the abnormalities of blood gases, disturbances of fluid and acid-base balance, and hemodynamic derangements, every effort should be made to identify and properly treat the underlying disease and precipitating factors. Management of various pulmonary or extrapulmonary disorders leading to respiratory failure has been discussed in appropriate chapters and is not repeated here.

The factors that precipitate or contribute to acute respiratory failure are numerous (see page 373). Many of these disorders are treatable and often preventable. Respiratory tract infection seems to be the common culprit in this regard. It may be viral, bacterial, or, rarely, fungal in origin. Its prevention, early diagnosis, and treatment are crucial in the management of respiratory failure.

Increased tracheobronchial secretions, changes in their characteristics, and difficulty in their elimination due to various factors may result in airway obstruction, particularly in patients with COPD. As was emphasized before, proper tracheobronchial hygiene is one of the most important measures in management of these patients.

Congestive heart failure and other circulatory disorders are common precipitating events; they should be identified and treated appropriately. Bronchospasm, particularly in patients with a background of asthma, may be a significant reversible factor contributing to respiratory failure, which will respond to bronchodilators. Corticosteroids are often used in this and other situations in which the anti-inflammatory effects of these drugs are considered to be beneficial.

Organic or metabolic disorders affecting the CNS or neuromuscular function should always be considered when investigating the precipitating causes of respiratory decompensation. Sedative, hypnotic, and, particularly, narcotic drugs are poorly tolerated by patients with chronic ventilatory insufficiency and may precipitate an acute episode of respiratory failure. The use of these agents should be discontinued and, in case of narcotic drug intake, a proper antidote should be administered. Indiscriminate use of oxygen, which may aggravate CO_2 retention or even result in CO_2 narcosis, should be avoided.

The presence of air or fluid in the pleural cavity may significantly impair ventilation; their removal may result in dramatic improvement in some patients. Abdominal distention, which may cause compression of the lung bases and interference with diaphragmatic movement, should be adequately treated and prevented from recurring. Use of respirator bags without a tracheal tube frequently results in distention of the stomach with air; this should be emptied by a nasogastric tube.

Respiratory impairment due to trauma and surgery, which may lead to or precipitate a bout of acute respiratory failure, is discussed in Chapter 23. Limitation of the thoracic wall movement, ineffective cough, immobility, and lack of deep breathing are among factors that contribute to respiratory difficulty under these circumstances.

Fever and other causes of heightened metabolism, which by increasing oxygen demand and CO_2 production contribute to respiratory failure, should be properly treated.

Fatigue of the respiratory muscles, especially the diaphragm, has been recognized as an important contributory factor in almost all forms of ventilatory failure. Its early recognition and treatment are essential parts of the management of respiratory failure. Resting these muscles by mechanical ventilatory support is the most effective measure in restoring their contractility. Aminophylline and beta-adrenergic agonists are known to improve the contractile force of the diaphragm and delay its fatigue. Among disorders of electrolyte balance, deficiencies of serum phosphates, potassium, and calcium are known to impair respiratory muscle function. They should be properly identified and adequately corrected.

Prevention of Potential Complications and Their Early Detection. Respiratory failure is frequently associated with various complications during its course and treatment. Because most of them occur in mechanically ventilated patients, they are discussed in Chapter 28 and are not repeated here.

Nutritional Support. Nutritional deficiency is known to contribute to respiratory failure through different mechanisms, such as the impairment of respiratory muscle function, reduction of ventilatory drive, and weakening of pulmonary defenses. Malnourished patients usually have a reduced diaphragmatic muscle mass. Ventilatory response to hypoxemia is diminished following inadequate nutrition. Impaired immunologic defenses, especially from an alteration of cell-mediated immunity, in malnourished patients predisposes them further to various infections including nosocomial pneumonia. Poorly nourished subjects have significant difficulty in being weaned off mechanical ventilatory support, necessitating prolonged and complicated hospitalization in critical care units. It is, therefore, essential that in the management of patients in respiratory failure, proper nutritional assessment and adequate nutritional support be steadfastly pursued. In most patients, enteral alimentation is preferred over parenteral feeding. Enteral feeding seems to be important for maintaining bowel wall integrity.

As most calories in usual nutritional formulas are derived from carbohydrates, patients receiving them have a high respiratory quotient (ratio of CO_2 production to O_2 consumption). The increased CO_2 production may contribute to hypercapnic respiratory failure and may become an obstacle against a successful weaning from mechanical ventilation. High lipid formulas, however, result in lower respiratory quotient and, therefore, may be more suitable for the nutritional support of patients in hypercapnic respiratory failure.

Periodic Assessment of the Course, Progress, and Response to Therapy. Patients in acute respiratory failure are usually critically ill and often medically unstable. Close observation, preferably in an intensive care unit, is necessary for proper evaluation of their progress and response to therapeutic measures. Among many clinical and laboratory parameters, ABGs are particularly important for this purpose. When there is no evidence of hypercapnia or other acid-base abnormalities, monitoring arterial oxygen saturation by pulse oximetry would obviate the need for frequent measurements of ABGs. In ventilatory failure, however, pulse oximetry alone cannot be relied on for the assessment of respiratory status and response to treatment.

Determination of a Need for Mechanical Ventilatory Support. A patient who is not already on a respirator may at a certain period in the clinical course require mechanical ventilatory support. In most patients the decision for instituting mechanical ventilation is made after a period of close observation while they are being treated by more conservative measures. Indications and other aspects of mechanical ventilation are discussed in Chapter 28.

BIBLIOGRAPHY

Bégin P, Grassino A. Inspiratory muscle dysfunction and chronic hypercapnia in chronic obstructive pulmonary disease. *Am Rev Respir Dis.* 1991; 143:905–912.

Bennett DA, Bleck TP. Diagnosis and treatment of neuromuscular causes of acute respiratory failure. *Clin Neuropharmacol.* 1988; 11:303–347.

Curtis JR, Hudson LD. Emergent assessment and management of acute respiratory failure in COPD. *Clin Chest Med.* 1994; 15:481–500.

Grassino A, Macklem PT. Respiratory muscle fatigue and ventilatory failure. *Annu Rev Med.* 1984; 35:625–647.

Green KE, Peters JI. Pathophysiology of acute respiratory failure. *Clin Chest Med.* 1994; 15: 1–12.

Heffner JE. Airway management in the critically ill patient. *Crit Care Clin.* 1990; 6: 533–550.

Juan G, Calverley P, Talamo C, et al. Effect of carbon dioxide on diaphragmatic function in human beings. *N Engl J Med.* 1984; 310: 874–879.

Leisure GS, Stone DJ, Spiekermann BF, Bogdonoff DL. Airway management of the chronically intubated patient. *Respir Care.* 1995; 40:1279–1286.

O'Connor BS, Vender JS. Oxygen therapy. *Crit Care Clin.* 1995; 11:67–78.

Pinard B, Geller E. Nutritional support during pulmonary failure. *Crit Care Clin.* 1995; 11:705–715.

Pingleton SK. Enteral nutrition in patients with respiratory disease. *Eur Respir J.* 1996; 9:364–370.

Rochester DF. Respiratory muscles and ventilatory failure. *Am J Med Sci.* 1993; 305: 394–402.

Roussos C. Respiratory muscle fatigue and ventilatory failure. *Chest.* 1990; 97(3 Suppl): 89S–96S.

Viires N, Aubier M, Murciano D, et al. Effects of aminophylline on diaphragmatic fatigue during acute respiratory failure. *Am Rev Respir Dis.* 1984; 129:396–402.

Weinberger SE, Schwartzstein RM, Weiss JW. Hypercapnia. *N Engl J Med.* 1989; 321: 1223–1231.

Zucker AR. Therapeutic strategies for acute hypoxemic respiratory failure. *Crit Care Med.* 1988; 4:813–830.

27.

Acute Respiratory Distress Syndrome

Acute respiratory distress syndrome (ARDS) is a distinct form of acute respiratory failure resulting from diffuse pulmonary injury of various causes, characterized by rapidly progressive dyspnea, tachypnea, refractory hypoxemia, diffuse pulmonary infiltration, and reduced lung volumes and compliance. Originally, the first letter in ARDS was intended to represent "adult" rather than "acute." Because the syndrome may also occur in children and adolescents, the latter is a more appropriate qualifier. This change was adopted by the 1992 American–European Consensus Conference on ARDS. Prior to 1967, when ARDS was first introduced to medical literature, the syndrome was known by various names (Table 27–1).

Etiology and Risk Factors. Numerous clinical disorders are known to cause ARDS or to contribute to its development. As the basic underlying lesion in ARDS from all causes is acute lung injury

(ALI), any condition that results in such an injury is a risk factor for or potential etiology of this syndrome. ALI and, therefore, ARDS can develop as a consequence of various disorders that directly or indirectly affect the lung parenchyma in a diffuse fashion. These disorders include

- Sepsis
- Pulmonary aspiration
- Thoracic trauma; pulmonary contusion
- Severe extrathoracic trauma, including head injury
- Extensive burns
- Inhalation of toxic fumes or gases, including smoke inhalation
- Circulatory shock from different causes
- Diffuse pulmonary infection (viral pneumonias, *Pneumocystis carinii* pneumonia [PCP])
- Near drowning
- Oxygen toxicity

- Fat embolism
- Transfusion of a massive amount of banked blood
- Prolonged cardiopulmonary bypass
- Acute severe pancreatitis
- Amniotic fluid embolism
- Air embolism
- Heat stroke
- Eclampsia
- Drug-induced lung injury (narcotics, cocaine, aspirin, antineoplastic drugs)
- Disseminated intravascular coagulation (DIC)
- Ionizing radiation
- Acute paraquat poisoning

Among this diverse group of etiologic factors, sepsis is the most common condition associated with ARDS. Most patients with septic shock develop this syndrome. Pulmonary aspiration and severe trauma are also major offenders. Although any of these causes can result in lung injury on preexistent pulmonary disease, most patients have no prior cardiorespiratory disorders. However, certain preexistent debilitating disorders and chronic dysfunction of organs such as the liver and kidney enhance the progression of ALI to ARDS. When more than one of the previ-

ously mentioned risk factors is involved, the likelihood of lung injury and ARDS is significantly increased.

Pathogenesis. Generally, acute diffuse injury of lung parenchyma in ARDS is initiated in two different ways. It may develop at the air–lung interface, in which causative factors enter the lungs through the airways, as in pulmonary aspiration and smoke inhalation. Initial insult may occur at the blood–lung interface via the bloodstream, as in fat embolism. Regardless of how it is started, the ensuing events result in a more or less similar pathologic and physiologic alteration of the lungs. Both endothelium and epithelium are damaged, resulting in leaky alveolar-capillary membrane. As part of the host defensive response and reparative effort, local and systemic inflammation develops. The inflammatory reaction itself causes further lung injury.

In conditions that result in lung injury directly, inflammation is secondary, whereas in sepsis the lung injury is the consequence of inflammation. Sepsis, which is the most common cause of ARDS, is defined as the systemic inflammatory response to infection that may be local or systemic (septicemia). Among the infectious agents, gram-negative bacteria are notorious for inciting severe systemic reaction. Endotoxin produced by these microorganisms is a major reason for their characteristic pathogenetic featurers. In addition to infection, other clinical conditions may also result in systemic inflammatory response syndrome (SIRS). They include multiple trauma, extensive burn, acute pancreatitis, and shock from noninfectious causes. When severe enough, SIRS affects the function of several organs including the lungs (multiple-organ dysfunction syndrome) and may even cause their failure (multiple-organ

TABLE 27–1. VARIOUS NAMES FOR ARDS[a]

Shock lung
Wet lung syndrome
White lung syndrome
Adult hyaline membrane disease
Da Nang lung
Progressive respiratory distress
Congestive atelectasis
Posttraumatic pulmonary insufficiency

[a] Prior to 1967.

system failure). Lung injury and ARDS almost always represent the predominant feature of these events.

Whether as a primary cause of or contributing factor in ALI, inflammation has been regarded as the major pathogenetic mechanism in ARDS. Despite extensive animal and human research in recent years, the exact mechanisms of lung injury by various inflammatory cells and mediators are not fully understood. Although many inflammatory cells and mediators of lung injury have been recognized, their exact role, the sequence of their involvement, and the degree of their importance have remained speculative. Among the cells involved, polymorphonuclear neutrophils (PMNs) play the central role in inflammation. They are sequestered in pulmonary microvasculature; become activated; and produce various proteolytic enzymes, toxic oxygen metabolites, and other inflammatory mediators. Other cells that participate in the process are macrophages, lymphocytes, and fibroblasts. They interact with the help of cytokines and produce various mediators of inflammation. Complement activation, involvement of coagulation factors, and participation of certain vasoactive substances (including nitric oxide), have also been considered to be important components of the pathogenetic process in ALI and ARDS. Table 27–2 shows some of the mediators implicated in acute lung injury.

ALI resulting from the initial event and sustained by subsequent inflammation is the basic mechanism of structural change and functional impairment characteristic of ARDS. In addition to accumulation of fluid and inflammatory cells in the lungs, other changes also take place. As a result of injury to alveolar cells and presence of edema fluid in the alve-

TABLE 27–2. MEDIATORS IMPLICATED IN THE PATHOGENESIS OF ALI

Cytokines (tumor necrosis factor, interleukins)
Oxidants (toxic oxygen metabolites)
Complement components
Activated coagulation factors
Arachidonic acid metabolite (prostaglandins, leukotrienes)
Nitric oxide (NO) and other vasoactive substances
Proteolytic enzymes
Platelet-activating factors
Growth factors
Neuropeptides

oli, surfactant is markedly reduced and becomes qualitatively abnormal. Some of the small vessels are obliterated from fibrin-platelet aggregation. Certain growth factors released by inflammatory cells result in early proliferation of fibroblast and beginning fibrous tissue formation.

Pathology. Although the underlying etiologic factors are quite varied, pathologic changes are almost similar. Diffuse alveolar damage with resultant changes secondary to alveolar-capillary leak and inflammatory reaction are the bases of morphologic abnormalities seen in the lungs of patients with ARDS. Early acute changes include destructive lesions and loss of endothelial and type I alveolar epithelial cells, edema, hemorrhage, infiltration with inflammatory cells, microatelectasis, and hyaline membrane formation. These changes are not homogeneous; whereas some alveoli are severely damaged or filled with proteinaceous fluid and cells, others may be more or less intact. Pathologic lesions have a predilection for dependent lung regions. Persistence of lung injury beyond 7 to 10 days usually results in chronic changes of organizing stage, in which type II alveolar cells proliferate. Increased number of fibroblasts denote beginning of fibrosis that may develop rapidly. At this stage, there are also changes in pulmonary microvasculature characterized by disruption of the vascular bed and thrombotic or embolic occlusion of some of the small vessels. Bronchoalveolar lavage (BAL) fluid recovered from patients with ARDS contains large numbers of PMNs. BAL fluid surfactant is deficient in its surface-tension lowering activity as a result of the alteration of its chemical composition.

Pathophysiology. Severe hypoxemia, an essential component of ARDS, is the result of marked maldistribution of ventilation and perfusion and their mismatching. Intrapulmonary shunting from perfusion of unventilated lung regions is the hallmark of pathophysiologic change of the syndrome. Alveolar and interstitial edema, inflammatory changes, reduced and ineffective surfactant, and early fibrotic changes are known causes of reduced lung compliance. Considering the

heterogeneity of lung injury, however, decreased compliance may be in large part from reduced volume of ventilating lung units. Such units, per se, may have normal compliance. This notion is important for understanding the deleterious effect of mechanical ventilation with large tidal volumes in ARDS.

Because of vascular disruption and obstruction of some of the small vessels, certain ventilated lung units may have reduced or no perfusion, resulting in increased dead-space ventilation. High minute ventilation, together with reduced lung compliance, markedly increases the work of breathing. Tachypnea is the result of increased minute ventilation and low tidal volumes. Pulmonary hypertension, a common occurrence in ARDS, is secondary to vascular obstruction and increased vascular tone from imbalance of vasoactive substances and hypoxia. Figure 27–1 schematically shows the pathophysiologic changes in ARDS.

In addition to pathologic changes in

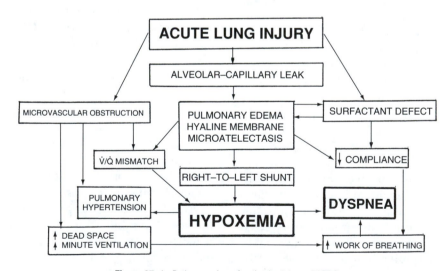

Figure 27–1. Pathogenesis and pathophysiology of ARDS.

the lungs, abnormality of gas exchange and transport may be from commonly associated circulatory impairment in ARDS. Myocardial dysfunction, systemic hypotension, impaired renal function, and metabolic disturbances of acid-base balance frequently occur in many conditions that are the cause of ARDS.

Clinical Manifestations. The clinical manifestations of many of the causes of acute pulmonary injury leading to ARDS are discussed in the appropriate chapters of this book. The onset of the syndrome, which usually occurs within 24 to 48 hours following serious injury or illness, is heralded by progressively severe dyspnea and tachypnea. Cough, with or without frothy and blood-tinged sputum, is common. Physical findings on examination of the chest may be surprisingly scant. Bronchial breath sounds and crackles may be heard. Respiration is rapid and the minute ventilation is markedly increased. The patient is usually cyanotic and appears distraught and apprehensive.

As the clinical settings for the development of ARDS are different, a variety of associated disorders will be present. Systemic hypotension, fever, changes of central nervous system (CNS) function, evidence of sepsis, signs of trauma to various sites, or manifestations of failure of other organs may be evident.

Radiographic Findings. Radiographic examination of the chest is an essential part of the evaluation of patients with respiratory failure, especially when ARDS is being considered. It is important not only for its diagnosis, but also for determination of its severity, assessment of its course, response to therapeutic measures, and detection of complications. In a full-blown case, a standard chest x-ray film shows evidence of diffuse bilateral interstitial and airspace densities characteristic of pulmonary edema (Fig. 27–2). Normal heart size, absence of significant pleural effusion, and lack of enlarged vessels differentiate ARDS from cardiogenic pulmonary edema. Despite diffuse appearance on plain radiograph, thoracic computed tomography (CT) shows that the process is patchy and heterogeneous, with dependent areas being more predominantly involved.

Laboratory Findings. The most consistent laboratory finding in ARDS is arterial hypoxemia refractory to the administration of high oxygen concentrations. There is often associated hypocapnia. Arterial blood pH may be high, at least initially. However, metabolic acidosis is a frequent occurrence. The most common acid-base disturbance is a combination of respiratory alkalosis and metabolic acidosis. Various biochemical and hematologic abnormalities are often present. Underlying causes of ARDS and concomitant

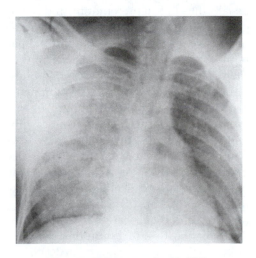

Figure 27–2. Pulmonary edema in ARDS.

dysfunction of other organs are usually reponsible for these abnormalities. Because sepsis is a common cause of ARDS, blood culture is an important component of laboratory studies.

Diagnosis. The diagnosis of ARDS with typical clinical, radiographic, and laboratory pictures is not difficult. A history of catastrophic event in a patient without chronic cardiopulmonary disorders is usually obtained. Diffuse, progressive, and bilateral pulmonary infiltration on chest x-ray film and refractory hypoxemia are among the essential criteria for the diagnosis of ARDS. As ALI causes hypoxemia of varying severity, a rather arbitrary degree of impairment of oxygenation is often chosen to define ARDS. There is no consensus in this regard. The PaO_2/FIO_2 ratio appears to be a better indicator of oxygenation rather than absolute level of PaO_2. The American–European Consensus Conference on ARDS has accepted a PaO_2/FIO_2 of 200 as the cutoff point for the definition of the syndrome. An important differential diagnosis is with cardiogenic pulmonary edema. Although usually the clinical presentation and radiographic picture in heart failure are quite distinctive, in critically ill complicated patients with multiple-organ system failure, the distinction is not always easy. In questionable cases, a flow-directed pulmonary artery catheter would be helpful in differentiating noncardiogenic from cardiogenic pulmonary edema and may also help in proper management of some patients with ARDS. As ARDS may result from numerous clinical conditions, making a diagnosis of ARDS without identifying the underlying cause is inadequate. Every diagnostic effort should be made to discover the primary cause of ARDS, because proper management of this dreadful syndrome should always include adequate treatment of its underlying cause.

Management. The principles of management of ARDS are the same as those of acute respiratory failure in general (page 379). In view of the severity of hypoxemia and difficulty of its treatment, every effort should be made to improve oxygenation without resorting to the administration of a toxic concentration of oxygen. Although in the early stage conservative treatment with oxygen without intubation and mechanical ventilation may succeed, progressive hypoxemia and failure to respond to this approach are indications for tracheal intubation. Continuous positive airway pressure (CPAP) or expiratory positive airway pressure (EPAP) may be tried first before considering intubation and mechanical ventilatory support. Various modes and proper settings of mechanical ventilation suitable for ARDS are discussed in Chapter 28. It should be stressed that the diffusely injured lung in ARDS is susceptible to further damage by inappropriate application of positive pressure ventilation and administration of excessive oxygen concentration. The main purpose of ventilatory support in ARDS is maintaining adequate tissue oxygenation while the underlying cause and associated disorders are being treated.

Other interventions are also known to enhance arterial blood oxygenation, which may be especially useful in intractable hypoxemia that does not adequately improve by O_2 supplementation and mechanical ventilatory support with an optimal positive end-expiratory pressure (PEEP) level. Hypoxemia in ARDS is largely from perfusion of poorly ventilated atelectatic and edematous lung regions. It has been shown that such regions are mostly in the dependent (dorsal in a supine patient) areas. Placing the patient in a prone position results in increased perfusion of lung regions that are better ventilated and at the same time causes reduced blood flow to poorly ventilated areas; consequently, $\dot{V}/\dot{Q}$ mismatch and intrapulmonary shunting are decreased. Almitrine is a drug known for its improvement of ventilation–perfusion matching by increasing pulmonary vascular response to regional hypoxia. This drug is not yet approved for clinical use in the United States. From the European studies, almitrine seems to improve arterial blood Po_2 in ARDS as well as in chronic obstructive pulmonary disease (COPD). As hypoxemia from shunting or $\dot{V}/\dot{Q}$ mismatch is aggravated by low venous oxygen content, efforts to improve oxygen delivery and/or reduce oxygen consumption will increase venous oxygen. Extracorporeal membrane oxygenation (ECMO) has not been shown to improve mortality from severe ARDS. Other modalities of extrapulmonary gas exchange with modified mechanical ventilation seem to be more promising.

Measures known to improve oxygen transport should be a major part of the management of ARDS. Optimizing cardiac output, maintaining adequate circulating volume, and normalizing blood hemoglobin level are essential for adequate oxygen delivery to tissues. Reduction of oxygen consumption is accomplished by controlling infection and fever and decreasing the work of breathing. Optimizing hemodynamic and fluid states is not only important for adequate oxygen delivery, but is also critical for preventing further fluid accumulation in the lungs. Because of the leakiness of the alveolar-capillary membrane in ARDS, any increase in pulmonary capillary pressure

or overhydration increases pulmonary edema. Treatment with inotropic agents and diuretics may be necessary. Monitoring pulmonary artery pressures with a Swan-Ganz catheter is often recommended for assessment of cardiac function and optimizing fluid therapy. Correction of anemia with transfusion of packed red blood cells is important for improvement of tissue oxygenation.

Infection, systemic or local, is often the underlying cause of ALI. It is also an important complicating factor in ARDS. Proper treatment and prevention of infection are essential in the management of this syndrome. Increased work of breathing in ARDS results in significant elevation of oxygen consumption. As discussed in Chapter 28, mechanical ventilation with adequate sedative and, sometimes, proper neuromuscular blockade is often the only way to contend with this important cause of increased oxygen consumption.

Diagnosis and treatment of the underlying cause, especially sepsis and primary pulmonary infection, constitute a major part of ARDS management. In recent years, as the importance of inflammation and various mediators of ALI are recognized, therapeutic strategies to control the inflammatory process have been under intense investigation. Corticosteroids have long been proved to be of no benefit in established ARDS. Antibodies against some of the inflammatory mediators, inhibitors of some others, and antioxidants are being tried in animal models and human subjects. Because of the importance of pulmonary hypertension in ARDS, various vasodilator drugs have been tried, but their effect on systemic blood pressure has limited their clinical usefulness. As inhaled nitric oxide (NO) exerts its vasodilating effect locally and preferentially reaches the better ventilated lung regions, it may improve ventilation–perfusion matching and, thus, oxygenation. Further prospective randomized studies are needed to prove the usefulness of these novel therapeutic approaches.

Although the benefit of surfactant replacement therapy in respiratory distress of the newborn is well known (Chapter 29), its benefit in human ARDS, despite reduced and/or ineffective surfactant, has not been enough for its routine use.

Course and Prognosis. Despite remarkable advances in the knowledge and understanding of ARDS and the availability of sophisticated therapeutic modalities, the survival rate of patients with this condition who require mechanical ventilation is only about 50%.

Generally, patients whose Pao_2 improves early in the course of the disease have a much better prognosis. Survivors from ARDS usually recover completely and have no significant pulmonary sequelae or abnormal respiratory function. ARDS secondary to sepsis syndrome has a worse prognosis. Death is usually due to multiple organ failure and intercurrent infection. With appropriate intensive care, death from respiratory cause is much less common.

BIBLIOGRAPHY

ACCP/SCCM Consensus Conference. Definitions for sepsis and organ failure and guidelines for the use of innovative therapies in sepsis. *Chest.* 1992; 101:1644–1655.

Anzueto A, Baughman RP, Guntupalli KK, et al. Aerosolized surfactant in adults with sepsis-induced acute respiratory distress syndrome. *N Engl J Med.* 1996; 334: 1417–1421.

Ashbaugh DG, Bigelow DB, Petty TL, Levine BE. Acute respiratory distress in adults. *Lancet.* 1967; 2:319–323.

Bell RC, Coalson JJ, Smith JD, Johanson WG Jr. Multiple organ system failure and infection in adult respiratory distress syndrome. *Ann Intern Med.* 1983; 99:293–298.

Bernard GR, Artigas A, Brigham KL, et al. The American–European Consensus Conference on ARDS: definition, mechanisms, relevant outcomes, and clinical trial coordination. *Am J Respir Crit Care Med.* 1994; 149:818–824.

Bigatello LM, Hurford WE, Kacmarek RM, et al. Prolonged inhalation of low concentration of nitric oxide in patients with severe adult respiratory distress syndrome: effect on pulmonary hemodynamics and oxygenation. *Anesthesiology.* 1994; 80:761–770.

Cerra FB. The multiple organ failure syndrome. *Hosp Pract.* 1990; 25(8):169–176.

Fulkerson WJ, MacIntyre N, Stamler J, Crapo JD. Pathogenesis and treatment of the adult respiratory distress syndrome. *Arch Intern Med.* 1996; 156:29–38.

Hanley ME, Repine JE. Pathogenetic aspects of the adult respiratory distress syndrome. *Semin Respir Crit Care Med.* 1994; 15:260–270.

Heffner JE, Repine JE. Pulmonary strategies of antioxidant defense. *Am Rev Respir Dis.* 1989; 140:531–554.

Hudson LD. New therapies for ARDS. *Chest.* 1995; 108(Suppl):79S–91S.

Kraff P, Fridrich P, Fitzgerald RD, et al. Effectiveness of nitric oxide inhalation in septic ARDS. *Chest.* 1996; 109:476–493.

Lewis JF, Jobe AH. Surfactant and the adult respiratory distress syndrome. *Am Rev Respir Dis.* 1993; 147:218–233.

Marinelli WA, Ingbar DH. Diagnosis and management of acute lung injury. *Clin Chest Med.* 1994; 15:517–546.

Murray JF, Matthay MA, Luce JM, Flick MR. An expanded definition of the adult respiratory distress syndrome. *Am Rev Respir Dis.* 1988; 138:720–723.

Niederman MS, Fein AM. Sepsis syndrome, the adult respiratory distress syndrome, and nosocomial pneumonia: a common clinical sequence. *Clin Chest Med.* 1990; 11:633–656.

Petty TL. Acute respiratory distress syndrome. *Dis Mon.* 1990; 36:7–58.

Prewitt RM, Matthay MA, Ghignone M. Hemodynamic management in the adult respiratory distress syndrome. *Clin Chest Med.* 1983; 4:251–268.

Repine JE. Scientific perspectives in adult respiratory distress syndrome. *Lancet.* 1992; 339:466–469.

Schuster DP. What is acute lung injury? What is ARDS? *Chest.* 1995; 107:1721–1726.

Sessler CN, Bloomfield GL, Fowler AA III. Current concepts of sepsis and acute lung injury. *Clin Chest Med.* 1996; 17:213–235.

28.

Mechanical Ventilation

All methods of artificial ventilation, in which a mechanical device replaces or assists the ventilatory function of the respiratory muscles, constitute mechanical ventilation. This chapter describes principles of positive-pressure ventilation and its clinical application, with particular focus on its use in management of acute respiratory failure. Unless stated otherwise in this chapter, mechanical ventilation denotes positive-pressure ventilation. Discussion of negative-pressure, high-frequency, and partial-liquid ventilatory methods is beyond the scope of this book.

Indications. The major indication for mechanical ventilation is acute respiratory failure. However, there are other clinical uses for tracheal intubation and mechanical ventilation. They are most frequently used as part of general anesthesia, especially when neuromuscular blocking drugs are administered. Other indications include management of unstable and critically ill medical or surgical patients, following cardiopulmonary resuscitation (CPR), support of other comatose patients, and

for the purpose of organ recruitment from persons who are brain dead.

Although acute respiratory failure is an important reason for administration of mechanical ventilation, in only a subset of patients with the following disorders is its indication clearcut:

- Severe intractable hypoxemic respiratory failure in patients with acute distress
- Severe acute respiratory acidosis in patients who fail to respond to intensive therapeutic measures or who present with altered mental state
- Intractable asthma in patients with evidence of exhaustion who do not respond to emergency therapeutic measures
- Respiratory muscle paralysis
- Markedly depressed respiratory center with hypercapnia
- Severe thoracic trauma with flail chest
- Hemodynamic instability in critically ill patients who have evidence of impaired respiratory function

The decision to mechanically ventilate patients in respiratory failure in most clinical situations is not easy, considering the fact that many such patients can be managed successfully without ventilatory support and there are risks and side effects of mechanical ventilation (see later in this chapter). Often the outcome of conservative management with oxygen supplementation, adequate tracheobronchial toilet, control of contributing factors, and treatment of the underlying cause is better than is the outcome with mechanical ventilation. The necessity for mechanical ventilation in questionable situations should be determined on an individual basis, taking into consideration several factors. Certain guidelines have been proposed that help in making the decision for ventilatory support in patients with acute respiratory failure. The widely used critical values are

- Tidal volume (V_T) less than 3 mL/kg of "ideal" body weight
- Respiratory rate more than 35/min
- Vital capacity (VC) less than 10 mL/kg of "ideal" body weight
- Minute ventilation less than 3 L or more than 20 L
- Maximum inspiratory pressure less than 20 cm of H_2O
- Pa_{O_2}, while on 50% oxygen by mask, less than 55 mm Hg
- Pa_{CO_2} more than 55 mm Hg *with* pH less than 7.25
- Ratio of dead space to tidal volume (V_D/V_T) of more than 0.6

Although these guidelines are helpful in determining whether or when to initiate mechanical ventilation, the trend of these values is more important than the absolute values. They should be used along with several other individual factors, including associated nonrespiratory conditions. Mechanical ventilatory support is often initiated when there is a good indication that the increased work of breathing necessary for adequate gas exchange cannot be sustained much longer, even with satisfactory arterial blood gases (ABGs). In rapidly progressive respiratory insufficiency, such as seen in posttraumatic cases, the decision for institution of ventilatory support is made before the previously mentioned parameters deteriorate to such abnormal levels, otherwise the patient may rapidly reach a moribund stage. Similarly, patients with central nervous system (CNS)-depressant drug overdose are usually ventilated with no, or only minimal, deterioration of their respiratory function. However, in acute respiratory failure superimposed on chronic pulmonary disease, although several of the previously mentioned criteria are met, conservative management (without mechanical ventilation) is often preferred.

As the main purpose of mechanical ventilation in respiratory failure is to maintain and tide the patient over during an acute episode, it is more appropriate medically when there are certain reversible disorders causing or contributing to respiratory failure. Patients with end-stage lung disease or irreversible degenerative neuromuscular disorders in whom respiratory failure is the result of the progression of their underlying condition, with no identifiable or treatable precipitating cause, pose a most difficult ethical and medical dilemma. It should be realized, and the patient and family informed, that mechanical ventilatory support will be indefinite and result in its lifelong dependency. The question of mechanical ventilation, as well as that of CPR, in patients with terminal and incurable disease who have no advanced directives (such as a living will) is also a difficult one, and cannot be answered without consideration of ethical, legal, socioeconomical, *and* medical issues. As the decision to discontinue ventilatory support is much more difficult and complicated, a great deal of circumspection should be exercised in deciding for the institution of artificial ventilation and/or CPR in such patients.

Beneficial Effects of Mechanical Ventilation. The major desired function of mechanical ventilation is to assist or replace the ventilatory work of respiratory muscles. As a result of this and other changes in the respiratory system consequent to positive-pressure ventilation, additional beneficial effects take place (Table 28–1). These effects of mechanical ventilation are interrelated. For example, better oxygenation may result from improved ventilation, reduced oxygen consumption, and reexpansion of atelectasis.

Undesired Effects of Mechanical Ventilation. The major complications of intubation and of mechanical ventilation are discussed later in this chapter (page 408) and are not repeated here. As an unphysiologic way of ventilating the lungs, positive-pressure ventilation results in certain expected side effects on the lungs and on hemodynamics. Increased pressures needed for the delivery of an adequate V_T into diseased lungs with nonhomogeneous lesions may result in alveolar

injury in more compliant lung regions. In lungs with obstructive airway disease, air trapping (dynamic hyperinflation) may occur, with consequent barotrauma and hemodynamic impairment. The latter side effect, which can also occur without air trapping, is a common cause of hypotension at the initiation of mechanical ventilation and is the result of substituting a normal negative mean intrathoracic pressure with an abnormal positive one.

Intubation. When the decision for mechanical ventilation is made, an airtight connection between the patient and a ventilator should be established. This is usually accomplished with an endotracheal (ET) tube that is inserted into the trachea through either the mouth or the nose. Tracheostomy is not the initial choice for tracheal intubation, except when there are certain types of upper airway obstruction or preexisting tracheostomy. With the improvement of ET tubes, particularly the adoption of soft and low-pressure cuffs, complications of prolonged endotracheal intubation are markedly reduced. It is now feasible to continue translaryngeal intubation for periods of 3 or more weeks. For longer ventilatory support, tracheostomy is usually performed while the translaryngeal tube is in place and the patient is being properly ventilated. Tracheostomy is usually performed earlier, when prolonged mechanical ventilation is anticipated. It is also done, regardless of duration of translaryngeal intubation, when because of increased tracheobronchial secretions and the patient's inability to clear them, frequent suctioning after the discontinuation of ventilatory support will be necessary.

The choice between orotracheal and nasotracheal intubation is less essential. The experience of the operator, ease of intubation, patient's acceptance and tol-

TABLE 28–1. SOME BENEFICIAL EFFECTS OF MECHANICAL VENTILATION

Assisting respiratory muscles for improving ventilation
Correcting respiratory acidosis
Improving hypoxemia
Resting respiratory muscles
Reducing oxygen cost of breathing, thus decreasing oxygen consumption
Relieving respiratory distress
Increasing lung volume, preventing and/or improving atelectasis
Allowing sedation and neuromuscular blockade

erance, and differences in sizes between the two tubes may influence their selection. Orotracheal intubation with a large tube is more desirable when secretions are troublesome and if bronchoscopy is anticipated. In CPR, because of necessity for speed in securing an airway, oral intubation is the procedure of choice. It is also preferred in patients with nasal obstruction or bleeding disorders.

In recent years, specially designed nasal and facial masks are being used in certain situations for administering mechanical ventilation. This so-called *noninvasive ventilation* may be used both on a short-term basis in acute respiratory failure and on a long-term basis for prolonged, mostly nocturnal, ventilatory support.

An artificial airway requires particular care to keep it safe and properly functioning. Securing the tube to prevent its

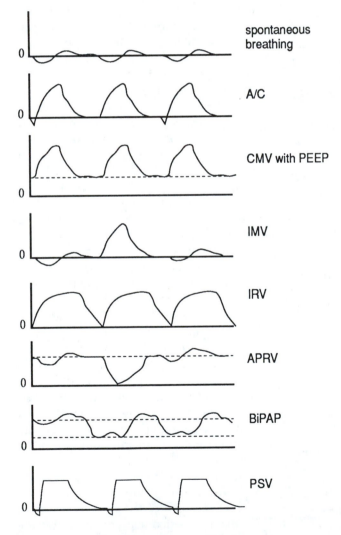

spontaneous breathing

A/C

CMV with PEEP

IMV

IRV

APRV

BiPAP

PSV

Figure 28–1. Airway pressures in various ventilation modes.

slipping in or out, avoiding its unnecessary movement, appropriate inflation of the cuff, its cleaning or occasional changing, and adequate humidification are some measures for its care.

Ventilation Modes

The method by which a ventilator delivers a desired V_T is referred to as *ventilation mode*. Currently, ventilation modes are divided into two categories: conventional and unconventional. Figure 28–1 shows airway pressure tracings representing various modes of positive-pressure ventilation.

Conventional (Standard) Modes. The following are standard modes of mechanical ventilation:

- **Assist/control (A/C) mode** is a combination of controlled and assisted ventilation. In controlled mechanical ventilation, which is rarely used alone, a preset V_T is delivered at a predetermined rate. In A/C mode, a preset V_T is delivered each time the patient makes an inspiratory effort, and there is additional backup controlled ventilation at a preset rate. The frequency of the patient's inspiratory efforts can exceed this rate. The A/C mode of ventilation usually results in a satisfactory patient–ventilator interaction and provides the needed ventilatory support. However, it may cause a significant fluctuation in the level of alveolar ventilation when the spontaneous respiratory rate changes as a result of an alteration of central respiratory drive or changes in pulmonary mechanoreceptor activity.
- **Intermittent mandatory ventilation (IMV) mode** allows the patient to breathe spontaneously between the "mandatory" ventilator breaths, the rate and volume of which are preset. In contrast to the A/C mode, in which the V_T delivered by the patient's inspiratory effort during the assist breath is the same as the controlled V_T, the V_T between IMV breaths is determined by the strength of the patient's inspiratory effort. The IMV was originally intended as a method of weaning from mechanical ventilation (page 414), but it has now become the preferred ventilation mode for the management of respiratory failure in most centers. Its advantages, especially if it is synchronized (SIMV), include better patient acceptance, ventilation with lower mean airway pressure, reduced need for sedation, and less wide fluctuation of the level of alveolar ventilation.

In some ventilators, *mandatory* or *minimum minute ventilation* (MMV) may be used with IMV to ensure a minimum minute ventilation with low IMV rates in case the spontaneous ventilation becomes inadequate.

- **Pressure support ventilation (PSV)** is basically the addition of a set amount of positive pressure to the spontaneous breaths during inspiration. It differs from the intermittent positive-pressure breathing in that the pressure in PSV is maintained at a plateau as long as an inspiratory flow is occurring. Low-level pressure support may be used to overcome the artificial airway resistance—and, thus, to improve patient comfort—and to reduce the added respiratory workload of the spontaneously breathing patient with or without

IMV. With higher pressures, PSV plays the role of conventional ventilatory support. It has the advantage of a better patient–ventilator synchrony. PSV is also used as a weaning method (page 414). In some ventilators equipped with a servo-controlled system, MMV may be used with PSV mode to ensure a set minimum amount of minute ventilation. A "hybrid" mode of mechanical ventilation is a combination of IMP with PSV during spontaneous breaths.

Unconventional Modes. The following modes of mechanical ventilation are used occasionally:

- **Inverse ratio ventilation (IRV),** in which the inspiratory to expiratory (I : E) ratio is usually 2 : 1 or greater, is intended to keep the alveolar units open by not allowing enough time for them to collapse during the brief expiratory time. As an alternative to positive end-expiratory pressure (PEEP) discussed later in this chapter, IRV has the advantage of raising the mean airway pressure without increasing the peak inspiratory pressure. It usually necessitates a ventilator that can be pressure controlled and time cycled; and because of its poor patient tolerance, sedation and muscle paralysis are required.
- **Airway pressure release ventilation (APRV)** is a mode for mechanical ventilation for patients on continuous positive airway pressure (CPAP) in which intermittent and prompt discontinuation of positive airway pressure for a short time results in passive exhalation. This mode is in-

tended to enhance alveolar ventilation in patients on CPAP when there is evidence of inadequate ventilation. It occurs without an increase in airway pressure above the CPAP. APRV may be considered as a variant of IRV, except that during inflation the patient on APRV continues to ventilate spontaneously and sedation or muscle paralysis is not necessary. APRV may be applied by a CPAP mask.

- **Proportional assist ventilation (PAV)** is a positive-pressure ventilatory support in which the ventilator adjusts inspiratory pressure in proportion to the patient's inspiratory effort. It is, therefore, intended for spontaneously breathing patients. It differs from PSV in that the pressure assist in PAV, which depends on the patient's effort, is variable and therefore, delivered tidal volumes also vary. Preliminary studies have shown that PAV results in reduced peak airway pressure and increased patient comfort.
- **Independent lung ventilation (ILV)** is a rare mode of ventilatory support in which two ventilators with different settings are used to ventilate each lung independently. It requires a special double-lumen endotracheal tube. ILV allows a better ventilation and oxygenation when there is predominantly unilateral severe lung disease.
- **Bi-level positive airway pressure (Bi-PAP)** is a relatively simple method of ventilatory assistance that is used with a nasal mask. It is intended for periodic (mostly nocturnal) ventilatory support for patients suffering from chronic ventilatory insufficiency resulting mainly from tho-

racic deformity or neuromuscular disorders. Alternating levels (bi-level) of airway pressure, generated by a CPAP machine modified with a time-cycling device, results in a form of intermittent positive-pressure ventilation.

Ventilator Settings

The optimal mechanical ventilatory pattern is quite variable depending on the nature of the underlying disease and the characteristics of respiratory mechanics. In initiating mechanical ventilation, either A/C or IMV mode is usually employed. The choice is often an individual preference. Tachypneic patients, however, are ventilated more satisfactorily with IMV mode. The argument that the A/C mode, by reducing the work of breathing, is conducive to more respiratory muscle rest is not tenable, as IMV at high enough rates is equally effective for this purpose. Initial ventilator settings are often empirical. They are usually decided on the basis of clinical settings, respiratory system mechanics, ventilator mode, goals of ventilation, and patient's size. The settings are revised according to the patient's physiologic response. Throughout mechanical ventilation, especially during the initial stabilizing period, they are reassessed and adjusted if needed. As discussed later in this chapter, mechanical ventilation in various clinical settings necessitates somewhat different modes and settings of the ventilator. Regardless of underlying disease state, in every patient on a ventilator, close monitoring of respiratory and hemodynamic states, daily assessment of fluid balance, and periodic radiographic examination are important. They are essential for the evaluation of the appropriateness and adequacy of physiologic response to mechanical ventilation, for early detection of its complications, and for determination of the proper timing for its discontinuation.

Tidal Volume. In a volume-cycled ventilator, V_T has to be set, whereas in a pressure-cycled ventilator, the machine-delivered V_T depends on the selected target pressure and, therefore, varies according to respiratory system compliance and resistance. Rather large V_Ts (10–15 mL/kg) were commonly used in the past in most situations requiring mechanical ventilation. Although they are still considered to be appropriate in ventilatory patients with fairly normal respiratory system mechanics, it has been shown that V_Ts of this size may be injurious to diseased lungs, especially in acute respiratory distress syndrome (ARDS). Large V_Ts may also be a significant factor in the development of dynamic hyperinflation (autoPEEP) in obstructive airway disease (see the discussion on mechanical ventilation in ARDS and COPD later in this chapter). Therefore, in selecting an appropriate V_T setting, factors such as respiratory system compliance and resistance, the nature of underlying lung pathology, and ventilatory needs should be taken into account. In adults, selected V_T varies from 5 to 15 mL/kg, predicated by these and other factors.

Respiratory Rate. Except in strictly controlled mechanical ventilation, the respiratory rate set in ventilatory modes, such as A/C or IMV, is actually a backup or mandatory rate. At the initial setting, the respiratory rate, regardless of ventilation mode, should be high enough to ensure an adequate minute ventilation, especially when the patient is sedated and/or paralyzed. Obviously, factors such as V_T, metabolic rate, and acid-base status are important in determining the initial setting of respiratory rate. As with other settings, it may be changed in the course of mechanical ventilation. When pressure support is the ventilatory mode, there is no reason to set the rate.

Flow Rate. The peak inspiratory flow rate should be set to maintain a proper I : E ratio. It should allow the V_T to be delivered quickly enough to leave sufficient time for complete exhalation, otherwise air trapping will develop. This is particularly important in mechanical ventilation of patients with COPD in whom a higher flow rate is necessary. Peak inspiratory flow should preferably meet the maximum inspiratory demand of the ventilated patient in order to alleviate dyspnea and to reduce the activity of respiratory muscles. Flow-rate settings range from 40 to 100 L/min, depending on the amount of minute ventilation, airway resistance, and the patient's ventilatory drive. Some of the volume-cycled ventilators are capable of delivering inspiratory flows with different characteristics (ie, sine wave, decelerating, or square). There is no definite evidence for the practical superiority of one flow pattern over the other as long as mean flow rate is the same.

I : E Ratio. In most current ventilators the I : E ratio is not set, as it is a function of V_T, mean inspiratory flow, and respiratory rate. By changing one or more of these parameters, the I : E ratio can be adjusted to a desired level. Generally, a ratio of 1 : 2 is preferable and, unless the IRV mode of ventilation is intended, it should not be more than 1. In ventilating patients with COPD, a ratio of 1 : 3 to 1 : 4 may be indicated.

Trigger Sensitivity. The trigger sensitivity should be set at a level that is sensitive enough so as not to impose a resistive load to the patient and not so sensitive that it results in self-cycling. Generally, a sensitivity level of 1 to 2 cm H_2O is appropriate. When there is air trapping, positive airway pressure at the end of expiration (autoPEEP) necessitates additional negative inspiratory pressure by the patient to trigger the ventilator. This may be improved by adding external PEEP.

FIO$_2$. An effective tissue oxygenation is the most important immediate goal of mechanical ventilation. Selection of *inspiratory oxygen concentration* (FIO$_2$) is often arbitrary at the beginning of artificial ventilation. However, the initial FIO$_2$ should preferably be set at 100% if there is uncertainty about oxygenation with a lesser concentration. After the arterial blood P_{O_2} is determined, the FIO$_2$ is then titrated downward to a level that maintains adequate arterial blood oxygenation (Pa$_{O_2}$ 60 mm Hg). The optimal FIO$_2$ will depend on the severity of the gas-transport abnormality. Measures directed to improve pulmonary oxygen transport reduce the need for high and potentially toxic oxygen concentrations.

PEEP/CPAP. PEEP is a set pressure applied during the expiratory phase of mechanically ventilated patient. CPAP is a pressure applied throughout a spontaneously performed respiration. Both result in an increase in lung volume at the end of expiration (functional residual capacity [FRC]) and prevention of early closure of the distal airways. As a result, FRC will become larger than the closing volume. Some of the collapsed lung units are recruited for gas exchange and, sometimes, pulmonary compliance is increased.

The major indication for application of PEEP is in mechanically ventilated patients with ARDS. It is usually used when, with an FIO_2 of 0.5 or more, arterial oxygen tension (PaO_2) remains less than 60 mm Hg. Improvement in oxygenation with PEEP is due to recruitment of nonfunctioning lung units and redistribution of lung fluid from inside alveoli to perivascular interstitial space. The benefit of PEEP may be offset, at least partly, by its effect on venous return and cardiac output. Tissue oxygenation depends not only on the oxygen content of blood but, even more importantly, on adequate perfusion. Therefore, an improvement in arterial oxygenation may not enhance tissue oxygenation if blood flow is diminished. Moreover, the effect of PEEP on arterial blood oxygenation is not always predictable; occassionally, it may fail to improve hypoxemia or may even make it worse. This occurs when the effect of PEEP on nonuniform pathologic changes of the lungs causes the blood flow to shift from the healthier lung units to less ventilated diseased areas. Therefore, the decision for the application of PEEP and selection of its level is made on an individual basis and with proper assessment of its risks and benefits. Usually at the beginning, a low-level PEEP (such as 5 cm H_2O) is tried and slowly increased if the beneficial effect is demonstrated by improvement in variables, such as PaO_2, alveolar-arterial oxygen gradient $P(A\text{-}a)O_2$, mixed venous oxygen content, shunt fraction, and respiratory system compliance. There are several terms that are used to characterize PEEP according to the objectives desired. They include

- Therapeutic PEEP: the range of PEEP levels used in clinical practice (5–20 cm H_2O)
- Optimal PEEP: a PEEP level with the lowest shunt fraction
- Best PEEP: a PEEP level causing highest respiratory system compliance
- Least PEEP: lowest PEEP level to reduce FIO_2 to nontoxic concentration
- Preferred PEEP: the level of PEEP that results in the highest oxygen delivery to tissues

The list demonstrates that the subject related to PEEP levels continues to remain controversial. As discussed in ventilation management of patients with COPD later in this chapter, PEEP is sometimes applied to counter the air trapping and the resultant difficulty of patients in triggering the ventilator.

Because CPAP is applicable to spontaneously breathing patients, in mechanical ventilation with IMV mode when PEEP/CPAP is used, mandatory breaths are under the effect of PEEP, whereas spontaneous breaths are subjected to CPAP. As discussed later in this chapter, before a patient is taken off a ventilator with a built-in CPAP capability, using a CPAP setting at zero is one method of determining the patient's ability to sustain spontaneous respiration.

Pressure Support. The use of pressure support as a mode of ventilation is mentioned earlier in this chapter and is discussed later as a weaning method. Sometimes a small amount of pressure support (around 5 cm H_2O) is applied in conjunction with the IMV mode of mechanical ventilation to help the spontaneous breaths by compensating for ET tube resistance.

■ MECHANICAL VENTILATION IN CERTAIN SPECIFIC CLINICAL SETTINGS

Normal Respiratory System Mechanics

There are several causes of ventilatory failure in which the lungs are fairly normal. They include various neuromuscular diseases involving the respiratory muscles such as myasthenia gravis, Guillain-Barré syndrome, muscular dystrophies, and amyotrophic lateral sclerosis; spinal cord disorders, such as high cervical spine injury; and conditions depressing respiratory drive, such as drug overdose. The main objectives in mechanical support are maintaining airway and providing adequate ventilation. The risk of barotrauma in these conditions is low and, therefore, relatively large tidal volumes (12–15 cm/kg) are preferred with or without a small amount of PEEP to prevent atelectasis. Adequate ventilation results in satisfactory oxygenation, thus there is no need for high FIO_2. With an easily reversible underlying condition, such as drug overdose, mechanical support is needed for a short time only and its discontinuation is accomplished without difficulty. However, mechanical ventilation in chronic progressive neuromuscular disorders, in which a prolonged and often lifelong ventilatory support will be needed, often presents complex medical, ethical, and socioeconomical problems.

COPD

Most patients with COPD with exacerbations who appear to benefit from mechanical ventilatory support can be managed conservatively with proper use of oxygen supplement, bronchodilators, antibiotics, and other measures to treat precipitating causes. Some patients may benefit from noninvasive ventilation via a nasal or facial mask for a short period of time. Decision for intubation for mechanical ventilation is made when the patient fails to respond to these measures, showing evidence of progressive respiratory acidosis, lethargy, or severe distress. The SIMV mode is often the preferred mode of ventilation in COPD.

In ventilating patients with COPD, it should be noted that most of them have *acute on chronic respiratory failure* (ACRF) and have elevated serum bicarbonate levels. Therefore, their ventilatory requirement will be rather modest to maintain arterial blood pH, but not to normalize its PCO_2. As expiratory flow obstruction is the major physiologic abnormality in COPD, expiration time should be maximized to ensure completion of exhalation, otherwise air trapping will easily occur. This rather common problem in mechanical ventilation of COPD patients is also known as *dynamic hyperinflation* or *autoPEEP*. Difficulties resulting from it include hemodynamic compromise, barotrauma, interference with triggering the ventilator, and other mechanical disadvantage resulting in increased patient discomfort and respiratory work. AutoPEEP, being the difference between pressures in alveoli and external airway at end expiration, can be determined by various methods. It is commonly measured by occluding the expiratory port of the ventilation circuit at the end of expiration and reading the pressure from the manometer. The patient should be entirely relaxed without active expiratory effort for this measurement to be valid. The presence of autoPEEP can also be demonstrated on the flow-time curve on the monitoring screen available on some of the modern ventilators.

To prevent or at least reduce air trapping, every attempt should be made to increase expiration time, which can be accomplished by increasing peak inspiratory flow rate, set sometimes at a level as high as 100 L/min. Reduction of V_T and minute ventilation should also be considered for this purpose. Sometimes it may be necessary to be content with higher than generally acceptable arterial $Paco_2$ provided that pH is maintained higher than 7.2–7.25. Known as *"permissive" hypercapnia,* this method is used in very severe airflow obstruction, when higher minute ventilation may result in unacceptable complications.

Asthma

As indications for and specific problems related to mechanical ventilation of severe asthma attack (status asthmaticus) are discussed in Chapter 6, they are not repeated here.

ARDS

The major objective of mechanical ventilation of patients with ARDS should be improvement of oxygenation without causing too much harm. Recent realization that large-volume ventilation causes injury to alveoli by overstretching their walls has resulted in reevaluation of earlier strategies of ventilating patients with ARDS. As changes in alveolar volume with positive-pressure ventilation is proportional to intra-alveolar pressure, controlling excessive alveolar pressure is an important measure for preventing further lung injury. Airway plateau pressure, which is the pressure at the end of inspiration with inflation hold, closely approx-

imates the alveolar pressure. It is generally recommended that plateau pressure be kept below 35 cm H_2O. It is usually accomplished by reducing V_T, which is often around 7 mL/kg. To achieve the goal of low plateau pressure, it may sometimes be necessary to let arterial Pco_2 rise ("permissive" hypercapnia). The addition of a novel method of tracheal gas insufflation (TGI) seems to make ventilation more efficient. This is done by a flow of fresh gas during expiration through a catheter placed in the trachea. By washing out part of the dead-space gas, alveolar ventilation is improved.

Application of PEEP is considered to be an important part of ventilatory support in ARDS for improvement of oxygenation. As discussed earlier in this chapter (page 404), excessive PEEP should be avoided to prevent or reduce its undesired effects. FIO_2 should not exceed concentrations that are known to be toxic (0.5–0.6), unless it is administered for a short period of time or is absolutely necessary. There is no need for Pao_2 to exceed 60 mm Hg when there is concern over oxygen toxicity. Measures that are effective in lowering oxygen consumption and/or increasing oxygen delivery can more than compensate for modestly low arterial oxygen tension.

A volume-cycled ventilator in A/C mode with adequate sedation is used most commonly for ventilating patients with ARDS. If properly applied and necessary measures are taken to prevent excessive alveolar distension, there is usually no need for other forms of ventilatory support. Mechanical ventilation modes, such as IRV or APRV, and the use of pressure cycled or high-frequency ventilators have not been conclusively shown to improve the outcome in adults with ARDS. Whether partial-liquid ventilation will have any significant positive impact in management of these patients remains to be proved.

■ COMPLICATIONS OF MECHANICAL VENTILATION

A host of complications may arise during mechanical ventilation that continue to be major causes of significant mortality and morbidity. Many of these complications are directly related to mechanical ventilation, although the combination of several factors, including various underlying diseases, may be responsible. Any sudden or unexpected changes in the patient's condition or ventilator mechanics are important warning signs for possible complications. Necessary measures for the prevention of such complications and their early recognition and treatment are essential for the proper management of patients in respiratory failure.

Complications Due to Tracheal Intubation

Difficult and traumatic endotracheal intubation, intubation of the right mainstem bronchus, excessive bleeding with tracheostomy, pneumomediastinum, and pneumothorax are complications that occur at the start of intubation or tracheostomy. Later in the course of intubated patients, insecure fixation of tubes results in their excessive movement and consequent injury to the larynx and the trachea. Self-extubation is a common occurrence, which may result in significant morbidity and even mortality. Kinking of the tube or mucous plugging can cause acute occlusion. Necrosis of the nose and sinusitis from lack of drainage of the paranasal sinuses are complications of prolonged nasotracheal intubation. Improper inflation or dislocation of the cuff, significant air leak from inability to seal around the tube, tracheal dilatation and tracheomalacia, and stomal infection of the tracheostomy are some other known complications that may occur while the tube is in place. The proper care of artificial airways is an important aspect of the management of patients on mechanical ventilators.

Immediate complications following extubation of the endotracheal tube include difficulty with phonation accompanied by laryngeal edema, which may be severe enough to cause stridor. Late complications are related to scarring of traumatic injury from the tube and/or its cuff and tracheostomy, which may cause significant stricture several weeks or even months after extubation. The use of low-pressure soft cuffs has significantly diminished the complications due to excessive cuff pressure.

Complications Related to Ventilator Malfunction

Machine disconnection is fairly common but easily noticeable with a properly functioning alarm system. Alarm failure, therefore, is one of the most serious mishaps and may result in a fatal outcome. Inadequate humidification may result from a defective ventilator humidifying system. Occasionally, overheating of the inspired air may occur. Other mechanical malfunctions are readily recognized by various monitoring and alarm devices.

Complications Related to Improper Machine Setup

The two major consequences of improper machine setup are alveolar hypoventilation and hyperventilation. There is a certain tendency to overventilate patients with hypercapnia to normalize the arterial blood P_{CO_2}, despite elevated serum bicarbonate. This may result in serious alkalosis.

Pulmonary oxygen toxicity may be caused by either inadvertent or intentional administration of high oxygen concentrations. With inappropriate settings of flow rates, air trappings or inordinately high airway pressures may result. As indicated in mechanical ventilation of patients with COPD, intrinsic or autoPEEP, in which the alveolar pressure at the end of expiration remains elevated from air trapping, occurs frequently in patients with predominantly obstructive airways disease. If significant, autoPEEP may result in the reduction of cardiac output and adversely affect the ventilation. Application of small amounts of external PEEP may help in preventing premature closure of small airways and in reducing the autoPEEP effect.

Barotrauma

Barotrauma is defined as the injury from mechanically induced positive airway pressure that results in air entry into the extra-alveolar tissues and spaces. Air can enter and dissect the interstitial tissue of the lung, causing interstitial emphysema. From there, it may track its way along the perivascular and peribronchial tissue and enter the mediastinum, resulting in pneumomediastinum. Subcutaneous emphysema develops when the air, usually from the mediastinum, enters the subcutaneous tissue. In rare instances, the air may find its way to the peritoneal space (pneumoperitoneum). However, the most common and serious complication of mechanical ventilation related to barotrauma is pneumothorax. As it is usually progressive and markedly impairs ventilation, its early recognition and prompt treatment are essential for effec-

tive management of these patients. Otherwise, it may rapidly progress into a tension pneumothorax. There is fairly good correlation between the airway pressures (both peak inspiratory pressure and mean airway pressure) and the occurrence of barotrauma. One of the disadvantages of PEEP is its association with this complication, although the underlying pulmonary disease for which PEEP is used is probably a more important predisposing factor.

Measures that result in the improvement of airway resistance and pulmonary compliance and proper ventilation settings will reduce the need for the use of high inflation pressures and, thus, diminish the incidence of barotrauma. More careful selection of patients for institution of PEEP and determination of optimal expiratory pressures will also be helpful in prevention of this complication.

As discussed earlier in this chapter in the section on mechanical ventilation in ARDS, ventilation with high V_T may result in injury to alveoli with a relatively normal compliance by overstretching their walls. This occurs because the pathologic changes in ARDS are not homogeneous and, therefore, some lung units remain fairly intact and by maintaining their normal compliance receive the bulk of delivered V_T. Known as *volutrauma,* this complication is prevented or, at least, reduced by keeping airway plateau pressure below 35 cm H_2O.

Pneumonia

Pulmonary infection not only plays a major role in causing respiratory failure, but also is a common complication in patients on prolonged ventilatory support. The subject of ventilation-associated pneumonia (VAP) has gained increasing attention in recent years, engendering extensive clinical research and numerous publications. As an important component of nosocomial infection, VAP results in a very high mortality rate. The factors predisposing to this complication, in addition to a critical underlying condition and presence of serious comorbidities, are numerous and include ready colonization of the respiratory tract by pathogenic organisms, inadequate protection of airways, impaired local and systemic defense mechanisms, use of antibiotics, contaminated equipment, and inadquate infection control.

Although VAP can occur in any mechanically ventilated patient, its incidence is much higher in patients with ARDS and is a major contributing factor for mortality from it. As discussed in Chapter 3 in the section on hospital-acquired pneumonia, gram-negative enteric bacteria and staphylococci are the most common organisms involved in VAP. The most feared infection, however, is caused by various organisms resistant to commonly used antibiotics. They include *Pseudomonas aeruginosa, Acinetobacter,* and methicillin-resistant *Staphylococcus aureus* (MRSA).

The diagnosis of nosocomial pneumonia in mechanically ventilated patients is a challenging problem because of difficulty in differentiating it from various other pulmonary lesions and identifying its cause by the usual methods. Among various diagnostic procedures, bronchoalveolar lavage (BAL) with appropriate bacteriologic study of the BAL fluid appears to be the most reliable method for diagnosis of VAP and identification of specific organisms involved. Even with correct diagnosis, treatment of VAP is often unsuccessful. Every effort should, therefore, be made to prevent this often-fatal complication of mechanical ventilation.

Cardiovascular Complications

Cardiac arrhythmias due to changes in acid-base and electrolyte balances and hypoxemia are common in patients with respiratory failure. Hemodynamic effects of positive-pressure ventilation, particularly when high volumes or pressures are used, are common. Reduced cardiac output at the initiation of mechanical ventilation is the cause of hypotension, which is frequently noted in these patients, especially when there is inadequate circulatory volume. Overhydration, fluid retention, and cardiac failure are not uncommon, but frequently overlooked. Patients on prolonged mechanical ventilatory support are prone to develop venous thrombosis and pulmonary embolism.

Gastrointestinal Complications

Distention of the stomach and intestines is common in patients on mechanical ventilators; it may be due to massive air swallowing and/or inhibition of gastrointestinal (GI) motility (ileus). Diarrhea from different causes may become a vexing problem in these patients. Significant abdominal distention may be a cause of restriction of proper ventilation. One of the common and serious complications of patients in respiratory failure, especially when on a mechanical ventilator, is the development of stress ulcers and subsequent upper GI bleeding. These patients should be prophylactically treated with an antiulcer medication. Because of the colonization of the stomach with microorganisms as a result of increased gastric pH from antacids or H_2 antagonists, the antiulcer drug sucralfate, which does not change the pH, is preferred in such patients.

Nutritional Deficiency

As discussed earlier (page 385), most critically ill patients on mechanical ventilation are known to suffer from inadequate and improper nutrition, which results in prolongation of their hospitalization and increased complications. One important cause of failure in weaning patients from mechanical ventilation is malnutrition, which is known to affect respiratory muscles. Enteral administration should be instituted as soon as possible.

Psychiatric Complications

It is understandable that many critically ill patients on respirators will develop psychiatric problems. Inability to communicate, complex intensive care unit (ICU) environment, sleep disturbances, sensory deprivation, and the use of various medications are among the factors that contribute to the development of such complications.

Other Complications

No body organ is spared from potential complications in patients with respiratory failure who require prolonged hospitalization on mechanical ventilation and who are subject to various diagnostic and therapeutic interventions. Renal, hematologic, endocrine, dermatologic, and neurologic complications are not uncommon in these vulnerable patients. The effect of neuromuscular blocking agents may persist long after their discontinuation in some patients, manifested by marked muscle weakness and/or reduced spontaneous ventilatory effort. Physicians and others involved in the care of these patients should always be aware of such possibilities and should make every necessary effort toward their prevention, early detection, and proper treatment.

■ DISCONTINUATION OF MECHANICAL VENTILATION

In many clinical situations, mechanical ventilation is necessary only for a short period of time when the underlying causes of respiratory failure are readily reversible. General anesthesia, drug overdose, and many postresuscitation cases are examples in which ventilatory support can be uneventfully terminated once the patients become alert. Such patients are extubated soon after mechanical ventilation is discontinued. The term *weaning* should be applied only when the withdrawal from mechanical ventilation is done in a gradual and stepwise fashion so that the patient can become *accustomed* to decreasing levels of ventilatory support until it is completely discontinued. Duration of weaning process depends, among other factors, on the length of time that the patient has been on ventilatory support.

Because weaning is an integral part of mechanical ventilation, it should be planned at, or even before, the initiation of mechanical ventilation. One important consideration in deciding for artificial ventilation is the question of feasibility of its eventual discontinuation. With increasing use of SIMV and PSV for mechanical ventilatory support, the exact time in which weaning begins is becoming more difficult to define. Successful weaning will depend primarily on how well the underlying conditions leading to respiratory failure and its precipitating factors are controlled. The same causes of respiratory failure that compel the institution of mechanical ventilatory support will also prevent its successful withdrawal. The process of discontinuation of the ventilator should, however, be initiated as early as possible, because the very nature of prolonged artificial ventilation contributes to the difficulty in weaning. Disuse and discoordination of the respiratory muscles, alteration of sensitivity of the respiratory center, psychological dependency, malnutrition, and other complications are well-known consequences of protracted mechanical ventilation. A vicious circle between prolonged ventilation and difficult weaning, is often established: the more prolonged the ventilation, the more difficult the weaning, and vice versa.

Discontinuation of mechanical ventilation will be feasible in patients with a stable clinical condition if the following interrelated basic respiratory derangements are corrected or ameliorated:

1. Increased work of breathing due to reduced pulmonary and/or thoracic compliance, elevated airway resistance, increased wasted ventilation, and high metabolic requirement.
2. Decreased respiratory muscle strength resulting from poor nutrition, disuse, neuromuscular disease, use of certain drugs, and respiratory muscle fatigue.
3. Depressed respiratory center due to CNS lesions, metabolic abnormalities, and depressant drugs.
4. Marked $\dot{V}/\dot{Q}$ abnormality and intrapulmonary shunting from severe pulmonary pathology.

Evaluation of these abnormalities by various methods, as in deciding for the institution of mechanical ventilation, will determine the suitable time and proper way for weaning. So-called *weaning parameters* that are often associated with successful withdrawal of mechanical ventilatory support are depicted in Table 28–2. The power of prediction of these measurements is increased when two or more of them are combined. A predictive index resulting from the ratio of respiratory rate to V_T during 1 minute of spontaneous breathing appears to have a fairly good predictive accuracy. With a ratio under 100, the chances of successful weaning are significantly increased. Although these measurements are quite helpful for making a decision concerning weaning, none will replace good clinical assessment and consideration of other factors specific for individual cases.

These measurements and various predictive indexes should be used only as guidelines. Satisfactory values do not always result in successful weaning, and they need not be present in every case. They are more useful in deciding to wean the patient whose overall condition has been stabilized, the functions of other organs are under control, and who have not been on ventilatory support very long (<7 days). Patients with poor control of their underlying disease process, unstable cardiorespiratory status, significant metabolic derangement, high fever, and failing of other organs should not be considered for weaning from ventilatory

TABLE 28–2. MEASUREMENTS FOR PREDICTING SUCCESSFUL WEANING (SPONTANEOUS RESPIRATION)[a]

Respiratory rate	≤ 25/min
Tidal volume	≥ 5 mL/kg
Vital capacity	≥ 10 mL/kg
Minute ventilation	≤ 10 L
Maximum inspiratory pressure	≥ 25 cm H_2O
Pao_2 with FIO_2 ≤ 0.5	≥ 60 mm Hg

[a] Most patients.

support until they are properly treated. It should also be noted that the "weaning parameters" may never be achieved in some patients with prolonged mechanical ventilation, especially in severe COPD, and they still could be successfully weaned. Therefore, the weaning is often a clinical experiment and is accomplished by trial and error.

Weaning Methods

Although there are different methods of weaning from mechanical ventilation, they are all based on the principle of allowing the patient to assume progressively increasing ventilatory work until he or she is able to carry it out without mechanical support. In *T-tube* or *T-piece* weaning, the patient is allowed to breathe spontaneously for a variable length of time determined by the clinical situation. Ventilators with a built-in CPAP capacity may be set to function as a T-tube system by using a CPAP setting at 0. However, it has the disadvantage of interposing an added resistance of the tubings. The addition of a small amount of pressure support (usually 5 cm H_2O) overcomes the added resistance of tubings. An adequately humidified oxygen mixture is administered at a concentration slightly higher than what the patient was receiving immediately before the initiation of weaning. The patient's cardiorespiratory status is closely and carefully monitored, with special attention given to the heart rate and rhythm, blood pressure, respiratory rate, and signs of respiratory muscle fatigue. The use of pulse oximetry during the weaning trial facilitates monitoring. With the development of significant changes in respiratory or cardiac status, such as tachypnea, increasing paradoxical abdominal-thoracic movement, tachycar-

dia, cardiac arrhythmias, change in blood pressure, alteration of mental status, and occurrence of hypoxemia, the patient is returned to full ventilatory support without delay.

Lacking any of these changes, the patient is allowed to breathe unassisted with the continuation of monitoring. A moderate rise in respiratory rate and transient paradoxical abdominal-thoracic movement immediately following the assumption of spontaneous breathing are common and should not be construed as evidence for respiratory muscle fatigue and indication of weaning failure. Depending on the underlying cause of respiratory failure, the length of ventilatory support, and the patient's tolerance of unassisted breathing trial, the weaning process may vary from being fairly rapid and uncomplicated to being most difficult and protracted. A patient with hypoxemic respiratory failure requiring short-term ventilatory support (< 7 days) usually tolerates spontaneous breathing better and can often be weaned successfully with little difficulty. If the patient appears comfortable off the respirator without evidence of significant cardiac or respiratory alteration for about 30 minutes and the ABGs remain satisfactory, he or she is usually ready for extubation.

In a patient with ventilatory failure requiring prolonged mechanical support, weaning becomes a challenging task, necessitating a much slower and more gradual approach. Initial short, spontaneous daytime breathing periods of 5 to 15 minutes between long rest periods are slowly increased in duration and frequency. In such a patient, a complete rest of respiratory muscles between unassisted breathing is essential. At night, the patient is put on uninterrupted ventilatory support for a restful sleep until he or she is able to tolerate spontaneous breathing throughout the day. By that time, the patient is usually able to assume spontaneous respiration at night as well and may be considered for extubation after 24 hours off the respirator.

Intermittent mandatory ventilation (IMV) has been increasingly used for gradual weaning from mechanical ventilation. This method allows the patient to breathe spontaneously between gradually decreasing rates of periodic, controlled mechanical ventilation with eventual resumption of the entire respiration. Because an increasing number of patients are being ventilated with an IMV mode (page 400), weaning with IMV has become the most commonly employed method. Although its superiority over a well-planned and properly executed T-piece weaning has not been proved convincingly, it appears to be a convenient, safe, and more comfortable method of achieving a smooth transition from artificial to spontaneous respiration. The IMV method, however, does not seem to accelerate the weaning process. At the start of weaning, the IMV rate is determined by the amount of ventilatory assistance necessary to sustain an adequate alveolar ventilation. The rate is then progressively reduced at intervals decided by the previously mentioned factors as well as the patient's tolerance. Complete weaning may be achieved within a short period of time if spontaneous respiratory efforts remain adequate while the IMV rate is being decreased. With satisfactory blood gases at the IMV rate of 0, the patient may be extubated. In weaning from a prolonged mechanical ventilation and difficult-to-wean patients, the IMV rate is reduced much more slowly, beginning once every 24 hours. As with T-tube weaning, it is recommended that the patient be returned to full ventilatory support during the night until he or she is able to breathe unassisted throughout the day.

Pressure support ventilation (PSV) as a weaning method may be useful in situations in which respiratory muscle fatigue prevails and prevents successful weaning by conventional methods. To initiate weaning by this method, a level of pressure support just enough to maintain adequate alveolar ventilation is used. Gradual reduction of pressure levels is undertaken in a way that results in increasing the activity of respiratory muscles while avoiding their fatigue. Minimum minute ventilation (MMV) may be added to assure an adequate ventilation with PSV, which is also used in conjunction with CPAP or IMV weaning.

BIBLIOGRAPHY

Abou-Shala N, Medure U. Noninvasive mechanical ventilation in patients with acute respiratory failure. *Crit Care Med.* 1996; 24:705–715.

ACCP Consensus Conference. Mechanical ventilation. *Chest.* 1993; 104:1833–1859.

Ashworth LJ. Pressure support ventilation. *Crit Care Nurse.* 1990; 10(7):20–25.

Benotti PN, Bistrian B. Metabolic and nutritional aspects of weaning from mechanical ventilation. *Crit Care Med.* 1989; 17:181–185.

Bone RC, Eubanks DH. The basis and basics of mechanical ventilation. *Dis Mon.* 1991; 37:327–406.

Bronchard L, Mancebo J, Wysocki M, et al. Noninvasive ventilation for acute exacerbation of chronic obstructive lung disease. *N Engl J Med.* 1995; 333:817–822.

Cassiere HA, Niederman MS. New etiopathogenic concepts of ventilator-associated pneumonia. *Semin Respir Inf.* 1996; 11:13–23.

Colice GL, Stukel TA, Dain B. Laryngeal complications of prolonged intubation. *Chest.* 1989; 96:877–884.

Coronel B, Mercatello A, Couturier JC, et al. Polyneuropathy: potential cause of difficult weaning. *Crit Care Med.* 1990; 18:486–489.

Criner GJ, Isaac L. Psychological issues in the ventilator-dependent patient. *Respir Care.* 1995; 40:855–865.

Downs JB, Stock MC. Airway pressure release ventilation: a new concept in ventilatory support. *Crit Care Med.* 1987; 15:459–461.

Epstein SK. Etiology of extubation failure and the predictive value of the rapid shallow breathing index. *Am J Respir Crit Care Med.* 1995; 152:545–549.

Feihl F, Perret C. Permissive hypercapnia. *Am J Respir Crit Care Med.* 1994; 150:1722–1737.

Glauser FL, Polatty RC, Sessler CN. Worsening oxygenation in the mechanically ventilated patient: causes, mechanisms, and early detection. *Am Rev Respir Dis.* 1988; 138:458–465.

Goldstone J, Moxham J. Weaning from mechanical ventilation. *Thorax.* 1991; 46:56–62.

Hamilton-Farrell MR, Hanson GC. General care of the ventilated patient in the intensive care unit. *Thorax.* 1990; 45:962–969.

Hirschl RB, Pranikoff T, Wise C, et al. Initial experience with partial liquid ventilation in adult patients with the acute respiratory distress syndrome. *JAMA.* 1996; 275:383–389.

Mac Intyre NR. Minimizing alveolar stretch injury during mechanical ventilation. *Respir Care.* 1996; 41:318–326.

Manthous CA, Hall JB, Kushner R, et al. The effect of mechanical ventilation on oxygen consumption in critically ill patients. *Am J Respir Crit Care Med.* 1995; 151:210–214.

Marcy TW, Marini JJ. Respiratory distress in the ventilated patient. *Clin Chest Med.* 1994; 15(1):55–73.

Marik PE. The cuff-leak test as a predictor of postextubation stridor. *Respir Care.* 1996; 41:509–511.

Marsh HM, Gillespie DJ, Baumgartner AE. Timing of tracheostomy in the critically ill patient. *Chest.* 1989; 96:190–193.

Mazzeo AJ. Sedation for the mechanically ventilated patient. *Crit Care Clin.* 1995; 11:937–955.

Peruzzi WT. The current status of PEEP. *Respir Care.* 1996; 41:273–284.

Pierson DJ. Complications associated with mechanical ventilation. *Crit Care Clin.* 1990; 6:711–724.

Prendergast TJ, Luce JM. Increasing incidence of withholding and withdrawal of life support from the critically ill. *Am J Respir Crit Care Med.* 1997; 155:15–20.

Ravenscraft SA. Tracheal gas insufflation: adjunct to conventional mechanical ventilation. *Respir Care.* 1996; 41:105–111.

Rello J, Torres A. Microbial causes of ventilator-associated pneumonia. *Semin Respir Care.* 1996; 11:24–31.

Schlichtig R, Sargent SC. Nutritional support of the mechanically ventilated patient. *Crit Care Clin.* 1990; 6:767–784.

Schuster DP. A physiologic approach to initiating, maintaining, and withdrawing mechanical ventilatory support during acute respiratory failure. *Am J Med.* 1990; 88:268–278.

Seneff MG, Zimmerman JE, Knaus WA, et al. Predicting the duration of mechanical ventilation. *Chest.* 1996; 110:469–479.

Tobin MS. Mechanical ventilation. *N Engl J Med.* 1994; 330:1056–1061.

Waldhorn RE. Nocturnal nasal intermittent positive pressure ventilation with bi-level positive airway pressure (BiPAP) in respiratory failure. *Chest.* 1992; 101:516–521.

Yang KL, Tobin MJ. A prospective study of indexes predicting the outcome of trials of weaning from mechanical ventilation. *N Engl J Med.* 1991; 324:1445–1450.

Younes M, Puddy A, Roberts D, et al. Proportional assist ventilation. *Am Rev Respir Dis.* 1992; 145:121–129.

Respiratory Distress Syndrome of the Newborn

Newborn infants may suffer from breathing difficulty as a result of a variety of causes, but *respiratory distress syndrome* (RDS), also known as *hyaline membrane disease,* is by far the most common acute pulmonary disorder of the newborn. RDS is characterized by respiratory failure following premature birth and is associated with severe atelectasis. Lack of maturation of the respiratory system in general and deficiency of pulmonary surfactant system in particular are the fundamental abnormalities.

Incidence and Risk Factors. As the leading cause of death in the neonatal period, RDS occurs in about 2% of live-born infants. Mainly because of successful resuscitation of growing numbers of premature infants with very low birth weight and gestational age, the incidence of RDS is increasing. There is direct relationship between the degree of prematurity and development of RDS,

reaching 80% for infants born at less than 28 weeks' gestation.

Although RDS is primarily a disease of premature infants, there are other added risk factors, including delivery by Cesarean section, complicated pregnancy, and maternal diabetes. It is more common in males and when there is a history of RDS in siblings. It rarely occurs in babies born at term except for infants born to diabetic mothers. Such infants actually have higher-than-normal birth weights.

Pathogenesis and Pathophysiology. Inadequate development prior to birth affects the respiratory function at birth through several mechanisms, which include a lack of growth of the respiratory units and a weak and compliant rib cage. However, the most important abnormality in RDS is a quantitative and qualitative deficiency of surfactant. Surfactant, made up of a mixture of phospholipids (mostly

417

lecithin) and proteins, is synthesized by and stored in the type II alveolar cells prior to its release into the alveoli during the last few weeks of a normal gestation. During this time, surfactant continues to fill the alveoli and the airways, partly spilling into the amniotic fluid. Its presence in this fluid is, therefore, an indication of its formation and release in the lung. Premature birth and defects in biosynthesis or lack of secretion of surfactant from other causes prevent its adequate accumulation in the alveoli.

Once the alveoli are filled with air following the baby's first breath, surfactant, by coating the alveoli and reducing their surface tension, is essential in preventing their collapse during expiration. The need for the surface tension–lowering effect of surfactant is greatest when the alveolar volume is small, and thus the potential for its collapse is increased. Normally the presence of surfactant on the alveolar lining lowers its surface tension further when the alveolar volume is decreased during expiration (Chapter 18). Therefore, this surface-active material is a potent antiatelectatic factor, and has the dual function of decreasing the pressure needed to distend the lung and of maintaining the alveolar stability. The lung that possesses this ability is considered to be mature and ready to assume its role of ventilation and gas exchange.

The lack of adequate amounts of surfactant in RDS is the major cause of failure of the respiratory system to adapt to the postnatal air-breathing state. Inadequate expansion of the lungs and *diffuse atelectasis* are basic mechanisms of this failure. In addition to atelectasis, premature lungs are predisposed to pulmonary edema because of increased permeability of alveolar-capillary membrane and inad-

equate fluid clearance. Lack of surfactant is also known to enhance pulmonary edema, which in turn impairs the function of surfactant. Surfactant deficiency is recognized to be a factor in predisposing lungs to infection. One of the characteristic features of RDS is hyaline membrane formation, which increases the effects of atelectasis and pulmonary edema on pulmonary compliance. With stiff lungs, the pressure necessary to expand the lungs will be too great for small and poorly developed immature infants to muster. Because of their supple and yielding chest wall, the amount of intrathoracic pressure that they can generate will be limited, causing further atelectasis.

Inadequate ventilation and gas exchange cause severe hypoxemia, hypercapnia, and acidosis, which increase the pulmonary vascular resistance. Elevated pressures in the right heart chambers and pulmonary artery keep the fetal communication between the two sides of circulation open (foramen ovale between the atria and ductus arteriosus between the pulmonary artery and aorta), resulting in right-to-left shunt, further hypoxemia, and reduced pulmonary perfusion. Hypercapnia is the result of reduced alveolar ventilation and ventilation–perfusion ($\dot{V}/\dot{Q}$) mismatching with markedly reduced tidal volume (V_T), dead-space ventilation is increased and, therefore, ventilatory effort is inefficient. With abnormal mechanics of lungs and chest wall, the work of breathing may be increased five-to sixfold, resulting in the baby's exhaustion. Ischemic injury to the alveolar capillary membrane causes leaking of fluid into the interstitial and alveolar spaces and formation of hyaline membrane. Injury to the surfactant-producing cells further impairs their function (Fig. 29–1).

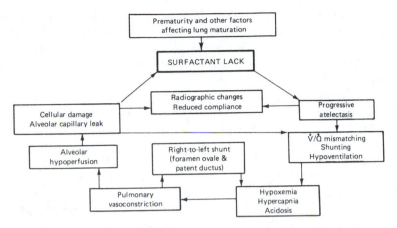

Figure 29–1. Schematic demonstration of pathogenesis and pathophysiology of respiratory distress syndrome of the newborn. The central abnormality is the lack of surfactant. Note several vicious circles in the scheme.

Pathology. On pathologic examination, the lungs look purplish red and liver-like, with extensive atelectasis, exudate, and hemorrhage. Pulmonary capillaries are congested or disrupted and lymphatics are engorged with fluid. Although most alveoli are collapsed, some are overdistended. Hyaline membrane is seen in cases in which death occurs less rapidly. In many cases, death occurs so fast that there is no time for hyaline membrane formation.

Clinical Manifestations. The breathing difficulty is usually evident from the time of birth, most often requiring resuscitative measures. The high inflating pressure necessary to open the alveoli for the first breath is also required for subsequent breaths; because of the inability of the lungs to hold residual air on expiration, they collapse with each expiration. Very immature infants (born between 26 and 30 weeks' gestation) develop the syndrome immediately. In some cases, when the lungs are more mature, they may function normally for a brief period of time and then fail. Rapid and shallow respiration heralds the onset of RDS. The

respiratory rate reaches 60 to 120/min, from a normal of 40 to 50/min. Expiratory grunting or whining is the result of breathing against a partially closed larynx, which is a feeble effort at preventing alveolar closure during expiration. Subcostal, intercostal, and suprasternal retraction signifies large intrathoracic pressure changes necessary for ventilation. The baby has a dusky color, and cyanosis may be severe and unresponsive to oxygen administration. Breath sounds are usually diminished; rales may be heard, but are not common. Infants with severe hypoxemia show evidence of circulatory collapse and are hypothermic.

Prenatal Evaluation for the Risk of RDS. A knowledge of the likelihood of the development of RDS is very important for proper planning for delivery and perinatal care. Prenatal diagnosis of lung immaturity, the most reliable predictor of RDS, can be suspected by gestational age, determination of fetal size (by ultrasound), and consideration of other risk factors. It can more reliably be determined by an examination of amniotic fluid sampled by amniocentesis or by collection of vaginal pool in case of ruptured membranes. Indirect estimation of surface active material in the fluid may be done by a simple test. Known as *shake test*, it depends on the ability of surfactant in the amniotic fluid to generate a stable foam in the presence of ethyl alcohol. The most commonly performed test, however, is the determination of licithin level and licithin/sphingomyelin ratio (L/S ratio). As this ratio increases with gestational age, it has an excellent predictive value. Normally, at term it is around 2.5. It should, however, be noted that in diabetic mothers, normal L/S ratio may not predict lung maturity.

Diagnosis. The diagnosis of RDS is made from the characteristic clinical presentation, chest roentgenogram, and arterial blood studies in infants born prematurely. The chest x-ray has diffuse granular appearance; air bronchogram is readily visible (Fig. 29–2). Arterial blood

gas (ABG) analysis shows marked hypoxemia; P_{CO_2} is usually elevated. Mixed respiratory and metabolic acidosis is common. Other causes of respiratory distress, such as pneumothorax, large diaphragmatic hernia, various congenital pulmonary or extrapulmonary anomalies, aspiration, heart failure, and pneumonia, should be properly ruled out. The most important differentiation of RDS is from streptococcal pneumonia of the newborn, which should be diagnosed promptly by bacteriologic studies and treated with appropriate antibiotics.

Preventive Measures. With the understanding of the cause of neonatal RDS, it is obvious that the prevention of premature births is the most important measure in reducing its incidence. In timing for Cesarean section or induction of labor, the determination of fetal age and the prediction of lung maturity are essential. Sometimes when premature labor develops, it may be necessary to intervene medically by the use of drugs known to stop labor (tocolysis). With determination of lung immaturity by antenatal testing of the amniotic fluid, fetal lung maturation can be accelerated by maternal use of a synthetic glucocorticoid such as betamethasone. The addition of thyrotropin-releasing hormone seems to further reduce the incidence of RDS.

Principles of Management of RDS. A detailed description of the highly specialized management of RDS is beyond the scope of this book; therefore, only certain principles are discussed. The most important and critical problem in infants with RDS is hypoxemia, which necessitates immediate attention and correction by appropriate means. Close monitoring of the temperature, cardiorespiratory function,

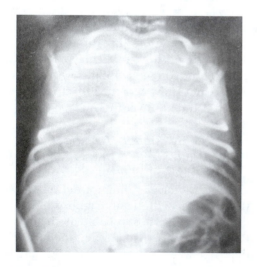

Figure 29–2. Radiograph of a newborn with severe acute RDS. Note bilateral pulmonary consolidation with marked air bronchogram.

blood gases, and acid-base status is important to forestall clinical worsening and complications. It should be stressed that premature infants are prone to develop retinal lesion with high *arterial* oxygen tension, in addition to their susceptibility to pulmonary oxygen toxicity with high *inspired* oxygen tensions. An adequately staffed and equipped neonatal intensive care nursery is essential for the optimal treatment of these infants. Their thermal environment should be properly controlled to prevent increased oxygen consumption.

In infants with mild to moderate hypoxemia, the administration of warm and humidified oxygen to bring the Pao_2 to 60 to 80 mm Hg is needed to improve oxygenation while minimizing the possibility of oxygen toxicity. In many cases, hypoxemia is more severe or progressive and measures to improve pulmonary oxygen transport are needed. The most effective measure in this regard is the application of *continuous distending airway pressure*. This is based on the knowledge of pathogenesis of the respiratory distress and hypoxemia. As discussed earlier, the lack of stability of the alveoli and their tendency to collapse and reduce the lung volume constitute the major problem. Maneuvers that result in increased resting lung volume would improve oxygenation. This is indeed the case in clinical trial of continuous distending airway pressure in this disease. This may be accomplished either by *continuous positive airway pressure* (CPAP) or sometimes by continuous negative pressure around the body. CPAP may be applied through an endotracheal tube or, to avoid tracheal intubation, it may be used with a head hood, head chamber, tight-fitting mask, or special nasal prongs. With constant distending pressure, the baby is breathing spontaneously a proper mixture of oxygen. It is the combination of appropriate pressure and the administration of nontoxic oxygen mixture that provides the optimal oxygenation.

Very ill babies who show evidence of severe respiratory distress, intractable hypoxemia, hypercapnia, acidosis, or prolonged apneic episodes are candidates for mechanical ventilatory support. The ventilator used in RDS should have the capability to deliver small V_T with a high respiratory frequency. It is usually time cyled and pressure limited. High-frequency (jet ventilation or oscillation) ventilators may sometimes be used.

Topical administration of surfactant is now possible with the availability of natural and synthetic preparations. Exogenous surfactant is used by intratracheal instillation via endotracheal tube. Prophylactic use immediately after intubation is intended to prevent atelectasis and edema in premature infants at a very high risk of developing RDS. For treatment purpose, these preparations are administered promptly if the infant develops RDS (rescue treatment). Surfactant therapy has been shown to be effective in reducing the risk of developing or worsening RDS and in decreasing its complications.

Complications. Infants suffering from RDS are prone to develop a variety of pulmonary and extrapulmonary complications, which are in part due to therapeutic interventions. Severe hypoxemia, acidosis, and other factors increasing pulmonary artery resistance may prevent timely closure of ductus arteriosus through which significant shunting between the pulmonary artery and the aorta takes place. Although with the improvement of respiratory status it may eventually close spontaneously, in some children it remains open (*patent ductus arteriosus*). The administration of high oxygen concentrations may result in *pulmonary oxygen toxicity,* which is enhanced bypositive-pressure ventilation. Infants requiring mechanical ventilation and high FIO$_2$s who survive the early acute stage of RDS may develop a chronic condition known as *bronchopulmonary dysplasia* (BPD). This condition is the result of extensive injury, repair, and remodeling of underdeveloped lungs. Instead of the usual improvement that most surviving infants show on the third or fourth day of their illness, these babies continue to have respiratory difficulty and require prolonged ventilatory support. The radiographic findings rapidly evolve from the consolidation of RDS to cystic changes, showing areas of atelectasis and hyperinflation with a spongelike appearance. After a long hospitalization and intensive respiratory care, many infants with BPD will survive and may even recover completely; however, pulmonary fibrosis, chronic respiratory failure, and cor pulmonale may develop from this complication.

BIBLIOGRAPHY

A multicenter, randomized trial comparing synthetic surfactant with modified bovine surfactant in the treatment of neonatal respiratory distress syndrome. *Pediatrics.* 1996; 97:1–6.

Caminiti SP, Young SL. The pulmonary surfactant system. *Hosp Pract.* 1991; 26(1): 94–117.

Golembeski D, Merritt TA. New strategies for prevention of neonatal respiratory distress syndrome: acceleration of fetal lung maturation and exogenous surfactant replacement. *Semin Respir Med.* 1990; 11:117–126.

Haas CF, Weg JG. Exogenous surfactant therapy: an update. *Respir Care.* 1996; 41: 397–415.

Horbar JD, Soll RF, Sutherland JM, et al. A multicenter randomized, placebo-controlled trial of surfactant therapy for respiratory distress syndrome. *N Engl J Med.* 1989; 320:959–965.

Jobe AH. Pulmonary surfactant therapy. *N Engl J Med.* 1993; 328:861–868.

Kendig JW, Notter RH, Cox C, et al. A comparison of surfactant as immediate prophylaxis and as rescue therapy in newborns of less than 30 weeks' gestation. *N Engl J Med.* 1991; 324:788–794.

Kopelman AE, Mathew OP. Common respiratory disorders of the newborn. *Pediatr Rev.* 1995; 16:209–217.

Moores RR, Abman SH. Bronchopulmonary dysplasia. *Semin Respir Med.* 1990; 11: 140–151.

Ryan CA, Finer NN. Antenatal corticosteroid therapy to prevent respiratory distress syndrome. *J Pediatr.* 1995; 126:317–319.

Surfactant for premature infants with respiratory distress. *Med Lett Drugs Ther.* 1990; 32:2–3.

Verma RP. Respiratory distress syndrome of the newborn infant. *Obstet Gynecol Surv.* 1995; 50:542–555.

Ward RM. Pharmacologic enhancement of fetal lung maturation. *Clin Perinatol.* 1994; 21:523–542.

XII

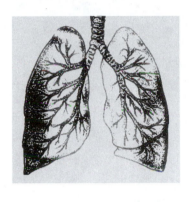

APPENDICES

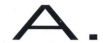

A.

Certain Symbols and Abbreviations Used in Respiratory Physiology

A	alveolar gas	C_aO_2	oxygen content in 100 mL of arterial blood
a	arterial blood		
A-aDO$_2$	alveolar-arterial oxygen gradient	C_cO_2	oxygen content in 100 mL of pulmonary capillary blood
(A-a)Po$_2$	alveolar-arterial oxygen tension gradient		
		C_L	compliance of lungs (static)
ATPS	ambient temperature and pressure saturated with water vapor	$C(L + T)$	compliance of lungs and thorax
BSA	body surface area	$C_{\bar{v}}O_2$	oxygen content in 100 mL of mixed venous blood
BTPS	body temperature and pressure saturated with water vapor		
		CVP	central venous pressure
C	content; concentration; compliance	**D**	diffusing capacity; dead-space gas
		DCO	diffusing capacity for carbon monoxide
c	capillary blood		
C(a-vDO$_2$)	arteriovenous oxygen content difference	D_LCO	diffusing capacity of lung for carbon monoxide

425

D_LO_2	diffusing capacity for oxygen
DO_2	oxygen delivery
E	expired gas
ERV	expiratory reserve volume
F	fractional concentration
f	frequency of breathing
FEF	forced expiratory flow
FEF_{25-75} or MMF	maximum midexpiratory flow
$FEF_{200-1200}$ or MEFR	maximum expiratory flow rate
FEV_T	forced expiratory volume over a given time
FIO_2	fractional concentration of oxygen in inspired gas
FRC	functional residual capacity
FVC	forced vital capacity
I	inspired gas
IC	inspiratory capacity
IRV	inspiratory reserve volume
MEFR	maximum expiratory flow rate
MMEF	maximum midexpiratory flow rate
mm Hg	millimeters of mercury
MPAP	mean pulmonary artery pressure
MVV	maximum voluntary ventilation
P	gas pressure
P_{50}	blood oxygen tension at which 50% of the hemoglobin is saturated
PA	pulmonary artery
$P(A-aDO_2)$	alveolar-arterial oxygen tension difference
Pa_{CO_2}	partial pressure of carbon dioxide in arterial blood
$P_{A}CO_2$	partial pressure of carbon dioxide in alveolar gas
Pa_{O_2}	partial pressure of oxygen in arterial blood
$P_{A}O_2$	partial pressure of oxygen in alveolar gas

PAP	pulmonary artery pressure
$P_E CO_2$	partial pressure of carbon dioxide in expiratory gas
PE_{max}	maximum expiratory pressure (static)
PFR	peak flow rate
PI_{max}	maximum inspiratory pressure (static)
$P_v O_2$	partial pressure of oxygen in venous blood
$P_{\bar{v}} O_2$	partial pressure of oxygen in mixed venous blood
PVR	pulmonary vascular resistance
PWP	pulmonary artery wedge pressure
Q	volume of blood
$\dot{Q}$	blood flow
$\dot{Q}_S$	blood flow through shunt
$\dot{Q}_T$	total blood flow (cardiac output)
R	respiratory exchange ratio or respiratory quotient ($\dot{V}_{CO_2}/\dot{V}_{O_2}$)
RA	right atrium
RAW	airway resistance
RV	residual volume, right ventricle
S	percent of saturation
STPD	standard temperature (0°C), 760 mm Hg pressure, dry
T	total; tidal; temperature
TLC	total lung capacity
Torr	Torricelli, mm Hg
TV	tidal volume
V	gas volume
$\dot{V}$	gas flow
v	venous blood
v	mixed venous blood
V_A	volume of alveolar gas
VC	vital capacity
$\dot{V}CO_2$	carbon dioxide elimination per minute

V_D volume of dead space

V_D/V_T ratio of dead space to tidal volume

V_E volume of expired gas

$\dot{V}_{max\ 50}$ maximum expiratory flow at 50% of expired vital capacity

$\dot{V}_{max\ 75}$ maximum expiratory flow at 75% of expired vital capacity

$\dot{V}O_2$ oxygen consumption or uptake per minute

$\dot{V}/\dot{Q}$ ventilation–perfusion ratio

V_T tidal volume

$\dot{V}O_{2\ max}$ maximum O_2 uptake

B.

Predicted Normal Values for Pulmonary Function Tests

■ LUNG VOLUMES

There are significant variations in lung volumes in normal individuals. They vary not only with age, race, sex, height, body surface area, and position, but also among members of a homogeneous group under standard conditions. Age is particularly important in relation to residual volume and the ratio of residual volume to the total lung capacity. Body height influences the total lung capacity, vital capacity, and functional residual capacity.

The following is an example of typical values for a hypothetical healthy young male; the figures are approximate and are shown for the purpose of comparison between various lung volumes and capacities.

Total lung capacity	6000 mL
Vital capacity	4800 mL
Inspiratory capacity	3600 mL
Functional residual capacity	2400 mL
Tidal volume	500 mL
Residual volume	1200 mL
Inspiratory reserve volume	3100 mL
Expiratory reserve volume	1200 mL

There are several equations and nomograms for calculation of *predicted* normal lung volumes from age, sex, height, weight, and body surface area. The following are some of the useful prediction formulas that are commonly used.

VITAL CAPACITY

Predicted normal values for vital capacity (VC) may be calculated from the following formulas:

For adult males:

$$VC \ (L) = 0.052 \times \text{height (cm)} \\ -0.022 \times \text{age} - 3.6$$

For adult females:

$$VC\ (L) = 0.041 \times height\ (cm) - 0.018 \times age - 2.69$$

TOTAL LUNG CAPACITY

Total lung capacity (TLC) is estimated by dividing the calculated predicted normal VC by 0.8 for the age group 15–34 years, by 0.75 for the age group 35–49 years, and by 0.65 for the age group older than 50 years. It may also be computed by one of the prediction equations, such as For adult males:

$$TLC\ (L) = 0.078 \times height\ (cm) - 7.30$$

For adult females:

$$TLC\ (L) = 0.0746 \times height\ (cm) - (0.013 \times age) - 6.2$$

RESIDUAL VOLUME

One of the prediction formulas for residual volume (RV) in adult males is

$$RV\ (L) = 0.027 \times height\ (cm) + 0.017 \times age - 3.45$$

For adult females:

$$RV\ (L) = 0.028 \times height\ (cm) + 0.016 \times age - 3.54$$

DEAD-SPACE VOLUME

Average normal dead-space volume for a young adult male is about 150 mL and the V_D/V_T ratio is 0.33. The regression of the dead-space/tidal volume ratio with age in seated normal subjects at rest is given by the following formula:

$$V_D/V_T = 24.6 + 0.17 \times age$$

■ FLOW RATES

From a simple forced expiratory spirogram, the most commonly used variables, including forced vital capacity (FVC), forced expiratory volumes (FEV_1, FEV_2, FEV_3), FEV_1/FVC, maximum midexpiratory flow rate (FEF_{25-75}), and maximum expiratory flow rate ($FEV_{200-1200}$), are compared with predicted normal values for height, age, and sex, derived from available tables, formulas, or nomograms. Figures B–1 and B–2 are prediction nomograms and formulas for normal men and women. Normal predicted values are determined by laying a straight edge between the height and the age of the individual and reading the values from the corresponding scales. It should be emphasized that there are significant variations among normal individuals with the same sex, height, and age, depending on other factors such as race and body build. In normal young adults, FEV_1/FVC ratio is 80% or higher.

■ DIFFUSING CAPACITY

The average normal diffusing capacity is about 25 mL CO/min/mm Hg. There are numerous prediction equations for CO diffusing capacity (D_LCO). The following prediction formulas are more commonly used.

Adult males:

$$D_LCO\ (mL/min/mm\ Hg) = 0.416 \times height\ (cm) - 0.219 \times age - 26.34$$

Adult females:

$$D_LCO\ (mL/min/mm\ Hg) = 0.256 \times height\ (cm) - 0.144 \times age - 8.36$$

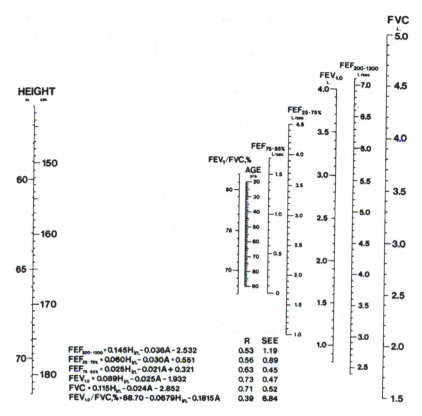

Figure B–1. Nomogram and formulas for determination of predicted values of expiratory flow rates for normal males. [Reprinted by permission from Morris JF. Spirometry in the evaluation of pulmonary function. *West J Med.* 1976; 125(8):110–118.]

Multiplying D_LCO by a factor of 1.23 will give diffusing capacity for oxygen (D_LO_2).

■ ARTERIAL BLOOD GASES

Normal arterial blood gases and pH for young adults at sea level are

PaO_2	95 ± 5 mm Hg
$PaCO_2$	40 ± 5 mm Hg
S_aO_2	$97 \pm 2\%$
pH	7.40 ± 0.02
HCO_3^-	24 ± 2 mEq

In normal subjects, the arterial blood PCO_2 does not change significantly with age; however, arterial blood PO_2 decreases with age. There are several regression equations for calculation of reference values of PaO_2. The most recently proposed formula, based on the study of large numbers of healthy people ages 40 to 90 years, is as follows:

$$PaO_2 = 108.75 - 0.39 \times age$$

In young healthy adults, on room air, the alveolar–arterial PO_2 difference is about

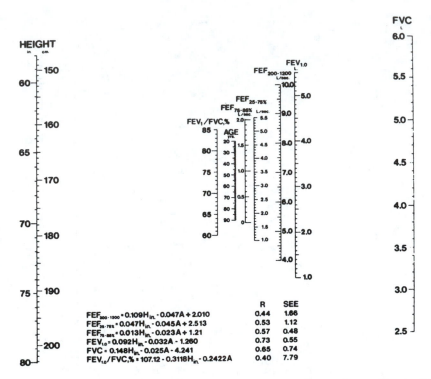

Figure B–2. Nomogram and formulas for determination of predicted values of expiratory flow rates for normal females. [Reprinted by permission from Morris JF. Spirometry in the evaluation of pulmonary function. *West J Med.* 1976; 125(8):110–118.]

9 mm Hg. This increases with age according to the following formula:

$$P(A\text{-}aDO_2) \text{ or } (A\text{-}a) \, P_{O_2} = 2.5 + 0.21 \times age$$

Normally, the ratio of arterial oxygen tension to alveolar oxygen tension ($Pa_{O_2}/P_{A O_2}$) is more than 0.8.

■ OXYGEN CONSUMPTION

Oxygen consumption (VO_2) can be determined from the workload in a bicycle ergometer by the following equation:

$$\dot{V}O_2 \, (mL/min) = 5.8 \times body \, weight \, (kg) + 101 \times workload \, (watts) + 151$$

■ COMPLIANCE

The normal values for static compliance are as follows:

Pulmonary compliance	0.166–0.246 L/cmH$_2$O
Chest-wall compliance	0.125–0.209 L/cmH$_2$O

Total compliance   0.072–0.110 L/cmH$_2$O

■ MAXIMUM RESPIRATORY PRESSURES

The following are predicted normal values for maximum inspiratory and expiratory pressures in adults (between the ages of 19 and 49 years).

Adult males:

PI$_{max}$	-127 ± 28 (cmH$_2$O)
PE$_{max}$	216 ± 45 (cmH$_2$O)

Adult females:

PI$_{max}$	-91 ± 25 (cmH$_2$O)
PE$_{max}$	138 ± 39 (cmH$_2$O)

Normal Compensatory Responses to Simple Acid-Base Disturbances

The following are relationships between changes resulting from primary acid-base disorders and corresponding secondary or compensatory changes (simple acid-base disorders). It should be noted that these relationships are not applicable when the acid-base abnormalities are extreme.

Primary disorders	Corresponding secondary changes
Metabolic acidosis	$\Delta P_{CO_2}(\text{mm Hg}) = 1.1{-}1.3 \times \Delta HCO_3^- (\text{mEq/L})$
Metabolic alkalosis	$\Delta P_{CO_2}(\text{mm Hg}) = 0.6{-}0.8 \times \Delta HCO_3^- (\text{mEq/L})$
Respiratory acidosis (acute)	$\Delta HCO_3^- (\text{mEq/L}) = 0.1 \times \Delta P_{CO_2} (\text{mm Hg})$
Respiratory acidosis (chronic)	$\Delta HCO_3^- (\text{mEq/L}) = 0.3{-}0.4 \times \Delta P_{CO_2} (\text{mm Hg})$
Respiratory alkalosis (acute)	$\Delta HCO_3^- (\text{mEq/L}) = 0.2 \times \Delta P_{CO_2} (\text{mm Hg})$
Respiratory alkalosis (chronic)	$\Delta HCO_3^- (\text{mEq/L}) = 0.5{-}0.6 \times \Delta P_{CO_2} (\text{mm Hg})$

The acid-base map in Figure C–1 shows, in different band forms, relationships between pH, P_{CO_2}, and HCO_3^- in simple acid-base disturbances. Each band represents the 95% confidence limits with the particular acid-base disturbance as indicated. Mixed acid-base disorders are usually, but not always, located outside these bands.

435

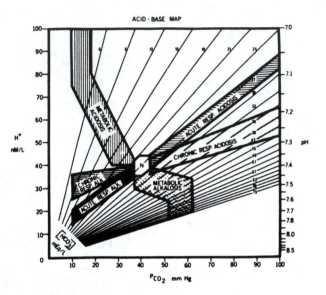

Figure C–1. Acid-base map. The bands show the six simple acid-base disorders. The numbered lines represent isopleths for bicarbonate levels. Mixed disorders are usually located outside the bands. (Reprinted by permission from Goldberg M, et al. Computer-based instruction and diagnosis of acid-base disorders: A systematic approach. *JAMA.* 1973; 223(3):270. Copyright 1973, American Medical Association.)

D.

Alveolar Air Equation: Alveolar-Arterial Oxygen Tension Gradient

When the inspired air enters the alveoli, it is warmed to the body temperature (37°C) and saturated with water vapor. At this temperature, the water vapor pressure is 47 mm Hg. Therefore, at sea level, the total pressure of the alveolar O_2, N_2, and CO_2 is $760 - 47 = 713$ mm Hg.

If the number of molecules of O_2 absorbed were equal to that of CO_2 entering the alveoli, the $P_{AO_2} = FIO_2 (713) - P_{ACO_2}$. However, because the respiratory exchange ratio (R, which is the ratio of the amount of CO_2 eliminated to the amount of O_2 consumed) is usually less than 1, a correcting factor of $[FIO_2 + (1 - FIO_2)/R]$ should be included in the previous equation for accurate calculation of alveolar oxygen tension:

$$P_{AO_2} = FIO_2(713) - P_{ACO_2}$$
$$\times \left(FIO_2 + \frac{1 - FIO_2}{R} \right)$$

A simplified form of the equation, which is commonly used for determining the alveolar oxygen tension, with an assumed R value of 0.8 is

$$P_{AO_2} = FIO_2 (713) - \frac{P_{aCO_2}}{0.8}$$

To determine the alveolar–arterial oxygen tension gradient, the arterial oxygen tension (P_{aO_2}) is subtracted from the alveolar oxygen tension (P_{AO_2}).

All calculations shown are for sea level. They should be corrected for the atmospheric pressure appropriate for the altitude in which they are being used.

E.

Calculation of Alveolar Ventilation

As all the CO_2 in the expired gas comes from alveolar gas, the volume of CO_2 will be equal to the alveolar ventilation multiplied by its fractional concentration (F_ACO_2):

$$\dot{V}CO_2 = \dot{V}_A \times F_ACO_2 \qquad (1)$$

or

$$\dot{V}_A = \frac{\dot{V}CO_2}{F_ACO_2} \qquad (2)$$

F_ACO_2 at atmospheric pressure of 760 mm Hg will be equal to $P_ACO_2/760$. Substituting F_ACO_2 by P_ACO_2, equation (2) becomes

$$\dot{V}_A = \frac{\dot{V}CO_2 \times 760}{P_ACO_2} \qquad (3)$$

However, this equation, which is based on STPD (standard temperature of 0°C, 760 mm Hg pressure, dry), should be corrected to BTPS (body temperature of 37°C and pressure saturated with water vapor). According to Charles' law, the volume of a gas increases proportionally to the absolute temperature. Therefore, equation (3) should be multiplied by a factor of $(273 + 37)/273$, or $310/273$. Thus,

$$\dot{V}_A = \frac{\dot{V}CO_2 \times 863}{P_ACO_2} \qquad (4)$$

As P_ACO_2 is practically the same as Pa_{CO_2}, the final equation will be

$$\dot{V}_A \text{ (mL/min, at BTPS)} = \frac{\dot{V}CO_{2(at\ STPD)} \times 863}{P_aCO_2} \qquad (5)$$

if V_A is calculated in L/min, the equation should change to

$$\dot{V}_A \text{ (L/min)} = \frac{\dot{V}CO_2 \times 0.863}{Pa_{CO_2}} \qquad (6)$$

Calculation of Physiologic Dead Space: Bohr's Equation

Tidal volume (V_T) is composed of two portions:

1. The portion made up of physiologic dead space (V_D), which has the same concentration of carbon dioxide as inspired air, that is negligible, and
2. the portion that participates in gas exchange and, therefore, is the source of carbon dioxide content of the expired tidal volume. The latter portion is equal to the difference between the tidal volume and the physiologic dead space ($V_T - V_D$).

Thus,

$$V_T \times F_E CO_2 = (V_T - V_D) F_A CO_2$$

in which $F_E CO_2$ and $F_A CO_2$ represent the concentration of carbon dioxide in expired air and alveolar air, respectively. The equation can be changed to

$$V_D = V_T \times \frac{F_A CO_2 - F_E CO_2}{F_A CO_2}$$

By changing the fractional concentration (F) to the partial pressure (P), the equation becomes

$$V_D = V_T \times \frac{P_A CO_2 - P_E CO_2}{P_A CO_2}$$

As the arterial $P CO_2$ is essentially the same as alveolar $P CO_2$, arterial $P CO_2$ ($Pa CO_2$) can be used to replace $P_A CO_2$. The final equation will be

$$V_D = V_T \times \frac{Pa CO_2 - P_E CO_2}{Pa CO_2}$$

which is known as *Bohr's equation*.

Normally, anatomic and physiologic dead spaces are almost equal, but in patients with ventilation–perfusion mismatch, physiologic dead space is higher than anatomic dead space.

441

Normal Hemodynamic Values in Recumbent Adults

Pressures (mm Hg)
Systemic artery
    Systolic (SBP)   90–140
    Diastolic (DBP)   60–90
    Mean (MAP)   70–105
Pulmonary artery
    Systolic (SPAP)   15–28
    Diastolic (DPAP)   5–16
    Mean (MPAP)   10–22
Pulmonary artery
    wedge Mean (PAWP)   6–15
Right ventricle
    Systolic (SRVP)   15–28
    End-diastolic (DRVP)   0–8
Right atrium (RAP)   0–8
    Central vein (CVP)   0–8
Resistance (dyne. sec. cm^{-5})
Total systemic (SVR)   900–1400

Total pulmonary
  (PVR) Flow
  (L/min)   150–250
Cardiac output (CO)   Varies with
                         body size
Cardiac index (CI)   2.8–4.2
Body surface area   1.4–2.1

SVR, PVR, and BSA are calculated using the following formulas:

$$SVR = \frac{(MAP - CVP) \times 79.9}{CO}$$

$$PVR = \frac{(MPAP - PAWP) \times 79.9}{CO}$$

$$BSA = \text{weight (kg)}_{0.425} \times \text{height (cm)}_{0.725} \times 0.0007184$$

H.

Venous-to-Arterial Shunt Equation

Arterial blood in a patient with venous-to-arterial shunt contains some mixed venous blood ($\bar{v}$) that bypasses the lungs and some well-oxygenated blood that passes through the pulmonary capillaries (c). The amount of O_2 in the arterial blood, therefore, equals the amount of oxygen in the pulmonary capillary blood plus the amount of this gas in the shunted venous blood:

$$\dot{Q}_T \times C_aO_2 = \dot{Q}_S \times C_{\bar{v}}O_2 + (\dot{Q}_T - \dot{Q}_S) \times C_cO_2 \qquad (1)$$

$\dot{Q}_T$ = amount of total blood flow; $\dot{Q}_S$ = blood flow through shunt; $\dot{Q}_T - \dot{Q}_S$ = blood flow through pulmonary capillary; C_aO_2 = concentration of O_2 in arterial blood; $C_{\bar{v}}O_2$ = concentration of O_2 in mixed venous blood; C_cO_2 = concentration of O_2 in pulmonary capillary blood.

Equation (1) can be rearranged to become

$$\frac{\dot{Q}_S}{\dot{Q}_T} = \frac{C_cO_2 - C_aO_2}{C_cO_2 - C_{\bar{v}}O_2} \qquad (2)$$

In situations in which Pa_{O_2} is high enough to ensure full saturation of hemoglobin (ie, Pa_{O_2} is 150 mm Hg or higher), the equation can be written as

$$\frac{\dot{Q}_S}{\dot{Q}_T} = \frac{P(A\text{-}aDO_2) \times 0.0031}{P(A\text{-}aDO_2) \times 0.0031 + C(a - \bar{v}DO_2)} \qquad (3)$$

$P(A\text{-}aDO_2)$ is the alveolar-arterial oxygen tension difference, and $C(a - \bar{v}DO_2)$ is the arteriovenous oxygen content difference. The shunt is usually calculated while the patient is breathing 100% oxygen.

I.

Essential Pharmacology of Respiratory Disease

■ BRONCHODILATORS

1. β-ADRENERGIC AGONISTS

Bronchodilation from adrenergic drugs occurs as a result of their effect on the receptors of the smooth muscles of the bronchial tree. As they are β2-adrenergic receptors, only drugs with β2 activity are bronchodilators. β1 receptors are the predominant adrenergic receptors of the heart. Drugs with β1 activity, therefore, stimulate the heart, increasing its rate and contractility. Isoproterenol, a potent β-adrenergic drug, has both β1 and β2 effects. Epinephrine, in addition to being a β1 and β2 agonist, has α-adrenergic effect (causing vasoconstriction). These two drugs were extensively used in the past for treatment of asthma. With the development of drugs with more selective β2 effect, the use of isoproterenol and epinephrine as bronchodilators is steadily declining.

The following is a list of bronchodilators with more or less selective β2-adrenergic effect. All of them are used as inhalers, but many are also used systemically (orally and parenterally).

- Isoetharine (Bronkosol, Bronkometer) is available as an inhalation solution for use with nebulizers and metered-dose inhaler (MDI). The degree of selectivity for β2-adrenergic receptors is less than the following drugs.
- Metaproterenol (Alupent, Metaprel) is available as an inhalation solution, an MDI, and an oral preparation. It is somewhat less β2 selective than are the following drugs.
- Terbutaline is available in the United States as an MDI (Brethaire), an oral preparation (Brethine, Bricanyl), and an injectible solution (Breathine, Bricanyl).

- Albuterol, also known as salbutamol (Proventil, Ventolin), is available as an MDI, an inhalation solution, and an oral preparation. There is also a dry powder form for inhalation (Ventolin Rotocaps) used with a special inhalation device (Rotahaler).
- Bitolterol (Tornalate) is available as an MDI and an inhalation solution.
- Pirbuterol (Maxair) is available as an MDI as well as a breath-activated actuator (Autohaler).
- Salmeterol (Serevent) is available as an MDI and is a $\beta2$-selective adrenergic drug with a prolonged duration of action (about 12 hours, versus 3–6 hours with most other inhalers). It has a relatively slow onset of action, and therefore is not suitable for prompt relief of bronchospasm. Long duration of action makes it more suitable for preventive therapy, mostly against nocturnal asthma.

2. ANTICHOLINERGIC BRONCHODILATORS

Ipratropium bromide (Atrovent) is a quaternary ammonium compound with local anticholinergic effect (blocking vagally mediated bronchospasm similar to atropine), but without systemic effect. It is available as an MDI and an inhalation solution. Its bronchodilatory effect is slow, with maximum effect developing in 30 to 60 minutes. It is used more in chronic obstructive pulmonary disease (COPD) than in asthma.

3. METHYLXANTHINES

Theophylline and aminophylline (theophylline ethylenediamine) are used mainly for their bronchodilatory effect. They are less potent than are $\beta2$-adrenergic drugs, and have significant toxicity requiring monitoring of blood drug levels. Theophylline is available as several regular or extended-release preparations for oral use. Only aminophylline is available for intravenous administration.

■ CORTICOSTEROIDS (GLUCOCORTICOIDS)

Corticosteroids are used both systemically and locally in pulmonary medicine, mainly for their anti-inflammatory effects. The common preparations for systemic use are

- Cortisol (hydrocortisone), available as oral and parenteral preparations.
- Prednisone and prednisolone, available in oral forms.
- Methylprednisolone, available as oral (Medrol) and parenteral preparations (Solumedrol).

Inhalational forms of glucocorticoids are available as MDIs. They have become important agents in the management of asthma. An increasing number of these pharmacologic agents are being investigated. Currently used inhaled corticosteroids are

- Triamcinolone (Azmacort)
- Beclomethasone (Beclovent, Vanceril)
- Flunisolide (AeroBid)
- Budesonide (Pulmicort), not available in the United States at the time of this writing
- Fluticasone (Flovent)

CROMOLYN AND NEDOCROMIL

Cromolyn and nedocromil are anti-inflammatory agents used for the preventive management of asthma. They inhibit antigen-induced bronchospasm and pulmonary mast-cell degranulation, preventing the release of mediators. They do not relieve established bronchospasm.

- Cromolyn sodium (Intal), available in capsule form and used with Spinhalor, MDI, and nebulizer solution.
- Nedocromil sodium (Tilade), available in MDI form.

LEUKOTRIENE RECEPTOR ANTAGONIST

Zafirlukast (Accolate) is the only leukotriene receptor antagonist approved for prophylaxis and chronic treatment of asthma in adults and children 12 years of age and older. It is an oral medication available in tablet form. By selectively blocking the effects of the important mediator leukotriene, it prevents both the early-phase and late-phase asthmatic response.

■ ANTIMICROBIAL AGENTS

The antimicrobial agents used in pulmonary infection include most of the antibiotics and various synthetic drugs against various bacterial, viral, fungal, and protozoal organisms that are known to cause respiratory tract infection (RTI).

1. ANTIBACTERIAL DRUGS

A. Betalactam Antibiotics

Betalactam antibiotics, with penicillin being a prototype, contain a β-lactam ring in their molecules. They interfere with bacterial cell wall synthesis. They are bactericidal.

Penicillins

- Penicillin G and penicillin V are active against streptococci, including *Streptococcus pneumoniae.* They become ineffective with the action of penicillinase (β-lactamase) produced by many organisms.
- Penicillinase-resistant penicillins are semisynthetic penicillins, which include nafcillin (intravenous [IV] and oral), oxacillin (IV and oral), cloxacillin (oral), and dicloxacillin (oral). These agents are active against *Staphylococcus aureus,* unless they develop resistance to them (methicillin-resistant *S aureus* [MRSA]).
- Aminopenicillins (ampicillin, amoxicillin) have an extended spectrum of effectiveness against some gram-negative organisms, including *Haemophilus influenzae.*
- Carboxypenicillins (carbenicillin, ticarcillin) and ureidopenicillins (mezlocillin, piperacillin) are effective against susceptible strains of *Pseudomonas aeruginosa.*

Combining of the semisynthetic penicillins with inhibitors of β-lactamase increases their spectrum of antibacterial activities. They include

- Ampicillin + sulbactam (Unasyn)
- Amoxicillin + clavulanic acid (Augmentin)
- Ticarcillin + clavulanic acid (Timentin)
- Piperacillin + tazobactam (Zosyn)

Cephalosporins

Cephalosporins have a broad spectrum of antibacterial activities against most gram-positive cocci and many gram-negative organisms. The number of these antibiotics continues to grow. They are classified by generations.

First-generation cephalosporins include cephalothin, cephalexin, and cefazolin. They have good activity against gram-positive cocci with only modest activity against gram-negative bacteria.

Second-generation cephalosporins include cefuraxime and cefoxitin. These antibiotics have better activity against gram-negative organisms than do the first-generation cephalosporins.

Third-generation cephalosporins include cefotaxime, ceftrioxone, and ceftazidime. These antibiotics are used mostly for gram-negative organisms. Ceftazidime has also antipseudomonas activity.

B. Aminoglycosides

Aminoglycosides interfere with bacterial protein synthesis and are bactericidal against gram-negative organisms. The commonly used aminoglycosides are gentamicin, tobramycin, and amikacin. Streptomycin, which is also an aminoglycoside, is primarily used as an antituberculosis agent.

C. Macrolides

Macrolides inhibit RNA-dependent protein synthesis. They are usually bacteriostatic but may be bactericidal in high doses against very susceptible bacteria. In addition to their activity against gram-positive cocci, they are useful against mycoplasma, legionella, and chlamydia. Commonly used macrolides in RTI are erythromycin, clarithromycin, and azi-

thromycin. The latter two have broader spectrum of activity than erythromycin.

D. Tetracyclines

Tetracyclines inhibit bacterial protein synthesis. They are bacteriostatic. These agents have a rather wide range of antimicrobial activity against aerobic and anaerobic bacteria. They are also effective against mycoplasma, legionella, and chlamydia infections. Because of their irritating affect on serous membranes, they are locally used for pleurodesis. Commonly used tetracyclines are doxycycline, minocycline, and tetracycline.

E. Quinolones

Quinolones are synthetic antimicrobial agents that have broad antibacterial activities. They inhibit bacterial DNA synthesis and are generally considered as bactericidal. Because of their rather poor in vitro activities against pneumococci and anaerobic organisms, their use in pulmonary medicine is limited. However, they are effective in respiratory tract infection from *H influenzae, Moraxella (Branhamella) catarrhalis, Chlamydia pneumoniae,* and *Mycoplasma pneumoniae.* Ciprofloxacin and ofloxacin are commonly used examples of the increasing numbers of quinolones.

F. Other Antibacterial Agents Used in Certain Lung Infections

Clindamycin suppresses bacterial protein synthesis. It is effective against gram-positive cocci and anaerobic bacteria. It is commonly used in lung abscess. It is also used in combination with primaquin as an alternative therapy for *Pneumocystis carinii* pneumonia (PCP).

Vancomycin inhibits bacterial cell-wall synthesis and is bactericidal against most gram-positive organisms, including MRSA.

Metronidazole (Flagyl) is active against a wide variety of anaerobic organisms. It interferes with DNA synthesis by these organisms. Its use in pulmonary medicine is limited to the treatment of anaerobic lung infection, especially lung abscess.

Trimethoprim–sulfamethoxazole (TMP–SMX) is also known as *cotrimoxazole*. This combination drug in 1 : 5 ratio is an excellent example of synergism in antimicrobial therapy. Together, they inhibit two consecutive steps in the biosynthesis of nucleic acids and proteins essential to most bacteria. TMP–SMX combination (Bactrim, Septra) is effective against most gram-positive and gram-negative organisms, including *H influenzae* and *S pneumoniae*. It is therefore a suitable antimicrobial for treatment of acute exacerbation in COPD. TMP–SMX is also a preferred agent for prophylaxis and treatment of PCP.

2. ANTITUBERCULOSIS DRUGS

Drugs for the treatment of tuberculosis (TB) are divided into primary and secondary categories. Primary antituberculosis drugs are as follows:

- Isoniazid (INH) is a bactericidal drug with an unknown mechanism of action. It is the most effective prophylactic agent. In drug sensitive TB, it is the major component of the combination drug regimen for the treatment of TB.
- Rifampin is also bactericidal. It interferes with RNA polymerase.
- Ethambutol's mechanism of action is unknown. It is always used in combination with other drugs.
- Pyrazinamide is bactericidal under

proper pH. It is used in combination with other antituberculosis drugs during the first 2 months of therapy for active TB.
- Streptomycin is bactericidal and is used sparingly because it is injectable. It is included in regimens for multidrug-resistant TB (MDRTB).

Secondary drugs are less effective and their use is limited for treatment of MDRTB or when primary drugs cannot be used for other reasons (ie, drug reaction or hypersensitivity). They include ethionamide, cycloserine, kanamycin, capreomycin, ciprofloxacin (or ofloxacin), amikacin, and clofazimine.

3. ANTIFUNGAL DRUGS

The antifungal drugs used in RTI are

- Amphotericin B is effective against all common fungal infections. It is used intravenously only.
- Fluconazole is a synthetic antifungal drug available as tablets and as solution for IV use. It is effective against cryptococcus.
- Ketoconazole is a synthetic broad-spectrum antifungal agent. It is effective against blastomycosis, histoplasmosis, and coccidiodomycosis. It is used orally.
- Itraconazole is effective as an oral antifungal agent against blastomycosis, histoplasmosis, and aspergillosis.

4. ANTIVIRAL DRUGS

Antiviral drugs useful in respiratory infection include

- Acyclovir for varicella pneumonia.
- Genciclovir for cytomegalovirus (CMV) infection.
- Ribavirin in aerosol form is used in

hospitalized children with respiratory syncytial virus (RSV), bronchiolitis, and pneumonia.

- Antiretroviral drugs for treatment of human immunodeficiency virus (HIV) infection.
- Zidovudine (ZDV, AZT) has high affinity for HIV reverse transcriptase (RNA-dependent DNA polymerase). The drug inhibits these enzymes.
- Didanosine (formerly known as ddI), zalcitabine (formerly known as ddC), and stavudine (formerly known as d4T) have mechanisms of action similar to zidovudine, although zidovudine remains the preferred inhibitor of HIV reverse transcriptase.

Recently approved antiproteinases block the effect of HIV proteinase, which cleaves the polyprotein (product of the viral mRNA produced by the host cell) into mature proteins essential to viral structure and replication. Their therapeutic effectiveness against HIV infection is promising.

■ ANTICOAGULANTS AND THROMBOLYTIC AGENTS

Anticoagulants used for the prophylaxis and treatment of pulmonary embolism (PE) are heparin for parenteral use and warfarin for oral use. Their mechanisms of action are different.

Heparin impairs the blood-clotting mechanism mainly by binding to antithrombin III (present in circulating blood). This combination inactivates the coagulation enzymes thrombin and activated factors X and IX; consequently, conversion of fibrinogen to fibrin is prevented. Heparin is administered either intravenously or subcutaneously. Its effect is monitored by a coagulation test known as partial thromboplastin time (PTT). It is used for treatment of established thromboembolism and also used in small subcutaneous doses for prophylaxis of deep-venous thrombosis (DVT).

Warfarin is an oral anticoagulant. It interferes with the synthesis of vitamin K–dependent coagulation factors (prothombin, factors VII, IX, and X). It is used for the prophylaxis and treatment of DVT and treatment of PE, usually following initiation of treatment with heparin.

Thrombolytic agents accelerate the normally occurring lysis of clot at the site of its formation or embolization. They are mainly indicated for the treatment of severe pulmonary thromboembolic disease, in which anticoagulation may not be adequate. Commonly used agents are as follows:

1. Streptokinase is a product of β-hemolytic streptococci. Despite its name, this drug is not an enzyme. By forming a complex with plasminogen or plasmin, it makes a highly effective enzyme activator for plasminogen, converting it to plasmin. Plasmin then degrades the fibrin in the clot, causing it to dissolve. It is administered intravenously.
2. Tissue plasminogen activator (tPA or alteplase) is produced by recombinant DNA technology. It has a strong affinity to plasminogen at the surface of fibrin clot and converts plasminogen to plasmin. It is considered to be a fibrin-specific thrombolytic agent. It is administered intravenously.

■ NICOTINE PREPARATIONS

Nicotine preparations are intended to be used as an aid to smoking cessation for the relief of nicotine withdrawal symptoms. There are three different systems for delivery of nicotine.

Nicotine gum, which was developed first, is a chewing gum containing nicotine bound to an ion-exchange resin. Known as nicotine polacrilex (Nicorette, Nicorette DS), the nicotine gum releases nicotine while being chewed, and it is absorbed primarily through buccal mucosa. Each piece of gum contains either 2 or 4 mg (double strength) of nicotine.

The more convenient transdermal system allows rate-controlled delivery of nicotine, included in a special patch, throughout the application period (usually 24 hours). The dose of nicotine on the label of each patch is the amount of nicotine absorbed by the user's skin. The rate of delivery of each system is proportional to the surface area of the patch. Transdermal systems are available under trade names of Habitrol, Nicoderm, Nicotrol, and Prostep.

A recently introduced nasal preparation enables faster delivery of nicotine. It will be available as Nicotrol NS.

■ MISCELLANEOUS DRUGS

Dornase alfa (Pulmozyme) is a solution of human deoxyribonuclease (DNase) produced by recombinant method. This enzyme is administered as an aerosol in patients with cystic fibrosis (CF) to break down the DNA that contributes significantly to sputum viscosity. It is not recommended for children younger than 5 years old.

Lung surfactant is used by intratracheal instillation as prophylaxis against respiratory distress syndrome (RDS) in the newborn with birth weight of less than 1450 g or any birth weight with evidence of lung immaturity. It is also used as rescue treatment of infants with established RDS. Two forms of lung surfactant are available for clinical use:

1. Natural bovine lung extract, which is reconstructed by adding surface lowering compounds to mimic natural lung surfactant (Survanta).
2. Protein-free synthetic surfactant (Exosurf).

Alpha$_1$-proteinase inhibitor, also known as *alpha$_1$-antitrypsin,* is prepared from pooled human plasma (Prolastin). It is used for chronic replacement therapy for patients with congenital deficiency of alpha$_1$-proteinase inhibitor with evidence of panacinar emphysema. It is administered intravenously once weekly.

Antitussive Drugs

Despite prevalence of cough as a symptom of respiratory disease, cough medications are only occasionally recommended because most coughs are either beneficial or have treatable causes. Codeine is a well-known drug for its antitussive effect. Most of the over-the-counter (OTC) cough medications contain dextromethorphan. This drug acts centrally by elevating the threshold for cough. Benzonatate (Tessalon) is believed to exert its antitussive effect on cough receptors in the lung. Hydrocodone and hydromorphone are also incorporated in several medications for their antitussive effect.

Respiratory Stimulants

- **Doxapram** (Dopram) produces respiratory stimulation through the peripheral chemoreceptors. In higher doses it also stimulates central chemoreceptors.
- **Almitrine,** a stimulant of chemoreceptors, is not yet available in the United States.
- **Theophylline,** in addition to its other pharmacologic effects, is a mild respiratory stimulant. It is used in Cheyne-Stokes respiration.
- **Naloxone** (Narcan) is a narcotic antagonist that reverses the effects of opioids, including respiratory depression. It is given intravenously.
- **Flumazenil** (Romazicon) antagonizes the actions of benzodiazepines on the central nervous system (CNS). It is known to increase benzodiazepine-associated depression of respiratory drive.

J.

Normal Values of Commonly Used Blood Tests

Chemistry

Albumin, serum	3.5–5 g/dL
Alpha₁-antitrypsin, serum	75–200 mg/dL
Anion gap, plasma	7–14 mEq/L
Bicarbonate, serum	21–27 mEq/L
Calcium (total), serum	8.5–10.5 mg/dL
Carbon dioxide, serum or plasma	23–29 mmol/L
Chloride, serum or plasma	98–106 mEq/L
Cholesterol, serum	140–200 mg/dL
Cortisol, serum or plasma (AM sample)	5–23 mcg/dL
Creatinine, serum or plasma	0.5–1.2 mg/dL

Glucose, serum (fasting)	70–105 mg/dL
Iron, serum	40–160 mg/dL
Lactate, blood	4.5–19.8 mg/dL or 0.5–2.2 mmol/L
Lactate dehydrogenase (LDH), serum	200–450 U/L (Wrobleski)
Osmolality, serum	255–295 mosmol/Kg
Oxygen saturation, arterial blood	90–95%
Oxygen tension, arterial blood	83–100 mm Hg
pH, arterial blood	7.35–7.45
Potassium, serum	3.5–5.1 mEq/L
Protein (total), serum	6.5–8.3 g/dL
Sodium, serum or plasma	136–146 mEq/L
Urea nitrogen, serum	10–20 mg/dL

Hematology

Activated partial thromboplastin time	25–35 sec
Blood volume	51–80 mL/Kg (male)
	50–75 mL/Kg (female)
Clotting time	5–8 min
Erythrocyte count (RBC)	4.5–5.9 million/mm^3 (male)
	4.0–5.2 million/mm^3 (female)
Erythrocyte indexes	
MCH	26–34 pg/cell
MCHC	31–37%
MCV	80–100 fL
Erythrocyte sedimentation rate	0–20 mm/hr

Hematocrit	41–53% (male)
	36–48% (female)
Hemoglobin	13.5–17.5 g/dL (male)
	12–16 g/dL (female)
Leukocyte (WBC) count	4500–11,000/mm^3
Leukocyte differential count	
Neutrophils	3000–5800
Lymphocytes	1500–3000
Monocytes	285–500
Eosinophils	50–250
Basophils	15–50
Platelet count	150,000–400,000
Prothrombin time (PT)	8.8–11.6 sec

BIBLIOGRAPHY FOR APPENDICES A THROUGH J

American Thoracic Society. Lung function testing: selection of reference values and interpretative strategies. *Am Rev Respir Dis.* 1991; 144:1202–1218.

Boren HG, Kory RC, Syner JC. The Veterans Administration–Army cooperative study of pulmonary function: II. The lung volume and its subdivisions in normal men. *Am J Med.* 1966; 41:96–114.

Cerveri I, Zoia MC, Fanfulla F, et al. Reference values of arterial oxygen tension in the middle-aged and elderly. *Am J Respir Crit Care Med.* 1995; 152:934–941.

The choice of antibacterial drugs. *Med Lett Drugs Ther.* 1996; 38:25–34.

Crapo RO. Reference values for pulmonary function tests. *Respir Care.* 1989; 34:626–634.

Crapo RO, Morris AH. Standardized single breath normal values for carbon monoxide diffusing capacity. *Am Rev Respir Dis.* 1981; 123:185–189.

Drugs for tuberculosis. *Med Lett Drugs Ther.* 1995; 37:67–70.

Forster RE II, Dubois AB, Briscoe WA, Fisher AB. *The Lung*, 3rd ed. Chicago: Year Book Medical Publishers, 1986.

Goldberg M, Green SB, Moss ML, et al. Computer-based instruction and diagnosis of acid-base disorders: a systematic approach. *JAMA.* 1973; 223(3):269–275.

Henningfield JE. Nicotine medications for smoking cessation. *N Engl J Med.* 1995; 333:1196–1203.

Kory RC, Callahan R, Boren HG, Syner JC. The Veterans Administration–Army cooperative study of pulmonary function: I. Clinical spirometry in normal men. *Am J Med.* 1961; 30:243–258.

Morris JF. Spirometry in the evaluation of pulmonary function. *West J Med.* 1976; 125:110–118.

New drugs for HIV infection. *Med Lett Drugs Ther.* 1996; 38:35–37.

Glossary

Accessory. supplementary, added to, or helping another with the same function.

Acetylcholine. a chemical neurotransmitter operating in many parts of the nervous system and neuromuscular junction.

Acetylcholinesterase. an enzyme, present at the sites of acetylcholine activity, that hydrolyzes acetylcholine and thus controls its effect.

Acidemia. a decrease in pH of the blood.

Acidosis. a disorder of normal acid-base balance resulting from accumulation of acid and/or reduction of bicarbonate in the blood or tissue.

Acinus. the portion of the lung distal to terminal bronchiole comprising respiratory bronchioles, alveolar ducts, alveolar sacs, and alveoli.

Acrolein. an aldehide (acrylic aldehyde) generated by decomposition of glycerin.

Adrenergic. related to epinephrine (adrenaline) or substances with similar activity; pertaining to or affecting the sympathetic nervous system.

Adventitious. associated with or added to something in a nonessential and extrinsic fashion.

Aerobic. occurring in the presence of molecular oxygen.

Agammaglobulinemia. absence of gamma globulins in the blood.

Agglutination. the process of the clumping together of antigen-bearing cells or substances in the presence of specific antibodies.

Air cyst or bulla. a thin-walled radiolucent area surrounded by more or less normal lung.

Alkalemia. an increase in pH of the blood.

Alkalosis. a disorder of normal acid-base balance resulting from excessive accumulation of base or excessive loss of hydrogen ion (acid).

Allergen. a substance capable of causing allergy or hypersensitivity reaction.

Allergy. a hypersensitivity state developing as a result of exposure to a substance (allergen), reexposure causing an exaggerated reaction.

Alpha interferon. an interferon produced by leukocytes (*see* Interferon).

Alveolar (air-space) density. results from the presence of denser substances replacing the air in the alveoli. Alveolar edema gives rise to this type of radiographic change. Pulmonary consolidation is a confluent air-space density.

Alveolitis. inflammation at the alveolar sites.

Alveolus. a small saclike dilatation; the smallest gas-exchanging unit of the lung outpouching from the respiratory bronchioles, alveolar ducts, or alveolar sacs.

Amyotrophic. pertaining to muscle atrophy.

Amyotrophic lateral sclerosis. a chronic neurologic condition resulting from degeneration of motor neurons in the spinal cord and brain stem causing progressive muscle weakness and atrophy.

Anaerobic. occurring in the absence of molecular oxygen.

Anaerobic threshold. the amount of exercise at which anaerobic metabolism begins.

Anaphylaxis. a severe, often life-threatening reaction resulting from an exaggerated allergic response to an antigen to which an individual is sensitized from previous exposure.

Angina pectoris. an acute, transient, and often recurring chest pain resulting from insufficient oxygen supply to the heart muscle to meet its metabolic demand.

Angiography. radiographic visualization of blood vessels following injection of contrast material.

Angiotensin. a polypeptide formed by the action of renin on its plasma precursor (angiotensinogen). Its activation by a converting enzyme results in the formation of a potent substance known as angiotensin II.

Anion gap. amount of unmeasured anions, difference between the total of measured cations and that of anions in a sample of serum.

Ankylosing spondylitis. inflammation of vertebrae that eventually results in their ankylosis.

Ankylosis. immobility of a joint resulting from fusion of component bones.

Anoxemia. lack of oxygen in the blood.

Anoxia. lack of oxygen in the tissue or cell.

Anthracite. hard coal.

Antibody. a specific protein molecule produced by special cells (plasma cells) as a result of their interaction with an antigen.

Anticholinergic. a substance that blocks the passage of impulses through the parasympathetic nerves.

Antigen. any substance capable of inducing an immunologic response or production of an antibody.

Antiprotease. a substance that checks the effect of proteolytic enzymes.

Antitussive. a drug used to relieve or suppress cough.

Aphonia. loss of voice.

Apnea. cessation of breathing.

Aromatic. characteristic of a chemical compound with a benzene ring.

Arthroconidia. spores formed asexually in close sequence in the hyphae of certain fungi.

Asbestosis. diffuse lung fibrosis resulting from exposure to asbestos fibers.

Atelectasis. incomplete or absence of expansion of a lung or part of it.

Atopy. a hereditary state of allergy predisposing to development of certain clinical conditions such as hay fever, asthma, and eczema.

Auscultation. the act of listening to the sounds produced within the body, usually with a stethoscope.

Autoantibody. an antibody against the body's own constituents.

Autoimmunity. a condition in which immunologic reaction occurs against the components of the body's own tissues or cells.

Bactericidal. capable of killing bacteria.

Bagassosis. lung disease due to exposure to moldy bagasse (the residue of sugar cane).

Barotrauma. injury resulting from changes in barometric pressure or high inflating pressure.

Bisulfite. an acid sulfite (salt of sulfurous acid).

Bituminous coal. soft coal.

Bleb. a blister; an air cyst in the lung adjacent to the pleura.

Blue bloater. a cyanotic patient with chronic respiratory failure, carbon dioxide retention, and right heart failure.

B lymphocytes. lymphocytes involved in humoral immunity (antibody production).

Bohr effect. facilitation of oxygen unloading at tissue sites by an increase in capillary blood P_{CO_2} (and decrease in pH).

Bradypnea. abnormally slow respiratory rate.

Bronchoconstriction. constriction or narrowing of the bronchi; bronchospasm.

Bronchogenic. originating in a bronchus.

Bronchogram. x-ray film demonstrating or outlining the bronchi, usually following instillation of a contrast material.

Bronchopulmonary dysplasia. a chronic lung disease of infants that usually develops following respiratory distress syndrome.

Bronchovesicular. pertaining to breath sounds with a quality between that of bronchial and vesicular sounds.

Buffer. a chemical system that prevents or attenuates changes in acid-base balance when an acid or base is added.

Bulla. an air cyst inside the lung.

Bullectomy. surgical excision of a bulla.

Byssinosis. pulmonary disease resulting from exposure to cotton dust.

Calcification. hardening of tissues by deposition of calcium salts.

Capilleritis. inflammation of blood capillaries.

Carbamino compounds. chemical compounds resulting from combination of carbon dioxide with amino ($-NH_2$) groups of hemoglobin or plasma proteins.

Carbonic anhydrase. an enzyme that catalyzes the chemical reaction between carbon dioxide and water, thus facilitating the transfer of carbon dioxide from tissues to blood and to alveolar air.

Carboxyhemoglobin. chemical compound of hemoglobin with carbon monoxide.

Carcinogenic. producing cancer.

Carina. a ridge; a ridgelike structure at the end of the trachea between the openings of two main bronchi.

Caseous. cheeselike.

Catecholamine. a group of compounds such as epinephrine and norepinephrine having a sympathomimetic action.

Cavity. a radiolucent lesion surrounded by denser tissue. It is due to a localized necrotic lung lesion that has sloughed off. It is the hallmark of the lung abscess. A fluid level may be seen inside a cavity.

Centrilobular. pertaining to the central portion of a pulmonary lobule or acinus; centriacinar.

Chemoprophylaxis. use of chemotherapeutic agents to prevent development of a specific disease.

Chemoreceptor. a receptor that senses the presence of chemical substances.

Chemotherapy. treatment with chemical agents that have a specific toxic effect on certain microorganisms (ie, tubercle bacilli) or neoplastic cells.

Cheyne-Stokes respiration. a waxing and waning of breathing with changing in its depth and rate at regular intervals.

Cholinergic. related to acetylcholine as applied to the nerve fibers with acetylcholine as their neurotransmitter, particularly the parasympathetic nerves; parasympathomimetic.

Cholinergic crisis. a critical worsening of muscular weakness in myasthenia gravis from excessive use of cholinergic drugs.

Chylothorax. presence of chyle (milky fluid of intestinal lymph) in the pleural cavity.

Cilia. hairlike vibrating processes projecting from the free surface of cells lining the airways or other similar structures.

Circadian. pertaining to rhythmic biologic cycles repeated at 24-hour intervals.

Coalescence. growing or blending together into one body.

Compliance. a quality of yielding to pressure; increase in volume per unit of pressure change.

Congestion. excessive accumulation of blood in the vessels of an organ.

Consolidation. process of becoming solid, as the lung becoming airless with accumulation of exudative fluid and cells in pneumonia.

Consumption. a wasting away of the body as applied to advanced tuberculosis.

Contusion. a traumatic lesion of an organ or tissue without breaking the overlying skin; bruise.

Coronal. related to a body plane passing longitudinally from side to side.

Costal. pertaining to ribs.

Costophrenic. pertaining to ribs and diaphragm, as applied to the angle between the rib cage and diaphragm in the chest x-ray film.

Croup. a condition resulting from an acute inflammation of laryngeal structures causing a characteristic barking cough.

Cyanosis. bluish or purplish discoloration of skin or mucous membrane usually from the presence of a high concentration of deoxygenated hemoglobin in the capillaries.

Cylindrical. shaped like a cylinder, describing a form of bronchiectasis.

Cyst. any saclike structure containing air or fluid.

Cytokine. a mediator released by a cell to cause action in a different cell.

Cytotoxic. having a toxic effect against cells.

Decortication. removal of a covering, usually applied to surgical excision of pleural peel from around the lung.

Deglutitory. pertaining to deglutition (swallowing).

Dermatomyositis. inflammation of skin and muscle.

Diffusion. random molecular movement by which a matter is transported from an area of higher to an area of lower concentration until equilibrium is reached.

Ductus arteriosus. a fetal blood vessel that connects the pulmonary artery to the aorta (it normally closes shortly after birth).

Dyskinesia. difficult or abnormal movement.

Dysphonia. abnormality of voice.

Dysplasia. abnormality of growth or development of an organ, tissue, or cell.

Dyspnea. difficulty in breathing.

Edema. accumulation of an excessive amount of fluid in an extracellular space resulting in swelling that usually pits on pressure.

Effector. an organ, tissue, or cell that responds to a chemical mediator.

Effusion. escape of fluid from its natural vessels into a body cavity.

Egophony. a characteristic change in sound on its transmission through the diseased lung and pleura; sound of a bleating goat.

Elastase. one of the proteases (enzymes that split the proteins) that preferentially attacks the elastic tissue.

Electrooculogram. a graphic tracing of the changes in electrical potentials resulting from eye movements.

Embolism. occlusion of a blood vessel by a matter (embolus) carried by the blood flow from another site.

Embolus. an undissolved matter carried in blood that lodges in a vessel and obstructs it.

Empirical. guided by practical experience.

Empyema. accumulation of pus in a body cavity, usually referring to the pleural space.

Endemic. present among a particular people or in a specified locality.

Endogenous. originating or growing from within.

Endoscopy. visual inspection of a body cavity or hollow organ with the help of an appropriate instrument (endoscope).

Epiglottitis. inflammation of the epiglottis.

Epithelioid. resembling the epithelium; applied to cells in granulomas (derived from monocytes or macrophages).

Ergometer. a device for measuring the amount of work performed.

Etiology. study of the causes of diseases.

Exacerbation. increase in severity of a disease, its symptoms, or its signs.

Exocrine. secreting externally.

Exogenous. originating or growing from outside.

Expectoration. the act of coughing up and spitting out materials from within the thorax.

Expiratory reserve volume (ERV). the maximum volume of air that can be exhaled after expiration of tidal volume.

Extrinsic. originating or operating from without.

Exudate. a fluid with a high protein content, and often with a high cell count, that has exuded from blood capillaries as a result of abnormal leakage, as with inflammation.

Exude. to ooze forth, to produce an exudate.

Ferrugenous. containing iron.

Fibroblast. a connective tissue cell that is involved in formation of fibrous tissue.

Fibroplasia. formation of fibrous tissue.

Fibrosis. development of excess fibrous and connective tissue in an organ or tissue.

Fibrothorax. a chronic pleural disease characterized by the formation of thick fibrous tissue and adhesion of the two layers of pleura.

Fick's method (principle). a method of measurement of cardiac output (L/min) by the oxygen consumption (mL/min) divided by the difference between the arterial and mixed-venous blood oxygen contents (mL/L).

Fremitus. a vibration felt by palpation.

Functional residual capacity (FRC). the volume of air remaining in the lungs at the end of expiration of tidal volume. *This is the resting end-expiratory position.*

Fusiform. shaped like a spindle.

Genioglossus. one of the muscles of the tongue originating from the inner surface of the mandible (mental spine) and attaching to the hyoid bone and the whole length of undersurface of the tongue.

Genomic. pertaining to a genome (the complete set of genetic factors).

Glomerulus. a tuft or cluster, used to describe the part of a microscopic unit of the kidney in which plasma filtation takes place.

Glossopharyngeal. pertaining to the tongue and pharynx, usually applied to the cranial nerve IX.

Glottis. the opening between the vocal cords.

Glutathione. a reduced form of tripeptide that is an important antioxidant against harmful effects of many toxic substances.

Granulocytopenia. reduced numbers of granulocytes (mainly neutrophils) in the blood.

Granuloma. a tumor-like pathologic structure composed of modified macrophages (epithelioid and giant cells) and usually surrounded by lymphocytes, resulting from chronic inflammation, as in tuberculosis or sarcoidosis.

Haldane effect. facilitation of carbon dioxide loading at the tissue site by unloading of oxygen (changing from HbO_2 to Hb).

Heat exhaustion. extreme weakness or fatigue from water loss or salt depletion.

Hectic. related to having undulating fever with wasting away, as in advanced tuberculosis.

Heliox. a mixture of helium and oxygen.

Hematoma. a localized swelling from accumulation of blood.

Hemithorax. one half (right or left) of the chest.

Hemodynamics. science or study of the movements of blood and related forces.

Hemopneumothorax. accumulation of blood and air in the pleural cavity.

Hemoprotein. a protein containing a heme molecule.

Hemoptysis. expectoration of blood.

Hemothorax. accumulation of blood in the pleural cavity.

Heterozygous. having dissimilar pairs of genes for any hereditary characteristic; opposite of homozygous.

Homogeneous density. characteristic of uniformly dense lesions, such as a solid tumor, fluid-containing cyst, or collection of fluid in the pleural space.

Honeycombing. coarse reticular density.

Hyaline. resembling glass; translucent or transparent.

Hydropneumothorax. collection of fluid and air in the pleural space.

Hydrostatic. pertaining to fluid in static equilibrium, often used to define pressure.

Hydrothorax. collection of watery fluid in the pleural space; pleural effusion.

Hypercarbia. excess of carbon dioxide in blood; hypercapnia.

Hypercoagulability. a state in which there is increased tendency to form a clot.

Hyperlucency. excessive radiolucency.

Hyperplasia. a nontumorous increase in the number of normal cells in normal tissue resulting in its enlargement.

Hyperreactivity. greater than normal responsiveness to stimuli.

Hypertrophy. a nontumorous increase in size of an organ or tissue as a result of the enlargement, but not increase in number, of its cells.

Hypocarbia. reduced carbon dioxide in blood; hypocapnia.

Hypopharynx. the lower part of the pharynx located between the upper edge of epiglottis and openings of larynx and esophagus.

Hypopnea. reduced rate and depth of breathing.

Hypoxemia. low blood level of partial pressure of oxygen.

Hypoxia. reduced oxygen in the tissue or cell.

Iatrogenic. induced in a patient by a physician's action, usually of adverse effect.

Idiopathic. of unknown origin or cause.

Idiosyncrasy. a structural or functional characteristic peculiar to an individual; an abnormal susceptibility to the effect of a drug, not from allergy.

Immune complex. combination of an antigen with its specific antibody.

Immunocompetent. capable of developing an immune response to antigenic exposure.

Immunocompromised. having a diminished or absent immune response as a result of pathologic conditions or the effect of certain drugs.

Immunodeficiency. a state of defective immune response, either humoral or cell mediated.

Immunosuppressive. an agent that prevents or reduces an immune response.

Immunotherapy. a treatment intended to alter the immune response by administration of a known antigen or allergen.

Indolent. causing little or no pain (or other symptoms or signs).

Induration. an abnormally hard lesion or reaction, as in a positive tuberculin skin test.

Infarction. formation of an area of necrosis as a result of failure of local blood supply (infarct).

Infiltration. penetration and accumulation in a tissue of substances or cells; radiodensity in the lung fields as a result of such an accumulation in lung parenchyma.

Inspiratory capacity (IC). the maximum volume of air that can be inspired from the resting end-expiratory position.

Inspiratory reserve volume (IRV). the maximum volume of air that one can breathe in after inspiration of tidal volume.

Interferon. a substance produced and released by certain cells infected by viruses, which inhibits viral replication in many cells throughout the body.

Interstitial. situated between essential parts or in the interspaces of a tissue.

Intractable. difficult to manage or alleviate.

Ischemia. local deficiency of blood supply due to vascular disorder.

Kussmaul's breathing. deep regular respiration in metabolic acidosis (particularly diabetic ketoacidosis) in which the accessory muscles of respiration are often utilized.

Kyphoscoliosis. combination of kyphosis with scoliosis; abnormal backward and lateral curvature of the spine.

Kyphosis. abnormal increase in curvature of the spine with backward convexity.

Laryngopharynx. hypopharynx.

Lecithin. a phospholipid that is a major constituent of surfactant.

Leukocytosis. an increase above normal (greater than $11,000/\text{mm}^3$) in the number of white blood cells in the blood.

Leukotrienes. chemical mediators of immediate hypersensitivity that include the slow-reacting substance of anaphylaxis (SRS-A).

Lobectomy. surgical resection of a pulmonary lobe.

Loculated. compartmented, as a space in a body cavity.

Lymphadenitis. inflammation of lymph nodes.

Lymphadenopathy. disease of lymph nodes, usually characterized by their enlargement.

Lymphokine. any of the chemical mediators released from the activated lymphocytes that affect other cells, especially during a cell-mediated immunologic reaction.

Lysis. disintegration of cells (red blood cells, bacteria, etc.) by dissolution.

Macrophage. any of the large mononuclear phagocytic cells that exist in many organs including the lungs (alveolar macrophages).

Macule. a small spot or blotch differing from its surroundings by virtue of its color.

Mediastinum. a partition containing intrathoracic structures between the lungs.

Melanoptysis. expectoration of black sputum, as in coal workers' pneumoconiosis.

Mesothelioma. a tumorous growth derived from the lining cells of serous cavities (pleura, pericardium, or peritoneum).

Metaplasia. change of normal tissue cells to a form abnormal for that tissue.

Miliary. characterized by lesions resembling millet seeds, as in miliary tuberculosis.

Mucosa. a mucous membrane.

Mucopurulent. containing mucus and pus, as applied to sputum.

Mucoviscidosis. an alternative name for cystic fibrosis, which characterizes the abnormally viscous mucus in this disease.

Myasthenia crisis. a critically severe worsening of muscular weakness in myasthenia gravis related to its exacerbation.

Mycelium. filamentous vegetative parts of a fungus; hyphae.

Mycosis. a disease caused by a fungus.

Myopathy. any disease of the muscle.

Nasopharynx. upper part of the pharynx located above the level of the soft palate.

Necrosis. death of a cell or tissue.

Necrotizing. causing necrosis, as in necrotizing pneumonia.

Neoplasm. a new growth of different or abnormal tissue, usually uncontrolled.

Nitrosamine. a compound formed by the combination of nitrates with amines with the type formula R_2N—NO.

Nodule. a small node or round lesion that can be palpated or visualized in a radiographic film.

Nomogram. a graph containing a number of parallel scales showing variables so that when a straight line connects two known values, the other related values are directly read at the points of intersection with their corresponding scales.

Normobaric. pertaining to normal atmospheric pressure.

Nosocomial. pertaining to or originating from a hospital, as a nosocomial infection.

Obtundation. dullness or obtuseness of sensorium.

Odynophagia. painful swallowing.

Oncotic pressure. colloid osmotic pressure.

Opportunistic. characterizing a microorganism that ordinarily does not cause disease but, with weakened body defenses, results in disease; describing a disease or infection caused by such an organism.

Oropharynx. part of the pharynx located between the levels of the soft palate and epiglottis.

Orthopnea. difficulty breathing on lying down, that is improved on sitting or standing.

Panlobular or panacinar. involving the entire lobule or acinus of the lung, as in panlobular emphysema.

Paradoxical. occuring contrary to the normal rule, as paradoxical chest wall or abdominal movement with breathing.

Paraneoplastic. occurring with or beside a neoplasm but not due to its direct effect; applied to syndromes associated with cancer.

Parapneumonic. occurring along with pneumonia; used to describe pleural effusion.

Parenchyma. essential functional elements of an organ.

Paroxysmal. occurring in sudden and usually violent attack, as in paroxysmal dyspnea.

Partial pressure. pressure exerted by each of the components of a gas mixture.

Pathogenesis. mechanism of development of a diseased condition.

Pathognomonic. diagnostic of a specific disease.

Pathophysiology. study or mechanism of disordered function in a disease.

PCR. an acronym for polymerase chain reaction used for amplification of DNA.

Pectus. chest, thorax, or breast.

Pectus carinatum. excessive prominence of the sterum; pigeon breast.

Pectus excavatum. excessive depression of the sterum; funnel breast.

Perfusion. the act of pouring over or through, as perfusion of tissue with blood; local blood flow.

Pericarditis. inflammation of the serous membrane enclosing the heart (pericardium).

Periphlebitis. inflammation around a vein.

Pertussis. whooping cough.

Petechia. a pinpoint purplish discoloration of skin or mucous membrane caused by intradermal bleeding.

Phagocyte. a cell that ingests and destroys microorganisms, foreign particles, or other cells.

Pharmacodynamics. biochemical and physiological effects of drugs and mechanism of their action.

Pharmacokinetics. movement of drugs in the body, including their absorption, distribution, binding, tissue penetration, biotransformation, and excretion.

Phlebitis. inflammation of a vein.

Phrenic. pertaining to the diaphragm.

Pink puffer. a patient with chronic obstructive pulmonary disease who maintains fairly normal blood gases despite significant dyspnea.

Plasmapheresis. removal of plasma from withdrawn blood and retransfusion of its cells with donor plasma or albumin; plasma exchange.

Platypnea. dyspnea occurring in upright position, but relieved by lying down.

Plethysmograph. an instrument for measuring and recording of changes in the volume of an organ or limb with blood flow, or determining changes in body volume with ventilation (body plethysmograph).

Pleural density. a radiodensity due to pleural inflammation, fluid, tumor, or scarring.

Pleuritis. inflammation of pleura; pleurisy.

Pleurodesis. creation of adhesion between the parietal and visceral pleurae by surgical or medical means.

Pneumoconiosis. pulmonary disease from exposure to aerosolized particulate matter (dust).

Pneumomediastinum. presence of air in the mediastinum; mediastinal emphysema.

Pneumonectomy. surgical resection of a lung.

Pneumonitis. inflammation of the lung; pneumonia.

Pneumotachograph. an instrument for recording the velocity of respired air.

Pneumotaxic. related to respiratory rate regulation.

Pneumothorax. accumulation of air in the pleural space.

Polyclonal. derived from different clones of cells.

Polycythemia. an abnormal increase in red cells in the blood.

Polymyositis. inflammation of many muscles at once.

Polynuclear. having several nuclei.

Polypnea. an increase in the respiratory rate; tachypnea.

Polysomnography. recording of several physiologic events during sleep.

Poudrage. application of a powder.

Prodrome. forewarning symptom(s) indicating that a disease is imminent.

Progenitor. ancestor, originator of a line of descent.

Prostaglandin. a group of naturally occurring chemicals that have multiple functions, including contraction and relaxation of smooth muscles.

Prostration. extreme physical exhaustion; a state of total helplessness.

Protease. any enzyme that acts on proteins; a proteolytic enzyme.

Proviral. related to provirus (the genome of a virus integrated into the chromosome of the host cell).

Psychogenic. originating from an emotional or psychologic process.

Pulmonary mass. a large (6 cm or more in diameter), demarcated radiodensity. It often indicates a neoplastic lesion. Mediastinal mass is a similar shadow in the mediastinum.

Pulmonary nodule. a circumscribed density of less than 6 cm in diameter, which may be single and then is called a solitary pulmonary nodule or "coin" lesion.

Purulent. consisting of, containing, or discharging pus.

Pyogenic. producing or able to produce pus.

Pyopneumothorax. collection of pus and air in the pleural space.

Pyothorax. collection of pus in the pleural space; thoracic empyema.

Pyrolysis. decomposition of an organic substance on exposure to very high heat in the absence of oxygen.

Radiodensity. state of being relatively resistant to the passage of x-radiation.

Radiolucency. property of permitting the passage of x-radiation.

Rale. an abnormal crackling respiratory sound; crackle.

Receptor. a specific chemical structure on the surface or within a cell that, on recognizing and binding with another chemical structure (ie, a hormone), causes a set of reactions culminating in a specific cellular response; a sensory nerve terminal that is specialized to respond to stimulating agents.

Residual volume (RV). the volume of air that remains in the lungs after a maximum expiration.

Resonance. prolongation and echoing of sound resulting from percussion over a relatively hollow structure.

Retrolental. behind the crystalline lens of the eye.

Rhonchus. an abnormal respiratory sound resulting from bronchial narrowing; a wheeze.

Saccular. shaped like a sac, as saccular bronchiectasis.

Sagittal. related to a plane, passing the body longitudinally from front to back, parallel to the median plane.

Sclerosis. a hardening of a tissue or part.

Scoliosis. an abnormal lateral curvature of the spine.

Sigmoid. shaped like the letter "S."

Sign. any objective evidence of a disease as detected by examination.

Situs inversus. transposition of the organs from right to left and vice versa.

Spectrophotometry. measurement of the intensity of light of a definite wavelength transmitted by a substance in solution, by which the quantity of the substance in the solution is determined.

Spherule. a small sphere; a round structure of the parasitic stage of *Coccidioides immitis* containing multiple small endospores.

Spherulin. an antigenic substance extracted from spherules of *Coccidioides immitis*, used for skin testing.

Sphingomyelin. a phospholipid present in alveolar surfactant.

Spondylitis. inflammation of vertebrae.

Squamous. scaly, as squamous epithelium.

Sternotomy. an incision through the sternum; sternal splitting.

Stridor. a harsh, grating sound heard during inspiration in association with upper airway obstruction.

Superoxide dismutase. an enzyme that catalyzes the conversion of the highly reactive oxygen radical (superoxide) to less toxic substances.

Suppurative. producing pus.

Supraglottitis. inflammation of structures above the glottis; epiglottitis.

Surfactant. a surface active agent; any substance that in solution lowers the surface tension between it and another liquid, usually referred to phospholipids in pulmonary alveoli.

Sympathomimetic. an agent producing effects similar to those produced by stimulation of sympathetic nerves.

Symptom. a subjective evidence of disease as perceived by the patient.

Syndrome. a set of symptoms and signs occurring together and characterizing a particular condition or disease.

Tachycardia. excessively rapid heart rate.

Tachypnea. excessively rapid respiratory rate.

Tactile. pertaining to touch.

Tamponade. pathologic compression of an organ resulting in its malfunction, as cardiac tamponade from pericardial effusion.

Taxonomy. classification of organisms.

Tension hydrothorax. large pleural effusion causing increased intrapleural pressure and affecting circulation and ventilation.

Tension pneumothorax. a large pneumothorax causing increased intrapleural pressure and affecting circulation and ventilation.

Tetraplegia. quadriplegia (paralysis of all four extremities).

Thermistor. an electric thermometer able to measure extremely small changes in temperature.

Thoracentesis. puncture of chest wall and pleural space for removal of pleural fluid; pleural tap.

Thoracoplasty. collapsing of chest wall by surgical removal of ribs.

Thoracotomy. surgical opening of the thoracic cavity.

Thrombocytopenia. low platelet count in blood.

Thromboembolism. obstruction of a blood vessel with a clot carried by the blood flow from its site of origin.

Thrombophlebitis. inflammation of a vein associated with blood clot formation.

Thrombosis. formation of blood clot (**Thrombus**) inside a blood vessel.

Tidal volume (TV). the volume of air inspired and expired with each normal breath.

T lymphocyte. thymus-dependent lymphocyte, being the major effector cell in cell-mediated immunity.

Tocolysis. pharmacologic elimination of uterine contraction in premature labor.

Tomography. special radiographic study in which the x-ray picture of selected plane of the body is recorded.

Total lung capacity (TLC). the volume of air in the lungs at the end of a maximum inspiration.

Tracheomalacia. softening and dilatation of tracheal cartilages.

Transaxial. positioned at a right angle to the longitudinal axis of the body.

Transbronchial. through the bronchial wall, as transbronchial lung biopsy.

Transcriptase. an enzyme that helps the synthesis or polymerization of RNA (also known as RNA polymerase).

Transcutaneous. through the skin.

Transthoracic. through the chest wall.

Transtracheal. through the wall of the trachea, as transtracheal aspiration.

Transudate. a fluid with a low protein content that has passed from blood capillaries through a serous membrane as a result of alteration of hydrostatic and colloid osmotic pressure balance.

Transude. to pass through, to produce a transudate.

Trepopnea. more comfortable breathing on lying on one side or the other.

Triad. a group of three entities; association of three symptoms or signs.

Trigeminal. pertaining to cranial nerve V.

Trophozoite. active, feeding, and motile stage of a protozoan.

Tubercle. a small granulomatous lesion resulting from infection with *Mycobacterium tuberculosis* (tubercle bacillus).

Tympanitic. drumlike; refers to the sound produced by percussion over a hollow organ, like a gas-filled stomach.

Unremitting. not abating or diminishing, as an unremitting symptom.

Vagus nerve. cranial nerve X, which supplies nerve fibers to the respiratory tract and other thoracic and abdominal viscera.

Varicose. related to a varix, usually of a vein; also describing a form of bronchiectasis.

Vesicular. related to vesicles or small sacs; quality of breath sounds considered to be originating from the alveoli.

Viremia. presence of virus in the blood.

Virion. complete viral particle.

Vital capacity (VC). the maximum volume of air that can be exhaled by forceful effort following a maximum inspiration.

Volume loss. reduction of volume of the whole lung or part of it as seen on a chest x-ray film.

Volutrauma. injury resulting from excessive inflation of lung tissue.

Wheezing. whistling sound made while breathing, caused by airway narrowing.

Index